Rapid Reference for Nurses

Karren E. Kowalski, RN, PhD, FAAN
Project Director
Colorado Center for Nursing Excellence

Adjunct Faculty
School of Nursing
University of Colorado
Denver, Colorado

Patricia S. Yoder-Wise, RN, EdD, CNAA, FAAN
Professor
Texas Tech University Health Sciences Center
Lubbock, Texas

JONES AND BARTLETT PUBLISHERS
Sudbury, Massachusetts
BOSTON   TORONTO   LONDON   SINGAPORE

World Headquarters
Jones and Bartlett Publishers
40 Tall Pine Drive
Sudbury, MA 01776
978-443-5000
info@jbpub.com
www.jbpub.com

Jones and Bartlett Publishers
Canada
6339 Ormindale Way
Mississauga, Ontario L5V 1J2
Canada

Jones and Bartlett Publishers
International
Barb House, Barb Mews
London W6 7PA
UK

Jones and Bartlett's books and products are available through most bookstores and online booksellers. To contact Jones and Bartlett Publishers directly, call 800-832-0034, fax 978-443-8000, or visit our website, www.jbpub.com.

Substantial discounts on bulk quantities of Jones and Bartlett's publications are available to corporations, professional associations, and other qualified organizations. For details and specific discount information, contact the special sales department at Jones and Bartlett via the above contact information or send an email to specialsales@jbpub.com.

The authors, editor, and publisher have made every effort to provide accurate information. However, they are not responsible for errors, omissions, or for any outcomes related to the use of the contents of this book and take no responsibility for the use of the products described. Treatments and side effects described in this book may not be applicable to all patients; likewise, some patients may require a dose or experience a side effect that is not described herein. The reader should confer with his or her own physician regarding specific treatments and side effects. Drugs and medical devices are discussed that may have limited availability controlled by the Food and Drug Administration (FDA) for use only in a research study or clinical trial. The drug information presented has been derived from reference sources, recently published data, and pharmaceutical research data. Research, clinical practice, and government regulations often change the accepted standard in this field. When consideration is being given to use of any drug in the clinical setting, the healthcare provider or reader is responsible for determining FDA status of the drug, reading the package insert, reviewing prescribing information for the most up-to-date recommendations on dose, precautions, and contraindications, and determining the appropriate usage for the product. This is especially important in the case of drugs that are new or seldom used.

Library of Congress Cataloging-in-Publication Data
Kowalski, Karren.
  Rapid reference for nurses / Karren Kowalski, Patricia S. Yoder-Wise.
    p. ; cm.
  Includes bibliographical references and index.
  ISBN 0-7637-3696-1 (pbk. : alk. paper)
  1. Nursing—Handbooks, manuals, etc.   2. Nursing services—Handbooks, manuals, etc.
  [DNLM: 1. Nursing—Handbooks.   2. Nursing Services—Handbooks. WY 49 K88r
  2006]   I. Yoder-Wise, Patricia S., 1941- II. Title.
  RT51.K68 2006
  617.73—dc22
                                                                              2005030597

6048

Production Credits
Acquisitions Editor: Kevin Sullivan
Production Director: Amy Rose
Associate Editor: Amy Sibley
Production Editor: Carolyn F. Rogers
Senior Marketing Manager: Emily Ekle
Manufacturing and Inventory Coordinator: Amy Bacus

Composition: ATLIS Graphics
Text Design: Paw Print Media
Cover Design: Kristin E. Ohlin
Printing and Binding: United Graphics
Cover Printing: United Graphics

Printed in the United States of America
10 09 08 07 06   10 9 8 7 6 5 4 3 2 1

BLS (Basic Life Support) Reminder

🖰 Note: The following information is intended as a rapid guide for people currently certified in BLS. Please check the current standards at www.americanheart.org for any updates.

The ABCs

- **A**irway: Keep the airway open and check for breathing. This may require tilting the head or thrusting the chin upward to open the airway. If individual is not on his/her back, log roll him/her to the back.
- **B**reaths: If the person is not breathing, use mouth-to-mouth, mouth-to-nose, or mouth-to-stoma, preferably with an assistive device (e.g., Ambu bag) or a barrier device (CPR mask). Look (rise and fall of chest), listen (air sound), and feel (cheek to airway, feel air exchange). Reposition if necessary. Remember that the smaller the body, the less air to use (puffs for infants, full breaths for adults).
- **C**ompressions: If no pulse is present, begin chest compressions. Remember that the smaller the body, the less depth for compression. Check pulse frequently, using a primary vessel such as the carotid. Be sure of finger (infant) or hand(s) placement over the sternum above the xiphoid process.

Using the Automatic External Defibrillator (AED)
The 1, 2, 3 Steps (Used if the person is unconscious, not breathing, and has no pulse.)

1. Turn the unit on.
2. Open the package with the self-adhesive patches and affix them as shown on the AED unit.
3. Follow the instructions/information printed on the screen. Press the shock button *only* if instructed.

Heimlich Reminder

Standing

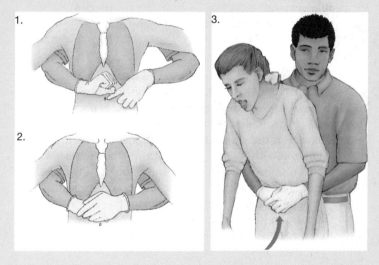

1. Tuck thumb into fist.
2. Place thumb side of fist against abdomen (midline below diaphragm). Cover fist with other hand.
3. Thrust up and in toward diaphragm.

Lying

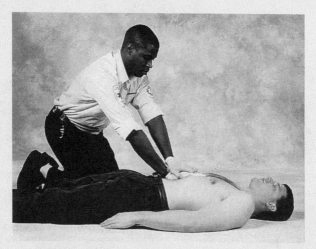

1. Straddle hips.
2. Interlock fingers.
3. Place heel of hand on abdomen.
4. Thrust heel of hand toward diaphragm.

Pediatric/Infant

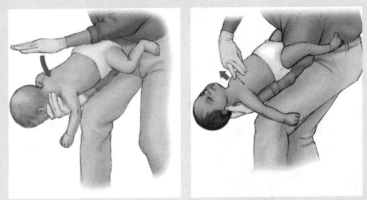

The key difference is to use less force with a child. With an infant, use gravity and back blows and chest thrusts (with fingers only), not abdominal thrusts.

ECG Reminder

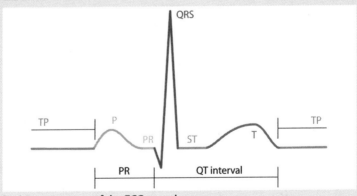

Basic components of the ECG complex.
Source: Garcia, T., & Holtz, N. (2001). *12-lead ECG: The art of interpretation.* Sudbury, MA: Jones and Bartlett.

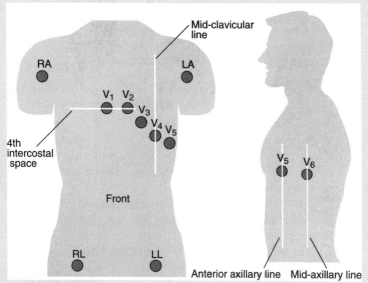

12 lead placement.
Source: Garcia, T., & Holtz, N. (2001). *12-lead ECG: The art of interpretation.* Sudbury, MA: Jones and Bartlett.

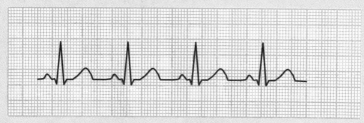

Normal sinus rhythm.
Source: Garcia, T., & Holtz, N. (2001). *12-lead ECG: The art of interpretation.* Sudbury, MA: Jones and Bartlett.

Standard (Universal) Precautions

Standard (or universal) precautions are designed to reduce disease transmission risk. The intent is to use the precautions in health care settings with all patients. The focus is on

- Blood and most body fluids
- Broken skin
- Mucous membranes

1. Use a *barrier protection* to protect skin and mucous membrane contamination. Use it at *all* times and with all substances. Examples include gloves, eye protection, face protection, and gowns.
2. Use *gloves* whenever there is the potential for contact with blood and body fluids or surfaces where such might be present.
3. Use *eye and face protection* when droplets of blood or body fluids are likely to be present.
4. Use *gowns* (disposable garments to cover regular clothing) when splashing of blood or body fluids is likely.
5. *Remove* gloves, eye and face protection, and gowns without touching skin to external surfaces. Dispose of items in designated safe disposal containers.
6. *Wash hands* and other exposed skin surfaces immediately after contact with blood or body fluids and immediately after gloves are removed. Use recommendations from the CDC regarding alcohol-based agents.
7. Use caution with *needles and other sharps*. Avoid accidents and dispose of needles, syringes, and other sharp items in a safe disposal device.

Source: Adapted from the National Institutes of Environmental Health Sciences.

Table of Contents

How to Use This Book

Rapid Reference for Nurses is designed as a quick source of information commonly needed by the profession of nursing in clinical settings. No element is designed to be comprehensive because providing that quantity of information would defeat the portability of this material. *Rapid Reference for Nurses* is designed to refresh memory, *not create it*. Regular textbooks and official Web sites should be the source for learning basic and specialty information. No procedures are contained in this book because most healthcare organizations have definitive policy and procedure manuals that are the expectations for practice within the specific organization. Therefore, users are expected to augment this reference with the applicable source documents within their organizations. Additionally, values such as those found in laboratory tests are included. However, they serve as a *general guide* rather than a definitive source. This means that if the organization in which the user is practicing or learning has a different definition of normal values, the values adhered to in that organization should be used in the care of patients.

The computer symbol, ⊖, is followed by a Web site address to connect users to the key source of information on a topic so that the latest information can be accessed. The information contained in this book reflects nursing knowledge up to and including that available in 2006. Because we know that knowledge affecting the practice of nursing has a half-life of approximately 18 months (meaning that about half of what we know today will be replaced or refined with new information within 18 months), it is important to update information on a regular basis. Some of the major changes that affect the practice of nursing can be found by searching reputable best-practice sites and through the following Web sites:

Agency for Healthcare Research and Quality (AHRQ)
www.ahcpr.gov
American Nurses Association (ANA) www.nursingworld.org
Centers for Disease Control and Prevention (CDC)
www.cdc.gov
Centers for Medicare and Medicaid Services (CMS)
www.cms.hhs.gov
Institute of Medicine (IOM) www.iom.edu
Joint Commission on Accreditation of Healthcare
Organizations (JCAHO) www.jcaho.org
National Quality Forum (NQF) www.qualityforum.org

Critical information is found in the orange colored "Reminder Section" immediately following the copyright page. A basic life support (BLS) guide, the Heimlich maneuver for both adults and children, and ECG reminders are found there. This allows a quick response to these events that occur infrequently in many healthcare settings. The computer symbol with BLS is designed to connect users with the most current BLS information. Standard (universal) precautions used with blood and body fluids, broken skin, and mucous membranes are also found in the orange Reminder Section. Appendix A lists commonly used medical symbols, and it is important to be absolutely accurate about what the symbol means before taking action. **Caution is urged in using symbols and abbreviations because they can lead to errors.**

Part 1, *Words and Meanings*, is designed as a source of general reference. It applies across all areas of nursing. Part 1 begins with prefixes and suffixes to increase the ability to combine parts of standard words to determine meanings of other words. Thus, it is possible to determine the general meaning of words other than those that appear here by identifying the root of the word and then the meaning of the prefix or suffix. The glossary is reflective of common terms needed to provide general clinical care, review, and record in health records and understand medical orders. The abbreviations and acronyms are those commonly found in most healthcare situations. Again, caution is urged in using abbreviations and acronyms because they can lead to errors.

Part 2, *Basic Processes*, highlights communication considerations, the nursing process, and select assessment strategies and guides. The assessment strategies and guides are those used across patient populations and in various settings. The final section of Part 2 focuses on common ways to document information.

Part 3, *Select Care Issues*, focuses on issues that cross various patient populations and settings and frequently are viewed as critical factors in creating quality care for patients and their families. For example, patient safety is of the utmost concern and dictates how care is delivered. Each of the items that is included here, such as pain management, medication administration, and violence, is a focus that crosses specialty considerations. Nurses can have a major effect on these issues.

Part 4, *Special Populations*, provides limited information about four patient populations because of the specialized knowledge that is associated with them. Because nurses work with people and their health needs in many family situations, it is important for nurses to have a broad, general understanding of these specialty areas. For example, nurses may see an elderly diabetic man who is accompanied by his pregnant granddaughter. Nurses may find that they need information about both gerontological health and obstetrical health.

Part 5, *Resources—Clinical*, includes common anatomy and physiology diagrams, measurements and conversions, standard laboratory tests and values, and nationally accepted classifications and general information about nutrition. Each of the elements in this part can be used to determine general interpretations (as in laboratory test values) or exact meanings. The expectation underlying this section is that the information is actually learned in depth in another source and that *Rapid Reference for Nurses* is used as a memory stimulus.

Part 6, *Resources—Professional*, provides key information about professional references that affect the practice of nursing on a broad basis. For example, *The Code of Ethics for Nurses* affects every nurse's practice, irrespective of specialty or setting. The same is true for the practice standards that serve as the organizing framework for all specially focused standards of practice. Key professional organizations and licensure agencies are noted with their Web site addresses. Both credentialing sources are included: licensure and certification. Additionally, the initials frequently seen following nurses' names are included to provide clarity about credentials.

Being able to find needed information quickly depends on the quality of the index, which means that information is listed in as many ways as possible to reflect real clinical life. Thus, the user does not need to think so much about to what something relates or what else something might be called.

The index is the best place to start unless you know you want to find a word. If nothing appears in the index, try the glossary; and if nothing appears there, try using the prefix and suffix lists to determine what the general sense of the word might be.

If the stimulus for seeking clarification derives from a patient record, try to stay in the general area of reference. For example, if some word appears in the assessment section of the record, determine if there is comparable information within this book. An example of that might be the use of the term *tibia* under *extremities* in the record. Looking for *tibia* in the illustrations related to the lower body might be the easiest way to connect with the general meaning of the word.

Finally, remember that this book does not substitute for more detailed texts and reliable Web sites related to a topic (such as anatomy and physiology). *Rapid Reference for Nurses* is designed as a quick reference source that is convenient and portable.

PART 1

Words and Meanings

Prefixes and Suffixes

Prefixes

a-, an-: without, lacking
ab-: away from
ad-: toward
adeno-: gland
adipo-: fat
aero-: air
amb-: both sides
ana-: again, up
andro-: male
anky-: bent, fused
ante-: precede, before
antero-: front, anterior
anti-: against
arterio-: artery
arthro-: pertaining to joints
aut-, auto-: self

bar-, baro-: pressure, weight
bi-: double, two
bili-: bile
blenn-, blenno-: mucus
blephar-, blepharo-: eyelid
brady-: slow

carcin-: cancer
cardi-: heart
cat-, cata-: under, against, lower
cephalo-: head
chole-: bile, gall
chondr-: cartilage
circum-: about, around
contra-: against, counter

cranio-: skull
cyno-: blue

de-: away or down from, remove
dextro-: right
dia-: across, apart, through
dis-: reverse, separate
dors-: back
dys-: difficult, painful, fault

e-, ec-, ex-: out of, from
ecto-: outside, on
em-, en-: in, on
endo-: in, within
entero-: intestine
epi-: additionally, upon
erythro-: red
etio-: causation
eu-: good, well, easy
exo-: outside
extra-: beyond, outside of

fibro-: fibrous tissue

gastro-: stomach
genito-: organs of reproduction
gingiv-: gums
gloss-: tongue
gyn-: female

hemi-: half
hepa-: liver
hetero-: other
histo-: tissue
homeo-: similar, like
homo-: same
hyper-: above, beyond

hypo-: below, under
hyster-: uterus

ideo-: mental image
ileo-, ilio-: ileum
im-, in-: in, on, into; also not
infra-: beneath
inter-: between, among
intra-: inside, within
intro-: within, into
ipsi-: self, same
iso-: equal, same

juxta-: close by, near

kera-, kerato-: horny substance
kines-: movement
kolp-: vaginal

lapro-: abdomen
laryng-: larynx
latero-: side
leuk-: white

macro-: excess, large, long
mal-: abnormal, bad
mamm-: breast
mast-: breast
med-, medi-: middle
mega-: large, abnormal largeness
melan-: black
meso-: intermediate, middle, moderate
meta-: after, beyond
micro-: small, minute
muc-, muci-, muco-: mucus
musculo-: muscle

myelo-: spinal
myring-: tympanic membrane

narco-: stupor, numb
necro-: dead
neo-: new, young, recent
nephro-: kidney
neuro-: nerves
non-: no, not
noso-: disease
noto-: the back

ob-: against
oculo-: eyes
olig-, oligo-: few, scant
onco-: tumor
oo-: ovum
ophthal-: eye
orch-: testicle
oro-: mouth
ortho-: straighten
os-: mouth
osteo-: bone
ot-: ear

pachy-: thick
pan-: all
para-: beside, beyond
path-: disease
ped-: foot
pedia-: child
per-: through
peri-: around
perineo-: perineum
peritoneo-: peritoneum
phago-: eat
phlebo-: vein
pleuro-: rib, pleura

pneum-: respiration
poly-: much, many
post-: after, subsequent
pod-: foot
postero-: after
pre-, pro-: before, in front of
presby-: old age
proct-: rectum, anus
pseudo-: fake, false
pulmo-: lung
py-: pus
pyelo-: pelvis
pyreto-: fever

recto-: rectum
reticul-: reticulum
retro-: behind, backward
rhino-: nose
roseo-: rose colored

sacro-: sacrum
salping-: auditory or fallopian
tube
sapro-: rotted, putrid
sarco-: flesh
scato-: fecal matter
schizo-: division
scirrho-, sclero-: hard
sebo-: fatty
semi-: half, part
soma-: body
sphygmo-: pulse
spondyl-: vertebra
steno-: narrow, contracted
stomato-: mouth
sub-, sup-: below, under
super-: above, on top of,
beyond

supra-: above, upon
sym-, syn-: together, with

tachy-: rapid, fast
thanato-: death
thermo-: hot
thrombo-: blood cot
tox-: poison
trans-: across, beyond, through
trich-: hair
troph-: nourishment

tympan-: eardrum

ultra-: beyond, excess
uretero-: ureter
urethro-: urethra
utero-: uterus

vaso-: vessel
veno-: vein
ventro-: abdomen
vesico-: bladder

Suffixes

-able, -ible: ability to, capable of
-aemia: blood
-al, -ar: related to
-algia: painful condition
-ary: related to, connected with
-ase: enzyme
-ate: state

-cele: hernia, tumor
-cle, -cule, -culum, -culus: small

-ectasia, -ectasis: dilated state,
    distended
-ectomy: excise, cut off
-emesis: vomit
-emia: blood
-esthesia: sensation

-form: structure, shape
-fugal: movement away from

-gen, -genic: production
-gram: record, written

-ia: condition, state
-ic: related to
-ile: related to, characteristic of
-ion: action, process
-ism: state, condition
-itis: inflammation
-ity: state

-lith: stone
-logy: study of, body of
    knowledge
-lysis: dissolve, disintegrate

-mania: frenzied

-odyne, -odynia: pain, related to
    pain
-oid: like, resembles
-ole, -olus: small
-oma: tumor
-or: agent
-ose: carbohydrate
-osis: condition

-ostomy: created outlet
-otomy: cut

-penia: deficiency
-pexy: fixed
-phil, -philia: craving
-phlagia, -phagy: ingest,
     consume, eat
-phobia: abnormal fear
-phoresis: transmit
-phylaxis: protection
-piesis: pressure
-plasia: growth
-plegia: paralysis
-poiesis: form, produce

-ptosis: prolapse, displacement
     downward

-rrhagia: break open, burst,
     discharge
-rrhaphy: suture in place
-rrthea: flow

-scopy: examination
-sis, -asis, -esis, -osis: state,
     condition, process

-tomy: cut, excise

-uria: urine

Glossary [CAUTION: AVOID ABBREVIATIONS]

abandonment: Unilateral termination of patient care by a health care professional.

abdominal: Pertaining to the part of the trunk lying between the thorax and pelvis and its functions and disorders.

abduction: Movement of a body part (usually the limbs) away from the midline of the body.

ABO incompatibility: Occurs when the mother's blood type is O and the baby's type is A, B, or AB and thus incompatible with the mother's; requires a transfusion for the baby shortly after birth.

abnormal: Not normal, average, typical, or usual; an irregularity.

abortion: Any loss of pregnancy, either accidentally or intentionally, before the 20th week or when the fetus weighs less than 500 grams; **complete abortion:** Both the fetus and all tissue/products of conception are expelled; **elective abortion:** Termination of pregnancy at the desire of the woman rather than for medical reasons; **habitual (recurrent) abortion:** Three or more successive pregnancy losses for no apparent cause; **incomplete abortion:** Some but not all products of conception are expelled spontaneously; **induced abortion:** Loss of pregnancy caused intentionally by health professionals or others; **inevitable abortion:** Imminent threat of loss of a pregnancy that cannot be prevented; **intentional termination of pregnancy (IT OP):** Loss of pregnancy based on specific personal actions; **missed abortion:** Products of conception remain in the uterus after the death of the fetus; **septic abortion:** Infection of the products of conception, creating the death of the fetus, often a result of attempted termination of early pregnancy; **spontaneous abortion:** Naturally occurring loss of the pregnancy from no known cause or intervention; also known as miscarriage; **therapeutic abortion:** Pregnancy which has been intentionally terminated for medical reasons.

abruptio placentae: Premature separation of the placenta from the uterine wall after 20 weeks of gestation.

abstinence: Temporary or permanent restraint from specific activities.

abscess: A swollen, inflamed area of body tissue in which there is a localized collection of pus.

absence: An epileptic seizure characterized by abrupt loss of consciousness for a few seconds, followed by a rapid, complete recovery.

absorption: Process by which a substance is made available to body fluids for distribution.

abstract thinking: Ability to derive meaning from an event or experience beyond the tangible aspects of the event itself.

acceleration: Increase in the speed or velocity of an object or reaction.

access to care: Opportunity to receive health care services.

accessibility: Degree to which an exterior or interior environment is available for use in relation to an individual's physical and/or psychological abilities.

accommodation: Process of adapting or adjusting one object or set of objects to another.

accreditation: A voluntary process of recognition through an external organization. Typically refers to programs or services.

accuracy of response: Percentage of errors and correct responses recorded.

achalasia: Failure of a circular sphincter or other muscle to relax and open (e.g., cardiac sphincter between the esophagus and the stomach).

achromatopsia: Color blindness.

acidosis: Increased hydrogen ion concentration resulting in a blood pH below 7.35.

acini cells: Milk producing cells in the breast.

acme: Highest point of a contraction.

acoustic stimulation test: Fetal heart rate response to sound performed by applying a sound source (usually a laryngeal stimulator) to the maternal abdomen.

acquaintance: A step in the attachment process where parents become familiar with their new infant.

acquired amputation: Person is born with all limbs, but after injury or accident, a limb is removed in part or total.

acquired immunodeficiency syndrome (AIDS): Condition caused by HIV (human immunodeficiency virus), which is spread by contact with body fluids and results in an inability to withstand infections, malignancies, and neurologic disorders.

acrochordons: Flesh colored skin tags.

acrocyanosis: Symmetric mottled cyanosis of the hands and feet, associated with coldness and sweating. A vasospastic disorder accentuated by cold or emotion and relieved by warmth. Occurs in most infants at birth and continues for 7 to 10 days.

acromion process: Outer projection of the spine of the scapula; considered to be the highest part of the shoulder, it connects laterally to the clavicle.

active labor: The second phase of the first stage of labor during which the cervix dilates from 4 to 8 cm.

active listening: Skills that allow a person to hear, understand, and indicate that the message has been communicated.

activin: Hormone releasing factor that assists production of follicular-stimulating hormone (FSH) at the pituitary.

activities of daily living (ADL): The self-care, communication, and mobility skills (e.g., bed mobility, transfers, ambulation, dressing, grooming, bathing, eating, and toileting) required for independence in everyday living.

activity: The nature and extent of functioning at the level of the person. Productive action required for the development, maturation, and use of sensory, motor, social, psychological, and cognitive functions.

activity theory of aging: Psychosocial theory of aging suggesting that successful aging occurs when the older person continues to participate in the satisfying activities of his or her earlier adulthood.

activity tolerance: The ability to sustain engagement in an activity over a period of time.

acuity: Ability of the sensory organ to receive information. Keenness, as of thought or vision.

acupressure: Use of touch at specific points along the meridians of the body to release the tensions that cause various physical symptoms. Based on the principles of acupuncture.

acupuncture: Chinese practice of inserting needles into specific points along the meridians of the body to relieve pain and induce anesthesia. Used for preventive and therapeutic purposes.

acute: Of short and intense duration. A very serious, critical period of short duration in illness. Intensification of need, or urgent.

acute myocardial infarction: Coronary artery blockage leading to loss of cardiac muscle.

adaptation: Satisfactory adjustment of individuals within their environment over time. Successful adaptation equates with quality of life.

adaptive devices: A variety of implements or equipment used to aid patients/clients in performing movements, tasks, or activities. Adaptive devices include raised toilet seats, seating systems, environmental controls, and other devices.

addiction: Dependence on substance or habit that becomes a driving force in life.

adduction (ADD): Movement toward the midline of the body.

adductor pads: Pads at the sides of a wheelchair that hold the hips and legs toward the midline of the body.

adenohypophysis: The anterior lobe of the pituitary gland.

adherence: Consistent behavior that is accomplished through an internalization of learning, enhanced by independent coping and problem-solving skills. Sticking to an object or thing.

adhesion: Soft tissue restrictions and scarring resulting from injury and inflammation. The product when two or more structures become attached, united, or stuck together.

adjustment reaction disorder: Characterized by reduced ability to function and adapt in response to a stressful life event. Disorder begins shortly after the event and normal functioning is expected to return when the particular stressor is removed.

administration: Management of activities; e.g., organizational, medications.

adnexa: Adjacent or accessory parts of a structure; **uterine adnexa:** Ovaries and fallopian tubes adjacent to the uterus.

adolescence: The period of transformation from childhood to adulthood, beginning with the appearance of secondary sex characteristics; approximately 11 to 18 years of age.

adrenal gland: A pair of endocrine organs lying immediately above the kidney, consisting of an inner medulla, which produces epinephrine and norepinephrine, and an outer cortex, which produces a variety of steroid hormones.

adrenocorticotrophic hormone (ACTH): A hormone released by the adenohypophysis that stimulates the adrenal cortex to secrete its entire spectrum of hormones.

adult respiratory distress syndrome (ARDS): Symptoms include decreased compliance of lung tissue, pulmonary edema, and acute hypoxemia. It is similar to respiratory distress syndrome in the newborn.

advanced directives: Living wills and care instructions in which a competent adult expresses his or her wishes regarding medical management in the event of a serious illness.

advanced practice: The service provided by nurses who are typically master's-prepared and function in one of the following roles: nurse practitioner, clinical specialist, nurse midwife, or nurse anesthetist.

adverse effects: Undesired consequences.

advocacy: Actively supporting a cause, an idea, or a policy (e.g., speaking in favor); recommending accommodations under the Americans with Disabilities Act.

aerobe: A microorganism that lives and grows in the presence of free oxygen.

aerobic activity/conditioning/exercise: Any physical exercise or activity that requires additional effort by the heart and lungs to meet the increased demand for oxygen by the skeletal muscles.

affect: Emotion or feeling conveyed in a person's face or body; the subjective experiencing of a feeling or emotion. To influence or produce a change in.

affection: Disease.

affective: Learning domain related to attitudes, values, and beliefs.

affective disorder: Marked disturbances of mood; typically characterized by disproportionately elevated mood (i.e., mania), extremely depressed mood (i.e., depression), or swings between the two (i.e., bipolar disorder/manic-depressive disorder).

afferent: Conducting toward a structure.

afferent neuron: A nerve cell that sends nerve impulses from sensory receptors to the central nervous system.

afibrinogenemia: Decrease or absence of fibrinogen in the blood so the blood does not coagulate.

afterbirth: Lay term for amniotic membranes and placenta expelled from the uterus during the third stage of labor.

afterbirth pains (afterpains): Painful uterine contractions or cramping of the uterus after the fetus and placenta are delivered which can occur for 2–3 days.

AGA: Appropriate (growth) for gestational age in newborns.

age-appropriate activities: Activities and materials that are consistent with those used by nondisabled age mates in the same culture.

ageism: Prejudice that one age is better than another.

agent: One who acts for another.

agenesis: Failure of an organ to develop.

agglutination: Act of blood cells clumping together.

aggressiveness: Forceful assertion, usually viewed as negative, which may harm or insult another.

agility: Ease of movement.

aging in place: Where older adults remain in their own homes, retirement housing, or other familiar surroundings as they grow old irrespective of changes in needs.

agnosia: Inability to comprehend sensory information due to central nervous system damage.

agonist: Muscle that is capable of providing the power so a bone can move.

agoraphobia: An abnormal fear of being in an open space.

agranulocytosis: Exceedingly low white blood cell level.

agraphia: Inability to write caused by impairment of central nervous system processing (not by paralysis).

airplane splint: A shoulder splint that stabilizes and maintains the shoulder in approximately 90° of horizontal abduction.

akathisia: Motor restlessness.

akinesia: Muscular weakness.

alanine aminotransferase: An intracellular enzyme essential to metabolism of carbohydrates; when blood levels are elevated, indicates necrosis or presence of disease.

albuminuria: Presence of detectable albumin in the urine.

alcoholism: A chronic disease characterized by an uncontrollable urge to consume alcoholic beverages to the point that it interferes with normal life activities.

aldosterone: A steroid hormone produced by the adrenal cortex gland, the chief regulator of sodium, potassium, and chloride metabolism, thus controlling the body's water and electrolyte balances.

alexia: Condition of being unable to read by impairment of central nervous system.

alkalosis: Abnormal body fluids characterized by an increase in pH, as from an excess of alkaline bicarbonate or decrease in acidity of the fluids.

allantois: The diverticulum from the hindgut of the embryo that appears around the 16th day of development, forming part of the umbilical cord and placenta.

allele: Alternative form of a gene coded for a particular trait.

allied health: Broad field of study encompassing diverse health professionals with special training in such fields as occupational therapy, physical therapy, respiratory therapy, speech pathology, and health information services, as well as laboratory, radiology, and dietetic services. Does not include physicians, nurses, dentists, or pharmacists.

allopathic medicine: Traditional Western medicine such as found in the United States.

alopecia: Absence or loss of hair; baldness.

alpha error (or Type 1 error): When the null hypothesis is rejected, the probability of being wrong or the probability of rejecting it when it should have been accepted.

alpha-fetoprotein (AFP): Nonhormonal plasma constituent in amniotic fluid that is used as a determinant of neural tube defects.

alternative/complementary therapies: Interventions to provide holistic approaches to the management of diseases and illnesses, such as acupuncture, massage, or specifically designed nutrition.

altruism: Unselfish concern for the welfare of others.

alveolar: A general term used in anatomical nomenclature to designate a small saclike dilatation, such as the sockets in the mandible and maxilla in which the roots of the teeth are held. The small outpocketings of the alveolar sacs in the lungs, through whose walls the gaseous exchange takes place.

amaurosis fugax: Temporary, partial, or total blindness often resulting from transient occlusion of the retinal arteries. May be a symptom of impending cerebrovascular accident.

ambulate: To walk from place to place.

ambulatory care: Care delivered on an outpatient basis.

amenorrhea: Absence or suppression of monthly menstruation; **primary:** menarche is delayed until after age 16 and/or secondary sex characteristics are absent after age 14; **secondary:** menses cease due to extreme mental or physical stress.

American Sign Language (ASL): Nonverbal method of communication using the hands and fingers to represent letters, numbers, and concepts.

amnesia: Dissociative disorder characterized by memory loss during a certain time period or of personal identity.

amniocentesis: A low-risk prenatal diagnostic procedure of collecting amniotic fluid and fetal cells for examination through the use of a needle inserted into the abdominal wall and uterus to determine the fetal maturity and genetic characteristics. Is performed after four months of gestation.

amnion: Innermost membrane enclosing the developing fetus and the fluid in which the fetus is bathed (i.e., amniotic fluid).

amnionitis: Inflammation of the amnion; frequently occurs after rupture of the membranes.

amniotic: Relating to the amnion; **amniotic fluid:** Fluid surrounding the fetus composed of maternal serum and fetal urine; **amniotic fluid embolism:** Embolism resulting from amniotic fluid entering the maternal bloodstream during labor or birth (after rupture of membranes). When embolism lodges in the lungs, often fatal to the mother; **amniotic fluid index (AFI):** Estimation of quantity of fluid, usually by ultrasound; **amniotic sac:** Membrane or "bag" which contains all the products of conception prior to birth.

amniotomy: Artificial rupture of the membranes (AROM), using an amnio hook or surgical clamp.

amplitude: The maximal height of a waveform, either from the baseline or peak to peak.

amputation: Partial or complete removal of a limb; may be congenital or acquired (traumatic or surgical).

anaerobe: A microorganism that grows in the absence of free oxygen.

anaerobic exercise/activity: Exercise or activity without oxygen; oxygen intake cannot keep up with level of exercise/activity, so oxygen debt occurs.

anakusis: Total hearing loss; deafness.

analgesia: Absence of pain sensitivity; patient may experience stimulus but it is not noxious.

analgesic: Type of medication for reducing pain. Some mild analgesics are nonsteroidal anti-inflammatory drugs (e.g., ibuprofen), and some analgesics are narcotics (e.g., morphine).

analog: Continuous information system (e.g., a clock with hands that move on a continuum, as opposed to a digital clock which moves as a minute passes).

analogue: Contrived situation created to elicit specific client behaviors and allow for their observation. Representing numerical values by physical quantities so as to allow the manipulation of numerical data over a continuous range of values.

analysis: An examination of the nature of something for the purpose of prediction or comparison.

analysis of covariance (ANCOVA): Controlling the effects of any variable(s) known to correlate with the dependent variable.

analysis of variance (or F ratio or ANOVA): Establishing whether or not a significant difference exists between the means of samples.

anaphylactic shock: Condition in which the flow of blood throughout the body becomes suddenly inadequate due to dilation of the blood vessels as a result of allergic reaction; may be fatal.

anaplasia: Reverting of a specialized cell to its primitive or embryonic state. Synonym: dedifferentiation.

anastomosis: Surgical formation of a passage between two open vessels.

anatomical position: Standing erect, arms at the sides, with palms facing forward.

anatomy: Area of study concerned with the internal and external structures of the body and how these structures interrelate.

andragogy: Art and science of helping adults learn.

androgens: Substances that produce or stimulate the development of male characteristics.

android pelvis: Male-type pelvis with heart-shaped inlet.

andropause: Male equivalent of menopause.

anemia: A condition in which there is a reduction of the number, or volume, of red blood corpuscles or the total amount of hemoglobin in the bloodstream, resulting in paleness and generalized weakness.

anencephaly: Congenital deformity characterized by absence of flat bones of the skull, cerebellum, and cerebrum.

anesthesia: Absence of sensibility to stimuli with or without loss of consciousness.

anesthetic: Type of medication that reduces or eliminates sensation. Can affect the whole body (e.g., nitrous oxide, a general anesthetic) or a particular part of the body (e.g., Xylocaine, a local anesthetic).

aneuploidy: Having an abnormal number of chromosomes.

aneurysm: A sac formed by local enlargement of a weakened wall of an artery, a vein, or the heart, caused by disease, anatomical anomaly, or injury.

angina pectoris: Chest pain due to insufficient flow of blood to the heart muscle.

angiography: Injection of a radioactive material so that blood vessels can be visualized.

angioneurotic edema: Edema of an extremity due to any neurosis affecting primarily the blood vessels resulting from a disorder of the vasomotor system, such as angiospasm, angioparesis, or angioparalysis.

anhedonia: Inability to enjoy what is ordinarily pleasurable.

ankle-arm index: A numerical comparison of the systolic blood pressures in the arm and ankle obtained by dividing the ankle pressure by the arm pressure. Values below 1.0 indicate varying degrees of ischemia.

ankle/foot orthosis (AFO): An external device that controls the foot and ankle and can facilitate knee positioning and muscle response.

ankylosis: Condition of the joints in which they become stiffened and nonfunctional. Abnormal immobility and consolidation of a joint.

anomaly: Pronounced departure from the norm. Malformed organ or in some way abnormal in structure or form or position.

anomia: Loss of ability to name objects or to recognize or recall names; can be receptive or expressive.

anorexia: Loss of appetite.

anorgasmic: Incapable of achieving an orgasm.

anosmia: Inability to smell.

ANOVA (analysis of variance): Abbreviation for the statistical method used in research to compare sample populations.

anoxemia: Absence or deficiency of oxygen in the blood.

anoxia/anoxic: Absence or deficiency of oxygen in the tissues. Can cause tissue death; synonymous with hypoxia.

antagonist: Muscle that resists the action of a prime mover (agonist).

antalgic: A compensatory behavior attempting to avoid or lessen pain, usually applied to gait or movement.

antenatal: During pregnancy.

antenatal glucocorticoids: Medications given 24 hours prior to a preterm birth (24–36 weeks gestation) to accelerate fetal lung maturity.

antepartum or antepartal: The period from conception to labor (also called prenatal).

anterior: Toward the front of the body.

anterior fontanel: Region of the head that is found as a membrane-covered portion on the top of the head, generally closing by the time a child reaches 18 months (the soft spot).

anterior horn cell: Motor neuron located anteriorly that is similar in shape to a pointed projection, such as the paired processes on the head of various animals.

ante version: Turning forward or inclining forward as a whole without bending; usually applied to the positional relationship between the head of the femur and its shaft.

anthropometric: Human body measurements, such as height, weight, girth, and body fat composition.

anthropoid pelvis: The anterior-posterior diameter of the pelvis is equal to or greater than the transverse diameter; an oval inlet.

antibacterial: An agent that inhibits the growth of bacteria.

antibiotic: Chemical substance that has the ability to inhibit or kill foreign organisms in the body.

antibody: A protein belonging to a class of proteins called immunoglobulins. A molecule produced by the immune system of the body in response to an antigen and which has the particular property of combining specifically with the antigen that induced its formation. Produced by plasma cells to counteract specific antigens (infectious agents like viruses, bacteria, etc.). The antibodies combine with the antigen they are created to fight, often causing the death of that infectious agent.

anticipatory grief: State of limited responses (social, emotional, and physical) due to an expected loss.

anticoagulant: A substance that prevents or retards blood clotting.

antigen: A substance foreign to the body. An antigen stimulates the formation of antibodies to combat its presence.

anti-inflammatory: Counteracting or suppressing inflammation.

antilymphocytic globulin: Antibody globulin used to reduce rejection of transplanted organs and tissues.

antimicrobial: Designed to destroy or inhibit the growth of bacterial, fungal, or viral organisms.

antineoplastic agents: Substances, procedure, or measures used in treating cancer, administered with the purpose of inhibiting the production of malignant cells.

antioxidant: A substance that slows down the oxidation of hydrocarbon, oils, fats, etc., and helps to check deterioration of tissues.

antisepsis: The prevention of sepsis by the inhibition or destruction of the causative organism.

antisocial personality disorder: Personality disorder resulting in a chronic pattern of disregard for socially acceptable behavior, impulsiveness, irresponsibility, and lack of remorseful feelings. Synonyms: sociopathy, psychopathy, or antisocial reaction.

antral: Relating to a body cavity.

anuria: Absence of urine excretion.

anxiety: Characterized by an overwhelming sense of apprehension; the expectation that something bad is happening or will happen; class of mental disorders characterized by chronic and debilitating anxiety (e.g., generalized anxiety disorder, panic disorder, phobias, and post-traumatic stress disorder).

anxiolytic: Anxiety-reducing drugs; formerly called tranquilizers.

aortic aneurysm: Aneurysm of the aorta.

aortic heart disease: A disease affecting the main artery of the body, carrying blood from the left ventricle of the heart to the main arteries of the body.

Apgar score: Assessment of the condition of the newborn expressed in numeric terms of 0 to 10 at 1 minute, 5 minutes, and 10 minutes.

aphakia: Absence of the crystalline lens of the eye.

aphasia: Absence of cognitive language-processing ability that results in deficits in speech, writing, or sign communication. Can be receptive, expressive, or both.

aphonia: Inability to produce speech sounds from the larynx.

apnea: Temporary cessation of breathing for more than 15 seconds; associated with cyanosis.

aponeurosis: Fibrous or membranous tissue that connects a muscle to the part that the muscle moves (bone or other tissue).

appendicular skeleton: Bones forming the limbs, pectoral girdle, and pelvic girdle of the body.

apprenticeship: Learning process in which novices advance their skills and understanding through active participation with a more skilled person.

apraxia: Inability to motor plan, execute purposeful movement, manipulate objects, or use objects appropriately.

apraxia of speech: Disruption of speech motor planning.

Apt test: A test to differentiate fetal and maternal blood when there is vaginal bleeding.

aquatherapy: The use of water as a therapeutic measure (e.g., hydrotherapy, whirlpools, pools for exercise).

arbitrary inference: Thinking error exhibiting a decision reached without facts or in spite of refuting facts.

arc: Any line wholly on a surface between two chosen points other than a chord.

architectural barrier: Structural impediment to the approach, mobility, and functional use of an interior or exterior environment.

arcus senilis: White fat deposit around iris. Does not interfere with vision.

areola: Darkened area around the nipple; **secondary areola:** A second faint ring of pigmentation seen around the areola during the 5th month of pregnancy.

arousal: Internal state of the individual characterized by increased responsiveness to environmental stimuli.

arrhythmia: Variation from the normal rhythm, especially of the heart-beat.

arterial: Pertaining to one or more arteries; vessels that carry oxygenated blood to the tissue.

arterial compliance: The property of healthy arterial walls to expand and contract with blood flow pulsations.

arterial embolism/thrombosis: The obstruction of an arterial blood vessel by an embolus too large to pass through it or a thrombosis caused by the coagulation and fibrosis of blood at a particular site.

arterial insufficiency: Inadequate blood supply in the arterial system usually caused by stenosis or occlusion proximal to the inadequately supplied area.

arterial pressure catheter: A Teflon intravenous catheter (usually 20 gauge) placed in an artery, connected to a monitor by a pressure line which provides continuous systolic, diastolic, and mean arterial blood pressures.

arteriolar vasospasm: A decrease in arteriolar vessel diameter that restricts blood flow to all organs and elevates blood pressure.

arterioles: The smallest arterial vessels (0.2 mm diameter) resulting from repeated branching of the arteries. Composed of smooth muscle only and conduct blood from the arteries to the capillaries.

arteriosclerosis: Thickening, hardening, and a loss of elasticity of the walls of the arteries.

arteriovenous: Designating arteries or veins or arterioles and venules.

arteriovenous fistula: An abnormal passage between the artery and the vein caused by an abscess at the junction of these vessels.

arteriovenous oxygen difference: The difference between the oxygen content of blood in the arterial system and the amount in the mixed venous blood.

arteritis: Inflammation of an artery.

arthritis: Inflammation of the joints that may be chronic or acute.

arthroclasia: Artificial breaking of an ankylosed joint to provide movement.

arthrography: Injection of dye or air into a joint cavity to image the contours of the joint.

arthrokinesiology: The study of the structure and function of skeletal joints.

arthropathy: Disease of a joint.

arthroplasty: Surgical replacement; formation or reformation of a joint; surgical reconstruction of a joint.

arthroscopy: Procedure in which visual equipment can be inserted into a joint so that its internal parts can be viewed.

articular cartilage: The tough, elastic tissue that separates the bones in a joint.

articulation: The joining or juncture between two or more bones. The process of moving a joint through all or part of its range of motion.

artifact: An artificial or extraneous feature introduced into an observation that may simulate a relevant feature of that observation.

asbestosis: Lung disease caused by inhaling particles of asbestos.

ASCII (American Standard Code for Information Interchange): Standardized coding scheme that uses numeric values to represent letters, numbers, symbols, etc. Widely used in coding information for computers.

ascites: Accumulation of fluid in the abdomen.

aseptic: Free from infection or septic material; sterile.

Asherman's syndrome: Intrauterine adhesions as a result of inflammation and infection; one cause of infertility.

aspermia: Lack of or failure to ejaculate semen.

asphyxia: Condition of insufficient oxygen; **perinatal asphyxia:** Decreased oxygen to the fetus in utero resulting in hypoxemia (lowering of PO_2), hypercapnia (increase in PO_2) and respiratory and metabolic acidosis (reduction of blood pH), all of which have a negative impact on the fetus/newborn.

aspirate: To inhale vomitus, mucus, or food (also for newborns, amniotic fluid with or with out meconium) into the respiratory tract.

aspiration: Inhaling fluids or solid substances into the lungs.

aspiration pneumonia: Inflammatory condition of the lungs due to inhalation of fluids or solids into the lungs.

assault: An act resulting in fear by an individual that another will touch him without consent.

assertiveness: Behavior aimed at claiming rights without denying the rights of others.

assessment: Process by which data are gathered, hypotheses formulated, and decisions made for further action; a subsection of the problem-oriented medical record. The measurement or quantification of a variable or the placement of a value on something (not to be confused with examination or evaluation).

assimilation: Expansion of data within a given category or subcategory of a schema by incorporation of new information within the existing representational structure without requiring any reorganization or modification of prior knowledge.

assisted-living facility: Medium-sized to large facilities that offer housing, meals, and personal care, plus such extras as housekeeping, transportation, and recreation. Small-sized facilities are known as board and care homes.

assisted reproductive therapies (ARTs): Infertility interventions including in vitro fertilization, embryo adoption, embryo hosting, and therapeutic insemination.

assisted suicide: Any service provided by another that results in the termination of life for the other person.

assistive devices: A variety of implements or equipment used to aid patients/clients in performing tasks or movements. Assistive devices include crutches, canes, walkers, wheelchairs, power devices, long-handled reachers, and static and dynamic splints.

assistive technology: Any item, piece of equipment, or product system that is used to increase, maintain, or improve functional capabilities of individuals with disabilities.

association learning: Form of learning in which particular items or ideas are connected.

associative intrusions: Inappropriate associations that interfere with normal thought processes.

associative network theory of memory: Theory that related memories are stored in networks and that the stimulation of a network will result in the recall of the memories in that network.

associative play: Play in which each child is participating in a separate activity but with the cooperation and assistance of the others.

assumption: Proposition or supposition; a statement that links or relates two or more concepts to one another.

astereognosis: Inability to discriminate the shape, texture, weight, and size of objects by touch.

asterixis: Involuntary muscle tremors, especially the hands and often associated with diseases of the liver.

asthenia: Chronic lack of energy and strength.

asthma: Respiratory disease in which the muscles of the bronchial tubes tighten and give off excessive secretions. Causes obstruction of the airway and results in wheezing; characterized by recurring episodes.

astigmatism: Refraction of light in the eye is spread over a diffuse area rather than focused on the retina.

asymmetrical: Lack of symmetry.

asymptomatic: Showing or causing no symptoms.

asynclitism: Oblique or synclitic presentation of the fetal head at the pelvic inlet; the pelvic planes and those of the fetal head are not parallel.

ataractics: Drugs that promote tranquility; tranquilizers.

ataxia: Poor balance and awkward movement.

atelectasis: Collapse or airless condition of the lung; particularly the alveoli.

atheroma: A deposit of fatty (or other) substances in the inner lining of the artery wall.

atherosclerosis: Deposits of fatty substance in arteries, veins, and the lymphatic system.

athetosis: Type of cerebral palsy that involves involuntary purposeless movements that fall into one of two classes: nontension involves contorted movements, and tension involves blocked movements and flailing.

atonicatony: Absence of muscle tone.

atopic dermatitis (ADD): A clinical hypersensitivity of the skin.

atresia: Absence of normally present passageway; **biliary atresia:** Absence of the bile duct; **esophageal atresia:** Esophagus ends in a blind pouch or narrows significantly thus forming no usable passage to the stomach.

atrial septal defect: An opening between the right and left atrium of the heart which is congenital and usually found in newborns.

atrioventricular block: Disruption in the flow of electrical impulse through the atrium wall of the heart leading to arrhythmias, brady-cardia, or complete cardiac arrest.

atrium: One of the two upper chambers of the heart. Right atrium receives unoxygenated venous blood from the body, left receives oxygenated blood from the lungs.

atrophy: The decrease in size of a normally developed organ or tissue due to lack of use or deficient nutrition.

atropine: Drug that inhibits actions of the autonomic nervous system; relaxes smooth muscle; treats biliary and renal colic; and reduces secretions of the bronchial tubes, salivary glands, stomach, and intestines.

attachment: Deep affective bond which ties one to another individual or a feeling that binds one to a thing, cause, ideal, etc.

attendant care: Services that provide individuals with nonmedical, personal health, and hygiene care, such as preparing meals, bathing, toileting, getting in and out of bed, and walking.

attention: Ability to focus on a specific stimulus without distraction.

attention span: Focusing on a task over time. Length of time an individual is able to focus or concentrate on a task or thought.

attitude: The position or posture assumed by the body; in connection with an action, feeling, or mood. One's disposition, opinion, or mental set; **fetal attitude:** Relation of fetal parts to each other in utero (e.g., all parts flexed except neck is extended).

auditory: Interpreting and localizing sounds, and discriminating background sounds; pertaining to the sense or organs of hearing.

auditory defensiveness: Oversensitivity to certain sounds (e.g., vacuum cleaners, fire alarms).

augmentation: The normal increase in the Doppler sound of venous flow upon compression distal to the Doppler probe or release of compression proximal to the probe. Augmentation resulting from the release of distal compression or the application of proximal compression indicates valvular incompetence.

augmentation of labor: Stimulation of ineffective uterine contractions with medication (e.g., Pitocin) after labor has begun.

augmentative communication: Method or device that increases a person's ability to communicate (e.g., nonelectronic devices, such as communication boards, or electronic devices, such as portable communication systems, that allow the user to speak and print text).

aura: Subjective sensation preceding a paroxysmal attack; a subtly pervasive quality or atmosphere seen as coming from a person, place, or thing.

auscultation: Process of listening for sounds within the body as a method of diagnosis. Stethoscope or other instruments may be used.

autism: Condition of inward attention to a fantasy world while ignoring reality of external world; little or no communication with others, can be accompanied with repetitive behaviors.

autocosmic play: Idea developed by Erikson in which a child plays with his or her own body during the first year of life.

autocratic: Leadership style reflected in leader making centralized decisions.

autocrine: Method of intracellular hormonal communication.

autogeneic drainage: Airway clearance through the patient's/client's own efforts (e.g., coughing).

autoimmunization: Antibodies developed against one's own tissue; e.g., a man may develop antibodies against his own sperm.

autoimmunity: Condition in which the body has developed a sensitivity to some of its own tissues.

autolysis: Disintegration or liquefaction of tissue or cells by the body's own mechanisms.

automatic process: Process that occurs with little, if any, attention effort.

automatic thoughts: Rapid, responsive thoughts with no rational basis.

automatization: When a learned motor skill is done with little conscious thought.

autonomic nervous system: Part of the nervous system concerned with the control of involuntary bodily functions.

autonomy: State of independence and self-control.

autosomal dominant: Genetic trait carried on the autosome. When one of a pair of chromosomes contains the abnormal gene, disorder appears. Passed on from the affected parent to half of the children.

autosomal recessive: Genetic trait carried on the autosome. Both asymptomatic parents must carry trait for disorder to appear.

autosome: Any chromosome other than the X and Y (sex) chromosomes.

aversion: A condition where the probability that a behavior will reoccur is diminished.

avocational: Leisure pursuits.

avoidance: Psychological coping strategy whereby the source of stress is ignored or avoided.

avoidance learning: Form of learning through stimuli avoidance and cause and effect (e.g., negative reinforcement).

avolition: Absence of interest or will to undertake activities.

axial skeleton: Bones forming the longitudinal axis of the body; consists of the skull, vertebral column, thorax, and sternum.

axilla: Area located dorsal to the humerus and glenohumeral joint. Site where cords of the brachial plexus pass through to innervate the muscles of the arm, superficial back, and superficial thoracic region.

axiology: Branch of philosophy concerned with the study of values related to ethics, aesthetics, or religion.

axis: A line, real or imaginary, running through the center of the body; the line about which a part revolves.

axon: Long part of a nerve cell that sends information away from the cell, across a synapse, to the dendrites of another cell.

azoospermia: Absence of sperm in the semen.

azotemia: Presence of nitrogenous bodies, especially urea, in the blood.

B cell: A type of lymphocyte capable of producing an antibody. White cell that is able to detect the presence of foreign agents. Once exposed to an antigen on the agent, it differentiates into plasma cells to produce antibodies.

baby boom generation: People born between the years of 1946 and 1964.

back disorder/injury: Injury to or disease of the lower lumbar, lumbosacral, or sacroiliac region of the back.

back school: A structured educational program about low back problems, usually offered to a group of patients/clients.

bacteremic shock: Septicemic shock that occurs when endotoxins are released from certain bacteria into the bloodstream.

bacterial diseases: Diseases resulting from infection by bacteria.

bacterial pneumonia: Inflammation caused by a bacterial infection in the lungs.

bactericidal: Able to kill bacteria. An agent that destroys bacteria.

bacteriostatic: An agent that is capable of inhibiting the growth or multiplication of bacteria.

bacteriuria: Presence of bacteria in urine.

bag of waters: Lay term for the membranes/sac containing the fetus and fluids.

balance: The ability to maintain a functional posture through motor actions that distribute weight evenly around the body's center of gravity, both statically (e.g., while standing) and dynamically (e.g., while walking).

ballottement: Mobility of a floating object (e.g., a fetus) which rebounds or moves away and then returns when pushed by the examiner's fingers.

barbiturate: Sedative that can cause both physiological and psychological dependence.

barriers: The physical impediments that keep patients/clients from functioning optimally in their surroundings, including safety hazards (e.g., throw rugs, slippery surfaces), access problems (e.g., narrow doors, high steps), and home or office design difficulties (e.g., excessive distance to negotiate, multistory environment). The point of restriction of a given movement.

Bartholin's glands: Two small glands situated on either side of the vaginal opening that secrete small amounts of mucus during coitus.

basal body temperature: The lowest body temperature in a healthy person taken prior to rising from bed first thing in the morning.

basal ganglia: A collection of nuclei at the base of the cortex, including the caudate nucleus, putamen, globus pallidus, and functionally including the substantia nigra and subthalamic nucleus.

basal metabolism: The energy used to support the functions of a body at rest.

baseline: The known value or quantity representing the normal background level against which a response to intervention can be measured.

base-of-support: The body surfaces, such as the plantar surface of the feet, around which the center of gravity is maintained via postural responses.

basic ADL: Activities of daily living tasks that pertain to self-care, mobility, and communication.

battering: Repeated physical assault.

battery: Nonconsensual touching of another individual.

battery of tests: Assessment approach or instrument with several parts.

bearing down effort: Energy exerted by a woman during contractions to push the baby out of the birth canal.

behavior modification: The process of reinforcing desirable responses; food, praise, and tokens may be used.

behavioral assessment: The assessment of activity, feeding, and sleeping patterns and the individual's responsiveness.

behavioral setting: Milieu in which the specific environment dictates the kinds of behaviors that occur there, independent of the particular individuals who inhabit the setting at the moment.

behavioral theory: Developmental theory that suggests that learning is a relationship between certain stimuli and their subsequent responses. Sees the individual as a result of present and past environments. Behaviorists believe learning occurs through the processes of classical or operant conditioning.

behaviorism: Theory of behavior and intervention that holds that behavior is learned, that behaviors that are reinforced tend to recur, and those that are not reinforced tend to disappear.

belief: Idea that is held to be true.

Bell's palsy: Peripheral paralysis of the facial nerve (cranial nerve VII); where the muscles of the unaffected side of the face pull the face into distorted positions.

belly: Midsection of a muscle (usually produces a bulge) between its two ends.

benchmark: Standard against which something else is judged.

beneficence: The quality of being kind or doing good; a charitable act or generous gift. Doing good resulting in benefit to others.

beneficiary: The recipient of some good deed, such as inheriting an estate.

benefit: Sum of money that an insurance policy pays for covered services under the terms of the policy.

benefit period: Time during which an insurance policy provides payments for covered benefits.

benign prostatic hypertrophy: Enlarged prostate gland that results in dysuria.

bereavement: Normal grief, depression, or sadness commonly associated with the death of a loved one.

beta error (or Type 2 error): When the null hypothesis is accepted, the probability of being wrong or the probability of accepting it when it should have been rejected.

bicornuate uterus: An anomaly of the uterus consisting of either two completely duplicated organs or one uterus with two horns.

bifurcation: The site of division into two branches, as in an artery, often the area of atherosclerotic deposits.

bilateral: Pertaining to or affecting both sides of the body.

bilingual: A person who speaks two languages fluently.

bilirubin: Yellowish or orange pigment in bile that occurs as a result of destroyed red blood cells that have completed their life cycle. The remains of the cells are carried to the liver where they are chemically transformed and excreted in the bile.

bimanual: Performed with both hands such as in an examination of a woman's organs where one of the examiner's hands is on the abdomen and fingers of the second hand are in the vagina.

binocular: Pertaining to both eyes.

binge and purge: Cycle of eating disorder, especially bulimia, where overeating is followed by use of laxatives or self-induced vomiting.

bioethics: Application of ethics to health care.

biofeedback: A training technique that enables an individual to gain some element of voluntary control over muscular or autonomic nervous system functions using a device that produces auditory or visual stimuli.

biological age: Definition of age that focuses on the functional age of biological and physiological processes rather than on calendar time.

biological warfare: Biologic agents designed to injure, incapacitate, or kill a person, animal, or plant. Biologics include bacteria, rickettsia, viruses, and bacterial toxins.

biomechanics: Study of anatomy, physiology, and physics as applied to the human body.

biophysical profile (BPP): Assessment of the fetus and its environment using ultrasonography and fetal monitoring (noninvasive) using the following indices: fetal breathing movements, total body movements, fetal tone, reactive fetal heart rate, and estimated amniotic fluid volume.

biopsy: Removal of a small tissue sample for microscopic evaluation and diagnosis.

biopsychological assessment: Evaluation used to determine how the central nervous system influences behavior and to understand the relationship between physical state and thoughts, emotions, and behavior.

biorhythm: Biological or cyclical occurrence or phenomenon (e.g., sleep cycle, menstrual cycle, or respiratory cycle).

biparietal diameter: The largest transverse diameter from one parietal bone to the other of the fetal head.

bipolar disorder: Disorder characterized by an unstable self-image, abrupt mood swings, and poor impulse control.

birth asphyxia: Interference in placental circulation (i.e., umbilical cord compression or premature separation of the placenta) resulting in too little oxygen.

birth cohorts: People born during the same general time period.

birth plan: A written tool by which parents designate their choices for birthing.

birth trauma: Injury during delivery of an infant.

birth rate: Number of live births per 1000 population.

Bishop score: An evaluation tool that scores the inducibility of the cervix; the higher the score, the more favorable or successful the endeavor.

bite reflex: Swift biting pathological reflex action produced by oral stimulation.

bittersweet grief: The intense feelings and emotions that occur when remembering the deceased loved one after the major mourning period has elapsed. Intense sadness and some joy and relief at being able to remember the loved one.

blanching: Becoming white with pressure; maximum pallor.

blastema: Immature substance from which cells and tissues are created.

blended family: Family that includes stepchildren and stepparents.

blepharorrhaphy: Suturing of an eyelid.

blister: Fluid accumulation in or below the epidermis.

blood borne pathogen: Infectious disease spread by contact with blood (e.g., HIV, hepatitis B).

blood pressure (BP): Pressure of the blood against the walls of the blood vessels. Normal in young adults is approximately 120 mmHg during systole and 70 mmHg during diastole.

bloody show: Vaginal discharge consisting of blood and mucus that comes from the dilating cervix.

boarding homes or board and care homes: Smaller-sized housing for older adults offering supervised housing, meals, and personal care, plus housekeeping, transportation, and recreational activities.

body boundaries: Area around the body that serves to separate the self from others or the nonself and provides a sense of safety.

body image: Subjective picture people have of their physical appearance.

body mass index (BMI): The index used to determine fitness/obesity; determined by dividing body weight in kilograms by body height in meters squared.

body mechanics: The interrelationships of the muscles and joints as they maintain or adjust posture in response to environmental forces.

body scheme: Acquiring an internal awareness of the body and the relationship of body parts to each other; perception of one's physical self through proprioceptive and interoceptive sensations.

body transcendence: One of the psychological development tasks of aging (Robert Peck). Focuses on cognitive and social skills to compensate for physical limitations.

bonding: The crucial attachment that develops between a mother, father, and their new baby after delivery.

bone graft: Transplantation of bone.

bone marrow: Tissue filling the porous medullary cavity of the diaphysis of bones.

bone mineral density (BMD): Test to determine density of bones and diagnose osteoporosis.

bone scan: Radiographic scan that evaluates skeletal involvement related to connective tissue disease.

borborygmus: Rumbling and gurgling sound made by the movement of gas in the intestines.

borderline personality: Disorder characterized by abrupt shifts in mood, lack of coherent sense of self, and unpredictable, impulsive behavior.

botulism: Fatal toxemia caused by ingestion of botulinum neurotoxin, which causes muscle weakness and paralysis.

boundaries: Physical and psychological space people define as their own.

boutonniere deformity: Abnormality that results from interruption of the ulnar and medial nerves at the wrist; causes metacarpal phalangeal joint hyperextension and interphalangeal joint flexion.

bowstringing: Spanning the shortest distance between two joints.

brachial palsy: Paralysis of upper-extremity muscles that occurs due to prolonged and difficult labor and a traumatic delivery.

brachial plexus: Network of nerves that originates as roots C5, C6, C7, C8, and T1 and terminates as nerves that innervate the upper extremity.

Bradley method: Father-coached childbirth using unique labor-breathing techniques with the father as the primary support person.

bradycardia: Slowness of heartbeat (e.g., less than 60 beats/minute).

bradykinesia: Slowness of body movement and speech.

Braille: Standardized system for communicating in writing with persons who are blind. Grade II Braille is standard literary Braille.

brain death: Irreversible destruction of the cortex and brainstem. Ways to determine are lack of responsiveness, apnea, absence of reflexes, dilation of pupils, flatline electroencephalogram, and absence of cerebral blood flow for a given period of time.

brain lateralization: Refers to the differentiation of function with the brain's two hemispheres. In most people, the left hemisphere controls the right side of the body, as well as spoken and written language, numerical and scientific skills, and reasoning. The right hemisphere controls the left side of the body and influences musical and artistic awareness, space and pattern perception, insight, imagination, and generating mental images to compare spatial relationships.

brain scan: Nuclear medicine diagnostic procedure used to detect tumors, cerebrovascular accidents, or other lesions in the brain.

brain tumor: Abnormal growth of cells within the cranium that may cause headaches, altered consciousness, seizures, vomiting, visual problems, cranial nerve abnormalities, personality changes, dementia, and sensory and motor deficits.

BRAT(Y): A diet consisting of bran, rice, apples and toast (and yogurt).

Braxton Hicks contractions: Mild intermittent contractions of the uterus during pregnancy. They do not represent true labor.

Brazelton assessment: Method for assessing the interactional behavior of the newborn.

breakthrough bleeding: Bloody discharge between menstrual periods most often seen in women using pharmaceutical methods of birth control.

breast self-examination (BSE): Self-examination of the breasts.

breast shells: Rigid plastic cups with holes in the middle which are inserted inside the bra to put pressure on the areola to help inverted nipples to take normal shape or to protect sore nipples from the pressure of clothing and to collect milk if they are leaking.

breech presentation: Describes the position of the fetus in which buttocks or feet are presented at the cervical opening and are born first. Occurs in approximately 3% of all births; **complete breech presentation:** Simultaneous presentation of buttocks, legs and feet; **footling breech presentation (incomplete):** Presentation of one or both feet; **frank breech presentation:** Presentations of buttocks with hips flexed and thighs against the abdomen.

bregma: The area of the anterior fontanel of the fetus/newborn which is the junction of the coronal and sagittal sutures of the skull.

brim: The inlet of the female pelvis.

bronchopulmonary dysplasia (BPD): A pulmonary condition seen in preterm infants who have been oxygen dependent for more than 28 days.

bronchiectasis: A chronic dilatation of the bronchi or bronchioles marked by fetid breath and paroxysmal coughing, with expectoration of mucopurulent matter.

bronchiolectasis: Dilation of the bronchioles.

bronchopneumonia: Inflammation of the bronchi accompanied by inflamed patches in the nearby lobules of the lungs. Also termed bronchiolitis.

bronchopulmonary dysplasia: A disordered growth or faulty development of bronchial and lung tissue.

brown fat: Source of heat unique to neonates. It has greater thermogenic capability than ordinary fat. Deposits found around some organs and thoracic structures and last for several weeks.

bruit: Soft blowing sound heard upon auscultation. Caused by turbulence as a result of deposits in the arterial lumen that alter normal hemodynamics.

bruxism: Grinding of teeth.

bulimia nervosa: Eating disorder characterized by binging (excessive consumption of calories) and purging (self-induced vomiting, use of diuretics or laxatives, excessive exercise, or severe caloric restriction).

bullous dermatosis: A large blister or cutaneous vesicle filled with serous fluid.

bunion: A swelling of the bursa mucosa of the first metatarsal head with callusing of the overlying skin and lateral migration of the great toe.

burn: A lesion caused by contact with heat.

burnout: State of mental fatigue that results in the inability to generate energy from one's occupational or personal performance areas.

bursa: Sac that contains synovial fluid. Bursae are located in superficial fascia, in areas where movement takes place and aid in decreasing friction.

bursectomy: Excision of bursae.

bursitis: Inflammation of a bursa resulting from injury, infection, or rheumatoid synovitis. It produces pain and tenderness and may restrict movement at a nearby joint.

bypass: A surgically created detour between two points in a physiologic pathway, often to circumvent obstructions. Similar to a shunt.

byte: Unit of information in computer programming equal to one character.

cachexia: Marked state of poor health and malnutrition secondary to disease, treatment, or poor nutrient intake.

calcification: The deposition of calcium salts in body tissues. A calcified substance or structure.

calcitonin: Peptide hormone that increases calcium and phosphate deposits in bone.

calibration: Determination of what the output of a measuring instrument means compared with known values.

callosities: Hardened, thickened places on the skin.

calorie: Unit of heat measurement.

calorimetry: Measurement of the energy produced by food when oxidized in the body.

cancer: Condition of abnormal cells multiplying and destroying normal cells.

candidiasis: Infection by fungi of the genus *Candida*, most commonly involving the skin, oral mucosa, respiratory tract, and vagina.

cane: Stick or short staff used to assist one during walking; can have a narrow or broad base depending on the amount of support needed.

cannabis: Substance derived from hemp that is used in marijuana or hashish.

cannulation: The process of inserting an artificial tube into a part of the body, such as an artery.

capacitance: Elastic capacity of vessels and organs of the body.

capacitation: Enzymatic process by which spermatozoon (sperm) is capable of penetrating the ovum.

capacity: One's best, includes present abilities as well as the potential to develop new abilities.

capillaries: Extremely narrow vessels forming a network between the arterioles and the veins. Walls are composed of a single layer of cells through which oxygen and nutritive materials pass out to the tissues, and carbon dioxide and waste products are admitted from the tissues into the bloodstream (osmosis).

capillary hydrostatic pressure: Pressure in the arterial capillary system that enables the movement of fluid across the semipermeable membrane of the capillary wall. This pressure is measured as the pulmonary capillary wedge pressure (PCWP).

capsular pattern: A proportional limitation of motion, characteristic for each joint, secondary to a lesion of the synovial membrane and/or the fibrous capsule.

capsular restriction: Limitation of mobility and range due to tightness or rigidity of the joint capsule.

caput: The portion of the fetal head, usually occiput, appearing at the vaginal introitus preceding the birth of the head; **caput succedaneum:** Edema of the tissue over the presenting part of the head.

carboxyhemoglobin: A compound formed from hemoglobin on exposure to carbon monoxide, with formation of a covalent bond with oxygen and without change of the charge of the ferrous state.

carbuncle: A painful bacterial infection deep beneath the skin having a network of pus-filled boils.

carcinogen: Any substance or agent that produces or increases the incidence of cancer.

carcinoma: Any of the several kinds of cancerous growths deriving from epithelial cells.

cardiac arrest: Cessation of effective heart action.

cardiac arrhythmia: Irregularity in the rhythm of the heart beat.

cardiac contusion: Bruising of the heart due to direct trauma or injury to the myocardium.

cardiac decompensation: Inability of the heart to maintain an adequate cardiac output.

cardiac output: Volume of blood pumped from the heart per unit of time. The product of heart rate and stroke volume.

cardiac tamponade: Acute compression of the heart due to effusion of the fluid into the pericardium or the collection of blood in the pericardium from rupture of the heart or a coronary vessel.

cardiomyopathy: A subacute or chronic disorder of heart muscle of unknown or obscure etiology, often with associated endocardial, and sometimes with pericardial involvement, but not atherosclerotic in origin.

cardiopulmonary: Pertaining to the heart and lungs.

cardiopulmonary resuscitation (CPR): Procedure instituted immediately upon cardiac arrest that seeks to restore heart and lung function. May include defibrillation, external cardiac compression, and mouth-to-mouth resuscitation.

cardiorrhaphy: Suture of the heart muscle.

cardiotonic: Drug that promotes the force and efficiency of the heart.

cardiovascular (CV): Pertaining to heart and blood vessels.

cardiovascular insufficiency: Inability of the cardiovascular system to perform at a level necessary for basic homeostasis of the body.

cardiovascular pump: Structures responsible for maintaining cardiac output, including the cardiac muscle, valves, arterial smooth muscle, and venous smooth muscle.

cardiovascular pump dysfunction: Abnormalities of the cardiac muscles, valves, conduction, or circulation that interrupt or interfere with cardiac output or circulation.

cardioversion: The use of electrical current to convert irregular rhythms or no rhythms to an active, regular, rhythmical heart beat.

care coordination: Key focus of nursing to assure individual appropriate care.

caregiver: One who provides care and support to a person.

carotid body: A small oval mass of cells and nerve endings located in the carotid sinus. These cells respond to chemical changes in the blood by altering the rate of respiration and other bodily changes.

carotid endarterectomy: Excision of the thickened, atheromatous tunica intima of the carotid artery.

carotid sinus: A slight dilatation at the point of carotid bifurcation. Contains cells and nerve endings that respond to a change in blood pressure by altering heart rate.

carpal tunnel syndrome: Pressure on the median nerve where it goes through the carpal tunnel of the wrist causing tenderness and weakness of the muscles of the thumb.

carpals: Bones of the wrist; there are eight carpal bones in each wrist.

carphologia: Picking at bedclothes; repetitive behavior typically observed in delirium.

carrier: Individuals who carry a gene that can be passed to children while they do not exhibit any of the characteristics associated with the gene. Also refers to an organism or substance conveying contagious diseases.

cascade effect: Ability of the blood to clot via multiple factors.

cascade system: Theoretical prototype used as a conceptual framework for providing educational services for children with disabilities. Children placed into the class that best fits their needs and is as close as possible to an everyday classroom.

case management: The use of a legally mandated case manager to oversee the coordination of services for a client. **case manager:** Individual who assumes responsibility for coordination and follow-up on a given client case, frequently a registered nurse. Roles may include helper, teacher, planner, and advocate; assists in facilitating the needs of a client and his or her family.

cataplexy: Sudden episode of loss of muscle function.

cataract: Abnormal progressive condition of the lens of the eye characterized by loss of transparency.

catastrophic thinking: View that the worse will happen when a more positive view is likely.

catatonia: Motor abnormality usually characterized by immobility or rigidity in which no organic base has been identified.

catecholamines: Active proteins epinephrine and norepinephrine.

categorization: Identifying similarities of and differences among pieces of environmental information; ability to classify; to describe by naming or labeling.

catharsis: A curative factor of group therapy.

cathartic: Drug that relieves constipation and promotes defecation for diagnostic and operative procedures.

catheter: A thin tube of woven plastic or other material to which blood will not adhere. Inserted into a vein or artery. Also inserted into the urethra for collection or drainage of urine.

cauda equina: Spinal nerves descending in the spinal column below the level of L2.

caudal: Away from the head or toward the lower part of a structure.

caul: Portion of the fetal membranes covering fetal head during birth.

causalgia: A condition of severe burning pain usually caused by a peripheral nerve injury.

cause and effect: When something occurs as a result of a motion or activity.

cauterization: Coagulation of blood by the application of chemicals or heat. Often used in surgery to reduce blood loss.

cell migration: Movement of cells in the wound repair process.

cellulitis: An inflammation of connective tissue, especially subcutaneous tissue. Inflammation of tissue around a lesion characterized by redness, swelling, and tenderness. Signifies infection.

centenarian: Person 100 years old or older.

center of gravity: Point at which the downward force created by mass and gravity is equivalent or balanced on either side of a fulcrum.

central nervous system (CNS): Consists of all the neurons of the brain, brainstem, and spinal cord.

central tendency: The typical, middle, or central scores in a distribution.

central venous pressure (CVP): The pressure representative of the filling pressure of the right ventricle, measured peripherally or centrally, corrected for hydrostatic pressure between the heart and point of measurement. Used to monitor fluid replacement.

centrifugal control: The brain's ability to regulate its own input.

centrifuge: Machine that separates components of blood for further testing through high-speed, rotational movement.

cephalad: Toward the head or upper portion of a part or structure. Synonym: superior.

cephalic: The head; **cephalic presentation:** The head as the presenting part of the fetus for delivery.

cephalocaudal pattern: Sequence in which the greatest growth always occurs at the top (i.e., the head) with physical growth in size, weight, and feature differentiation, gradually working its way down from top to bottom.

cephalopelvic disproportion: A condition in which the infant's head is unable to fit through the pelvic outlet and is an indication for cesarean delivery.

cerclage: A purse string ring suture placed around an incompetent cervix at the level of the cervical os at 12 to 14 weeks of gestation to prevent premature delivery from an incompetent cervix.

cerebellar ataxia: Disorder of the brain that results in total or partial inability to coordinate voluntary bodily movements, as in walking.

cerebellar degeneration: Deterioration or loss of function or structure of brain tissue.

cerebral angioplasty: Injection of dye into the cerebral vascular system to observe its function.

cerebral atrophy: Deterioration of the cerebral tissue.

cerebral contusion: Bruising of brain tissue.

cerebral cyst: A saclike structure filled with fluid or diseased matter in the tissue of the brain.

cerebral degeneration: Deterioration or loss of function or structure in the cerebral region of the brain.

cerebral embolism: The obstruction of a blood vessel by a blood or other clot in the brain.

cerebral laceration: Torn or mangled cerebral tissue.

cerebrovascular: Pertaining to blood vessels and circulation in the brain.

cerebral vascular accident (CVA): Lack of blood and oxygen to a portion of the brain due to bleeding, embolus, or thrombus.

cerebrovascular insufficiency: A lack of oxygen in the brain due to restriction or blockage of cerebral vessels.

certification: Process developed to declare that a practitioner has met standards required for competent professional practice in an area, especially specialization (e.g., gerontological, pediatrics, family nurse practitioner).

cervical cauterization: Destruction of cervical tissue through the use of heat or electrical current.

cervical intraepithelial neoplasm (CIN): Progressive, usually rapid, abnormal growth of cervical cells.

cervical spondylosis: Dissolution of the cervical vertebrae.

cervical os: Opening of the cervix.

cervical ripening: Physical softening and distensibility of the cervix in preparation for labor and birth.

cervical vertebrae: Seven small neck bones between the skull and thoracic vertebrae that support the head and allow movement.

cervicitis: Cervical infection.

cervix: The neck of the uterus, which leads into the vagina and thins out and dilates during labor.

cesarean section: Delivery of a child by abdominal surgery.

cesarean hysterectomy: Removal of the uterus at the time of the birth of the baby.

Chadwick's sign: Increased vascularity of pregnancy that appears as a dark blue or violet coloration of the vaginal mucus membrane.

characteristic behavior: Behavior typical of one's performance under everyday conditions.

checklist: Type of assessment approach whereby a list of abilities, tasks, or interests is presented and those items meeting a designated criterion are checked.

chemical warfare: Chemicals in any form used to injure, incapacitate, or kill a person, animal, or plant. Includes such elements as nitrogen mustards and chlorine gas.

chemotherapy: The use of drugs or pharmacologic agents that have a specific and toxic effect on a disease-causing pathogen.

chest pain: Angina resulting from ischemia of the heart tissue.

chest physical therapy (physiotherapy): The use of vibration, shaking, or tapping techniques in various postural drainage positions to facilitate the expectoration of secretions in the lungs.

Cheyne-Stokes respiration: Breathing characterized by rhythmic waxing and waning and a fluctuation in the depth of breathing. May result in periods of apnea, especially seen in coma resulting from affection of the nervous system.

Chi: Healing energy flowing through meridian pathways, in Chinese medicine.

chickenpox (varicella): An acute, communicable disease caused by a virus and marked by slight fever and an eruption of macular vesicles that appear as a rash.

child abuse: Intentional physical or psychological injury inflicted upon children by caretaker(s).

child development play programs: Hospital play programs for children who have a long-term hospital stay; includes curricula ordinarily found in preschool or elementary school classrooms.

child neglect: Inadequate social, emotional, or physical nurturing of children.

chi-square (X^2): A statistical test used to establish whether or not frequency differences have occurred on the basis of chance.

chloasma: Pigmentation appearing on the forehead and cheeks of some pregnant women; can also be seen in some women when they begin oral contraceptives. Also called mask of pregnancy.

chloroform: Colorless, heavy liquid formerly used as a general anesthetic.

choanal atresia: Separation between the nose and the pharynx.

cholecystectomy: Removal of the gallbladder.

cholecystitis: Inflammation of the gallbladder.

choledocholithotomy: Incision into the bile duct for removal of gallstones.

cholelithiasis: Gallstones in the gallbladder.

cholestasis: Suppression or arrest of bile flow.

chondrocyte: Cartilage cell embedded in lacunae within the matrix of cartilage connective tissue.

chondromalacia: Softening of the articular cartilages.

chord: The shortest line (path) between any two points on a surface.

chorea: Abrupt irregular movements of short duration involving the fingers, hands, arms, face, tongue, or head.

chorion: The outermost membrane that encases the fetus.

chorionic villus sampling (CVS): Biopsy of the chorionic villus (fetal placental tissue) that determines chromosomal and metabolic abnormalities of the fetus from 9 to 11 weeks of gestation.

choreoathetosis: Type of cerebral palsy characterized by uncontrollable, jerky, irregular twisting movements of the arms and legs.

chromocytopenia: Edema containing blood from ruptured blood vessels between the skull bone and its external covering.

chromosome: Threadlike structure made up of genes; there are 46 chromosomes in the nucleus of each cell of a human.

chronic: Of long duration or frequent recurrence.

chronic bronchitis: Chronic inflammation of the bronchial tubes. A long-continued form, often with a more or less marked tendency to recurrence after stages of quiescence. Diagnosis made when a chronic cough for up to 3 months in 2 consecutive years is present.

chronic disorders: Characterized by slow onset and long duration; rarely develop in early adulthood, increase in middle adulthood, and become common in late adulthood.

chronic pain: Pain of unexpected duration, especially longer than 3 months.

chronic respiratory disease: Lung disease resulting from constrictive or obstructive conditions of the airways.

chronological: An individual's age; definition of age that relies on the amount of calendar time that has passed since birth.

chronotropic: Affecting the time or rate, applied especially to nerves whose stimulation or agents whose administration affects the rate of contraction of the heart.

chylothorax: The presence of effused chyle (pockets of milky fluid) in the thoracic cavity.

circadian rhythm: The 24-hour biological rhythm that influences various regulatory functions such as sleep, temperature, and activities.

cicatrix: Scar; the fibrous tissue replacing the normal tissues destroyed by injury or disease.

circulation: Movement in a regular or circuitous course, as the movement of blood through the heart and blood vessels.

circumcision: The surgical removal of foreskin from the male penis; **female circumcision:** Religious or cultural removal of a portion of the clitoris or labia, which can cause mutilation and problems in childbirth.

circumduction: Movement in which the distal end of a bone moves in a circle while the proximal end remains stable, acting like a pivot.

claiming process: Parents attaching or identifying their infant through the similarities, likenesses, differences, and uniquenesses to other family members.

clang associations: Speech characterized by choosing words based on the sounds, especially rhyming.

class: Group containing members who share certain attributes, such as economic status, social identifications, or cultural identity.

classical conditioning: Method of eliciting specific responses through the use of stimuli that occur within a period of time that permits an association to be made between them. Also called Pavlovian conditioning, after the Russian scientist who made the technique famous.

classification: Arrangement according to some systematic division into classes or groups.

claudication: Lameness, limping; usually caused by poor circulation of blood to the leg muscles; **intermittent claudication:** A complex of symptoms characterized by absence of pain or discomfort in a limb at rest or the commencement of pain, tension, and weakness with walking, which intensifies with continued walking and is relieved by rest. Usually seen in occlusive arterial diseases of the limbs.

clavicle: Bone that acts as a brace to hold the upper arm free from the thorax to allow free movement and serves as a place for muscle attachment. Synonym: collarbone.

cleansing breath: The breath taken at the beginning and end of a labor contraction to signal the support person to begin and end each breathing technique.

cleft lip: Congenital incomplete closure of the lip.

cleft palate: Congenital incomplete closure of the roof of the mouth or palate.

clients: Patients. Frequently used to refer to individuals who are basically well.

climacteric: Major turning point in a female's life from ability to reproduce to a state of nonreproductivity. Transitional phase of life leading to menopause.

clinical guidelines: Systematically developed statements to assist practitioner and patient decisions about appropriate health care for specific clinical circumstances.

clinical reasoning: Thinking that directs and guides clinical decision making; reflective thinking.

clinical pathway: Outcome-oriented plan with specific activities designated at specific time periods.

clinical trial: Studies with human subjects.

clinical utility: Factors such as clarity of instruction, cost, and facileness in using the assessment to determine the amount of the assessment's utility.

clitoris: Small, round-shaped organ at the anterior part of the vulva.

clonus: Spasmodic alternation of contraction and relaxation of muscles. A test for eclampsia in pregnancy measured in "beats."

closed question: Question that asks for a specific response (e.g., one that may be answered with a yes or no).

closed reduction: Situation in which a broken bone can be manipulated into its natural position without surgery. External manipulation.

close supervision: Contact that is daily, direct, and given on the work premises.

clubbing: A proliferative change in the soft tissues about the terminal phalanges of the fingers or toes with no osseous changes.

clubfoot: Birth defect in which the soles of the feet face medially and the toes point inferiorly; occurs in about one out of 1000 births and may be caused genetically or by the folding of the foot up against the chest during fetal development. Synonym: talipes and equino-varus.

clubhand: Medical condition seen in children in which the hand is radically displaced; the radius bone may be partially formed or may be absent.

coagulation: The process of blood clot formation.

coagulopathy: A pathological defect in coagulation of the blood.

coarctation: Literally a pressing together. In practice, a narrowing of a vessel, usually congenital in origin.

coccyodynia: Painful coccyx usually resulting from an injury whereby sitting is difficult.

coconsensus: A common center or agreement.

codeine: Highly addictive narcotic derived from the opium family.

code of ethics: Statement that a certain group follows; sets the guidelines so that a high standard of behavior is maintained, e.g., the Code of Ethics for Nurses.

codependence: Condition in which substance dependence is subtly supported by the codependent who meets some need through the continued dependence of the individual.

coefficient of contingency: A statistical test used on nominal data to determine correlation.

coefficient of determination (r2): Determining what proportion of information about y is contained in x.

coenzyme: Substance that promotes action of enzymes.

cognition: Mental processes that include thinking, perceiving, feeling, recognizing, remembering, problem solving, knowing, sensing, learning, judging, and metacognition. The act or process of knowing, including both awareness and judgment.

cognitive development: Process of thinking and knowing in the broadest sense, including perception, memory, and judgment.

cognitive disability: Physiologic or biochemical impairment in information-processing capacities that produces observable and measurable limitations in routine task behavior.

cognitive domains: Levels of performance abilities delineated in a hierarchy related to knowing and understanding.

cognitive learning: Form of learning that encompasses the forming of mental plans of events and objects.

cognitive stages in development: Jean Piaget's theory proposing that children's biological development is related to their environment, which enables children to progress through discreet age-related stages in forming cognitions.

cognitive therapy: Means of exploring how one thinks about events to affect resultant emotions and thus behavior.

cognitive theory: Theory that focuses on intelligence, reasoning, learning, problem solving, memory, information processing, and thinking as the tools that individuals use to understand environmental stimuli.

cohesiveness: Growth of interpersonal harmony and intimacy within a group.

cohort effects: Effects that are due to an individual's time of birth or generation but not to actual age.

coitus: Penile-vaginal sexual intercourse; **coitus interruptus:** Penis withdrawn from the vagina prior to ejaculation.

cold stress: Excessive loss of heat resulting in increased respirations and thermalgenesis to maintain core body temperature.

collagen: Main supportive protein of skin, tendon, bone, cartilage, and connective tissue.

collective variable: Fewest number of dimensions that describes a unit of behavior.

Colles' wrist fracture: Transverse fracture of the distal end of the radius (just above the wrist).

colloid osmotic pressure: The pressure exerted by substances capable of influencing osmosis of water across membranes.

colonized: Presence of bacteria that cause no local or systemic signs or symptoms.

color agnosia: The inability to recognize colors.

colostrum: Watery milk secreted from a woman's breasts during pregnancy and during the first few days postpartum.

colposcopy: Examination of the vagina and cervical tissue by colposcope.

colposcope: Instrument containing lens and camera to examine vaginal area for tears and abrasions.

coma: Abnormally deep unconsciousness with the absence of voluntary response to stimuli.

commitment: Degree of importance attached to an event by an individual based on his or her beliefs and values. An important element in motivation.

commitment procedures: Legal process by which persons are institutionalized.

communication: The act of transmitting thoughts or ideas. Giving or exchanging of information, signals, or messages by talk, gestures, or writing. A system of sending or receiving messages.

community: Group of people with some common interest and some dependence on each other.

community forum: A needs assessment technique that invites residents/members of the target population to discuss their concerns at open "town hall" type meetings.

comorbidity: Characterized by the presence of symptoms of more than one ailment (e.g., depression and anxiety).

competence: Achievement of skill equal to the demands of the environment; also a legal term referring to the soundness of one's mind.

complementary health: Practices that augment mainstream health care to enhance the total patient experience.

compliance: Subservient behavior that implies following orders or directions without self-direction or choice. Also related to respiratory mechanics with change in respiratory volume over pressure gradient. Refers to the elasticity and expandability of the lungs.

component: Fundamental unit; in relation to activities, refers to processes, tools, materials, and purposefulness.

compression therapy: Treatment using devices or techniques that decrease the density of a part of the body through the application of pressure.

compulsion: A repetitive, distressing act that is performed to relieve obsession-related fear.

computerized assessment: Assessment that includes the administration, scoring, and interpretation of test results done by a sophisticated computer program.

computer-axial tomography (CAT): Scanning procedure that combines X-rays with computer technology to show cross-sectional views of internal body structures.

conative hypothesis: Theory that autistic children choose not to play and interact with other children rather than their being unintellectual.

concentration: The ability to maintain attention for longer periods of time in order to keep thoughts directed toward completing a given task.

concept: Mental image, abstract idea, or general notion.

conception: Fertilization of the ovum by the sperm resulting in the formation of the one-celled zygote.

conceptional age: The number of completed weeks of the pregnancy since conception as related to fetal development. Estimated at two weeks less than gestational age.

conceptus: The product of conception including embryo or fetus, membranes, amniotic fluid, and the fetal portion of the placenta.

concrete-operational stage: Term coined by Jean Piaget to denote development of a group of skills acquired in middle childhood, including decentration, class inclusion, and taking another's perspective. In this stage, such mental operations can only be applied to "concrete" objects.

concrete thinking: Thoughts focused on specifics rather than generalities; nonabstract.

concussion: Resulting from impact with an object (usually to the brain).

conditioning: Learning process that alters behavior through reinforcements or associating a reflex with a particular stimulus to trigger a desired response. Also a cardiovascular effect related to exercise and the overall improvement of functional endurance.

condom: A mechanical barrier worn on the penis (or in the vagina) for contraception or protection from sexually transmitted infections.

conduction: Conveying energy (e.g., heat, sound, or electricity).

condyloma acuminatum: A wartlike growth of the skin usually near the external genitalia or anus caused by human papillomavirus (HPV).

confidentiality: Maintenance of secrecy regarding information confided by a client.

conflict of interest: Situation in which a person may have hidden or other interests that conflict or are inconsistent with providing services to a client or agency.

congenital: Present or existing prior to birth resulting from hereditary or prenatal environmental factors.

congenital adrenal hyperplasia: Congenital deficiency in enzymes necessary for production of adrenal cortical hormones and exhibited in ambiguous genitalia.

congenital amputation: Condition in which a child is born without part or all of a limb or limbs.

congenital anomalies/disorders: Structural abnormalities resulting from birth defects or genetic disorders.

congenital defects: Abnormalities or deformities of the muscular-skeleton system or any other major organ system usually occurring in the developing embryo.

congenital heart defect: A structural abnormality of the heart present at birth.

congenital rubella syndrome: Neonatal anomalies such as hearing defects, cardiovascular defects, or cataracts created by first trimester maternal rubella infection.

congregate housing: Housing for unrelated individuals, often older persons, usually sponsored by government or nonprofit organizations.

conjoined twins: Twins who are physically joined.

conjugate: Important diameter of the pelvis. **Diagonal conjugate:** Distance from the sacral promontory to the lower inner surface of the symphysis pubis and measures from 11.5 cm to 13 cm. **True conjugate:** Distance between upper margin of symphysis pubis and the sacral promontory and is usually 1.5–2.0 cm. Less than the diagonal conjugate.

conjunctivitis: Inflammation of the conjunctiva of the eye.

connective tissue: Structural material of the body that connects tissues and links anatomical structures together.

consent: Agree to participate.

conservation: Cognitive skill that requires the realization that a quantity of a substance remains constant regardless of changes in form.

conservator: Court-appointed individual with authority to make decisions for an incapacitated person.

constrictive pericarditis: Inflammation of the pericardium that results in constriction. The pericardium is covered with fibrinous deposits.

construct: Conceptual structure used in science for thinking about the factors underlying observed phenomena.

constructional apraxia: The inability to reproduce geometric designs and figures.

construct validity: In research, the extent to which a test measures the construct (mental representation) variables that it was designed to identify.

consultation: Process of assisting a client, an agency, or other provider by identifying and analyzing issues, providing information and advice, and developing strategies for current and future actions.

contact dermatitis: Inflammatory response of the skin due to contact with a toxic or caustic agent (e.g., chemical, poison ivy).

contamination: Soiling by contact or introduction of organisms into a wound.

context: Refers to the social, physical, and psychological milieu of a situation.

contingency contracting: Written document used to modify behavior with consequences specified.

continuing care retirement community: A place that provides the spectrum of care from independence through death.

continuity of care: Coordinated efforts from entrance to a service through discharge.

continuity theory of aging: Psychosocial theory of aging that focuses on the integration of the older person's past experiences, inner psyche, and the changes that occur with aging in such a way as to preserve the individual's sense of self.

continuous positive airway pressure (CPAP): Pressure applied to keep the airway open during expiration.

contraception: Prevention of conception and pregnancy.

contractile protein: A substance produced to remove waste at an intra- and extracellular level.

contractility: Capacity for becoming short in response to a suitable stimulus.

contraction: Tightening of a muscle to create stabilization or movement. Also, the pulling together of wound edges in the healing process. The development of tension within a muscle or muscle group with or without changes in its overall length.

contractions: Shortening and tightening of muscle fibers during and after labor; **duration:** Time from the beginning of the contraction to the end of the contraction; **frequency:** The time from the beginning of one contraction to the beginning of the next contraction; **intensity:** Strength of the contraction at its peak; **interval:** The rest period between contractions timed from the end of one contraction to the beginning of the next; **resting tone:** The tension in the uterine muscle between contractions.

contraction stress test (CST): Assessing fetal response through stimulating uterine contractions; healthy fetuses do not react to the contractions, but unhealthy fetuses experience fetal heart decelerations (late decelerations) that can indicate utero-placental insufficiency.

contracture: Static shortening of muscle and connective tissue that limits range of motion at a joint.

contraindication: Condition that deems a particular type of treatment undesirable or improper.

contralateral: Pertaining to, situated on, or affecting the opposite side.

contrast bath: The immersion of an extremity in alternating hot and cold water.

contrecoup injury: Usually more extensive damage on the opposite side of the brain from the point of impact during a strike to the head.

control group: Comparison group in research.

control stage: Second stage of group development; it includes a leadership struggle on a group and individual level.

contusion: A bruise.

convergence: The ability of the brain to respond only after receiving input from multiple sources.

convergent problem solving: Developing one correct solution by forming separate pieces of information.

conversion disorder: Disorder characterized by the presence of physical symptoms or deficits that cannot be explained by medical findings.

convulsion: Paroxysms of involuntary muscular contractions and relaxation; spasm.

Coombs' test: **indirect:** To determine presence of Rh-positive antibodies in the maternal blood; **direct:** To determine presence of maternal Rh-positive antibodies in fetal cord blood.

cooperative play: Goal-set form of play that involves two or more children striving for that goal.

coordination: Property of movement characterized by the smooth and harmonious action of groups of muscles working together to produce a desired motion.

coping: Process through which individuals adjust to the stressful demands of their daily environment.

copious: Large amounts. Used, for example, when referring to respiratory secretions during chest physical therapy.

cor pulmonale: Right-sided heart failure, usually as result of chronic lung condition.

coronary artery bypass graft (CABG): Creating new circulation to an area of the heart where an obstruction occurred by using a graft (a vessel or a synthetic).

corporal potentiality: The ability to screen out vestibular and postural information at conscious levels in order to engage the cortex in higher-order cognitive tasks.

copulation: Sexual intercourse.

corpus luteum: Endocrine body that produces progesterone and develops in the ovary at the site of the ruptured ovarian follicle. If impregnation occurs, hormones continue to be produced until the placenta can begin the function.

correlation coefficient: The relationship among two or more variables.

cortically programmed movements: Movements that are based on input from structures in the cortex (motor strip or basal ganglia).

corticorubrospinal pathway: Descending pathway that serves limb control; from the motor cortex through the red nucleus in the brainstem and onto the spinal cord.

corticospinal pathway: Oversees the finely tuned movements of the body by controlling finely tuned movements of the hands; this pathway travels from the motor cortex to the spinal neurons that serve the hand muscles.

cortisone: Hormone produced in the cortex of the adrenal gland that aids in the regulation of the metabolism of fats, carbohydrates, sodium, potassium, and proteins.

cosmesis: A concern in rehabilitation, especially regarding surgical operations or burns, for the appearance of the patient/client.

counterculture: Subculture that rejects important values of the dominant society.

counterpressure: Pressure to the sacral area during uterine contractions to alleviate the pressure created as the presenting part presses against the back during the descent.

coup injury: Brain contusions and lacerations beneath the point of impact when the head is struck.

couplet care: One nurse, appropriately educated and oriented, cares for both the mother and the infant (also known as mother–baby care).

cotyledon: One of the visible segments of the placenta on the maternal side composed of fetal vessels, chorionic villi, and intervillous spaces.

Couvade syndrome: When expectant fathers' experience pregnancy-like symptoms.

Couvelaire uterus: Hemorrhage of the myometrium after premature separation or abruption of the placenta from the uterus. Symptoms include purplish-blue discoloration and boardlike rigidity of the uterus.

covert sensitization: Aversion technique to modify behavior.

crackle: Abnormal, short, sharp, respiratory sound heard upon auscultation. Superficial crepitation heard in the early stages of acute fibrinous pleurisy.

cradle cap: Common dermatitis of infants appearing as thick, yellow, scales on the scalp.

cramp: A painful muscle contraction brought on by involuntary use of that muscle or muscle group.

cranial nerve: Nerve extending from the brain.

crater: Tissue defect extending at least to the subcutaneous layer seen in wounds.

creatinine: Substance found in body fluids and muscle; the levels in maternal urine correlates with fetal size and thus fetal muscle mass.

credentialing: The broad term to encompass licensure, certification, and accreditation.

creep: A measure of the deformation in a material as a result of a constant load applied over a specific time interval.

crepitus: Dry, crackling sound or sensation, such as made by the ends of two bones grating together.

cretinism: Condition in which an individual is small, unusual looking, and has severe mental retardation as a result of the lack of thyroid hormone.

crib death: Lay term for sudden and unexpected death of a healthy and apparently normal infant occurring during sleep with no apparent disease. Also known as sudden infant death syndrome (SIDS).

Cri-du-chat syndrome: Congenital disorder diagnosed at birth from presence of kitten-like cry, low birth weight, microcephaly, "moon face," wide-set eyes, strabismus, and low set misshapen ears. Associated with hypotonic and heart defects and mental and physical retardation. Also called "cat-cry" syndrome.

crisis: Psychological disequilibrium resulting from inadequate problem-solving resources.

criterion: Particular standard or level of performance or expected outcome.

criterion-referenced tests: Goal of these tests is to evaluate specific skills or knowledge where the criterion is full mastery of them.

criterion validity: A measure of how well one variable or set of variables predicts an outcome based on information from other variables.

critical inquiry: Important investigation or examination.

critical path: Optimal sequencing and timing of diagnosis or procedure-based intervention.

critical period: Fixed time period very early in development during which certain behaviors optimally emerge.

cross-addiction: Addiction to a variety of chemical substances.

cross-linking: Theory that aging is caused by a random interaction among proteins that produce molecules that make the body stiffer.

cross-sectional research: Nonexperimental research sometimes used to gather data on possible growth trends in a population.

croup: An acute viral infection usually involving the larynx, trachea, and bronchi that usually occurs between 6 months and three years of age accompanied by a barking cough (sounding like a seal) and varying degrees of respiratory distress that can lead to hypoxia and hypercapnia.

crowning: When the top of the fetal head (or the presenting part) is visible at the vaginal opening; sometimes refers to the time at which the widest diameter of the presenting part distends the vulva.

crusted: Dried secretions found in wound care.

cryosurgery: Local freezing and removal of tissue with minimal blood loss and little or no damage to adjacent tissue. Done with a cryoprobe, using liquid nitrogen.

cryotherapy: Therapeutic application of cold (e.g., ice).

cryptomenorrhea: Monthly signs of menstruation without blood flow.

cryptorchidism: Failure of one or both testicles to descend. Also called undescended testicles.

crystal arthropathies: Diseases of the joints that result in crystallization, such as gout and pseudogout.

crystallized intelligence: Accumulation of knowledge and experience over time that results in abilities that are stable throughout adulthood.

cue: Subjective and objective input that serves as a signal to do something. A secondary stimulus that guides behavior.

cueing: Hints or suggestions that facilitate the appropriate response.

cuirass: A firm covering for the chest.

Cul-de-sac of Douglas: Rectouterine pouch located between the rectum and posterior wall of the uterus formed from a fold of the peritoneum.

culdocentesis: Obtaining specimens for diagnostic reasons from the cul-de-sac of Douglas by aspiration or surgical incision through the vaginal wall.

Cullen's sign: Faint, irregular, blue-black patches of skin around the umbilicus often seen in ruptured ectopic pregnancy or acute pancreatitis.

culture: Patterns of behavior learned through the socialization process, including anything acquired by humans as members of society; system of meanings and customs shared by some identifiable group or subgroup and transmitted from one generation of that group to the next; reproduction of microorganisms in special media.

curative care: Care directed toward eliminating symptoms and problems.

Curandera: Female folk healer in Hispanic/Latin cultures.

Curendero: Male folk healer in Hispanic/Latin cultures.

curettage: Scraping with a curet to remove the endometrial lining of the uterus. Used to remove growths and polyps in the uterus, in incomplete abortions, to produce abortion, or to obtain specimens.

curvature of the spine: Structural deformity of the spine resulting in scoliosis, kyphoscoliosis, lordosis, or kyphosis.

custom: Habitual practice that is adhered to by members of the same group or geographical region.

cyanosis: Blue discoloration of the skin and mucous membranes due to excessive concentration of reduced hemoglobin in the blood.

cycle of battering (cycle of violence): Three-phased predictable behavior of battering: period of tension building, acute battering episode, period of calm, love, and respite.

cyclodialysis: Formation of an opening between the anterior chamber and the suprachoroidal space for draining the aqueous humor.

cyclothymia: Condition of hypomania and depression of insufficient duration and severity to meet criteria for diagnosis of bipolar disorder.

cyst: Closed sac or pouch with a definite wall that contains fluid, semi-fluid, or solid material.

cystic fibrosis: Congenital autosomal recessive disease that manifests in the lungs, pancreas, and GU system and causes chronic obstructive pulmonary disease.

cystocele: Downward and forward displacement of the bladder toward the vaginal opening, often related to weakness or traumatized muscles from childbirth.

cytokine: A soluble factor produced by myriad cells involved in communication between immune cells. Many cytokines are growth factors.

cytomegalovirus (CMV): One of a group of highly host-specific viruses that infect man, monkeys, or rodents, with the production of unique large cells bearing intranuclear inclusions; **cytomegalic inclusion disease:** Disease caused by cytomegalovirus and seen in infected infants as anemia, thrombocytopenia, purpura, macrocephaly, and abnormal mental or motor development with a 50% mortality rate; infants are infected from mothers who carry virus.

cytology: Study of cells; science dealing with the origin, formation, structure, function, and pathology of cells.

cytostatic: The ability to inhibit cellular growth.

cytotoxic: The ability to kill cells.

daily fetal movement counts (DFMCs): Assessment of fetal activity or number of times the fetus moves within a specific timeframe counted by the mother and reported to caregivers.

database: Collection of data organized in information fields in electronic format.

date rape: Sexual assault between a dating couple without the consent of one of the participants.

death: Cessation of all vital functions; **fetal death:** Intrauterine death of a fetus weighing at least 500 gm or more than 20 weeks gestation with an unknown cause; **infant death:** Death during the first year of life; **maternal death:** Death due to pregnancy or pregnancy-related problem; **neonatal death:** Newborn death within the first 28 days of life; **perinatal death:** Death of fetus or infant during the timeframe of 20 weeks gestation to 28 days of age.

death rates: Number of deaths occurring within a specific population during a particular time period, usually in terms of 1000 persons per year.

debility: Weakness or feebleness of the body.

debridement: Excision of contused and necrotic tissue from the surface of a wound; **autolytic:** Self-debridement (i.e., removal of contused or necrotic tissue through the action of enzymes in the tissues); **sharp:** Debridement using a sharp instrument.

debris: Remains of broken down or damaged cells or tissue.

decatastrophizing: In cognitive therapy, assisting client to examine validity of negative automatic thought and appropriate coping strategies.

decidua: Mucous membrane lining the uterus (or endometrium) that changes in preparation for pregnancy and is sloughed off during menstruation and during postpartum.

decision making: The process of making decisions (e.g., the choice of certain preferred courses of action over others).

declarative memory: The registration, retention, and recall of past experiences, sensations, ideas, thoughts, and knowledge through the hippocampal nuclear structures or the amygdala that result in long-term memory.

decompensation: Failure of heart to maintain sufficient circulation to maintain life.

deconditioning: The physiologic changes in systemic function following prolonged periods of rest and inactivity.

decorticate rigidity: Exaggerated extensor tone of the lower extremities and flexor tone of the upper extremities resulting in abnormal posturing due to damage to the brainstem.

decortication: Removal of portions of the cortical substance of a structure or organ, as of the brain, kidney, lung, etc.

decrement: Stage of decline (after the peak) in uterine contraction.

decubitus ulcer: Open sore due to lowered circulation in a body part. Usually secondary to prolonged pressure at a bony prominence.

dedifferentiation: *See* anaplasia.

deductive reasoning: A serial strategy in which conclusions are drawn on the basis of premises that are assumed to be true.

deep tendon reflexes (DTRs): Reflex action created by stimulation of elbow, wrist, knee, triceps, or ankle tendons.

deep vein thrombosis: A blood clot in a deep vein.

defamation of character: Sharing information about a person that could be detrimental to his or her reputation.

defense mechanisms: Unconscious processes that keep anxiety-producing information out of conscious awareness (e.g., compensation, denial, rationalization, sublimation, and projection).

defibrillation: The stoppage of fibrillation of the heart.

defibrillator: An apparatus used to counteract fibrillation by application of electric impulses to the heart.

defibrination syndrome: A syndrome resulting from a deprival of fibrin.

deficiency: The quality or state of being deficient; absence of something essential; an incompleteness, a lacking, or a shortage.

deficiency disease: A disease caused by a dietary lack of vitamins, minerals, etc., or by an inability to metabolize them.

deficit: Inadequate behavior or task performance. A lack or deficiency.

deglutition: The act of swallowing.

degrees: In reference to the measurement of range of motion, the amount of movement from the beginning to the end of the action.

degrees of freedom: The options or directions available for movement from a given point in statistics.

dehydration: Absence of water. Removal of water from the body or a tissue. A condition that results from undue loss of water.

deinstitutionalization: Transfer to a community setting of patients who have been hospitalized for an extended period of time, usually years.

delay of gratification: Postponement of the satisfaction of one's needs.

delirium: Characterized by confused mental state with changes in attention; hallucinations, delusions, and incoherence.

delirium tremens (DT): Condition caused by acute alcohol withdrawal, characterized by trembling and visual hallucinations; may lead to convulsions.

delivery (birth): Assisted or spontaneous delivery of the infant and placenta and membranes by the mother and care givers.

delusion: Inaccurate, illogical beliefs that remain fixed in one's mind despite having no basis in reality.

delusional disorder: Psychosis characterized by the presence of persistent delusions often involving paranoid themes in an individual whose behavior otherwise appears quite normal.

demand feeding: Feeding a newborn every 2–4 hours or whenever it cries to be fed.

demarcation: Line of separation between viable and nonviable tissue.

dementia: State of deterioration of personality and intellectual abilities, including memory, problem-solving skills, language use, and thinking, that interferes with daily functioning.

demography: Scientific study of human populations particularly in relation to size, distribution, and characteristics of group members.

demyelinating disease: Disease that destroys or damages the myelin sheath of the nerves.

demyelination: The destruction of myelin, the white lipid covering of the nerve cell axons. The loss of myelin decreases conduction velocity of the neural impulse and destroys the "white matter" of the brain and spinal cord.

denial: State of refusing to accept a real situation as real.

dentofacial anomalies: Relating to abnormalities of the oral cavity and surrounding facial musculature and joints.

dendrite: Short processes found on the end of a nerve cell that send or receive information from another neurotransmitter.

dendritic growth: New evidence indicating growth (rather than the common descriptions of decline) in the brains of the elderly.

denude: Loss of epidermis.

deontology: Prioritization of ethical principles to resolve a dilemma.

dependence: Need to be influenced, nurtured, or controlled; relying on others for support.

dependent: Person who can be claimed on insurance.

depersonalization: Altering one's feelings to neutralize an experience.

depolarization: The process or act of neutralizing polarity, such as in a heart beat.

depression: Characterized by an overwhelming sense of sadness that may be brought on by an event or series of events, but lasts far longer than a reasonable time.

depth perception: Determining the relative distance between objects, figures, or landmarks and the observer, and changes in planes or surfaces; the ability to determine the relative distance between self and objects and figures observed.

derangement: To upset the arrangement, order, or function of a system. Clinically, it describes various affections—either intra-articular, extra-articular, or both—often caused by trauma or abnormal use, that interfere with the function of a joint.

dermal: Related to the skin or derma. Synonym: skin.

dermatome: Surgical instrument that thinly cuts layers of skin for use in transplantation, as with burn treatment.

dermatomyositis: Systemic connective tissue disease characterized by inflammatory and degenerative changes in the skin that lead to symmetric weakness and some atrophy.

dermis: The inner layer of skin in which hair follicles and sweat glands originate; involved in grade II to IV pressure sores.

DES (diethylstilbestrol): A synthetic estrogen preparation; can lead to reproductive tract malformations in female fetuses when ingested by pregnant woman.

descriptive ethics: Ethics used to describe the moral systems of a culture.

descriptive statistics: An abbreviated description and summarizing of data; nonexperimental.

desensitization: To deprive or lessen sensitivity.

desquamated interstitial pneumonitis: Pneumonia with cellular infiltration or fibrosis of the pulmonary interstitium with progressive dyspnea and a nonproductive cough; etiology unknown.

desquamation: Process by which old layers of skin cells (epidermis) are shed.

desquamation: Shedding of the epithelial cells (often in newborns) of the skin and mucus membranes.

detoxification: Withdrawal from a substance that has become habit forming.

detrusor muscle: The muscular component of the bladder wall.

developmental: Pertaining to gradual growth or expansion, especially from a lower to a higher state of complexity. Pertaining to development.

developmental assessment: Evaluation of an individual in comparison with the expected activities and behaviors of individuals of comparable age.

developmental crisis: Severe stress seen in persons unable to complete a specific psychosocial developmental stage and fails to move on to the subsequent stage.

developmental delay: The failure to reach expected age-specific performance in one or more areas of development (e.g., motor, sensory-perceptual). Wide range of childhood disorders and environmental situations in which a child is unable to accomplish the developmental tasks typical of his or her chronological age.

developmental disabilities: A physical or mental handicap or combination of the two that becomes evident before age 22, is likely to continue indefinitely, and results in significant functional limitation in major areas of life.

developmental milestones: Important skills associated with a specific age, such as sitting or crawling.

developmental tasks: Age-specific expectations about human growth responsibilities. May be physical, especially with young children, or emotional/life considerations.

developmental theory: Theoretical explanation of family development in which members experience phases from dependence to independence to interdependence.

deviance: Behavior that is in contrast to acceptable standards within a community or culture.

dexterity: Skill in using the hands or body, usually requiring both fine and gross motor coordination. Synonym: agility.

diabetes mellitus: Systemic metabolic disorder created by deficient insulin production with ensuing hyperglycemia from poor utilization of carbohydrates, fat, and protein.

diabetic retinopathy: Complication of diabetes in which small aneurysms form in retinal capillaries.

diabetitian: Health care provider specializing in care of clients with diabetes.

diadochal: A succession of two movements at an angle to each other.

diagnosis (Dx): Technical identification of a disease or condition by scientific evaluation of history, physical signs, symptoms, laboratory tests, and procedures.

diagnosis related groups (DRG): Classifications of illnesses and injuries that are used as the basis for prospective payments to hospitals under Medicare and other insurers.

Diagnostic and Statistical Manual of Mental Disorders (DSM): The nomenclature of emotional illnesses, including classifications, guidelines, and diagnostic criteria, published by the American Psychiatric Association. The number denotes the version of the manual.

diagnostic interview: Interview used by a professional to classify the nature of dysfunction in a person under care.

diagnostic tests: Tests to determine a disease condition.

dialect: Variation of a language; particular to a certain geographical region.

dialysis: The process of separating crystalloids and colloids in a solution by the difference in their rates of diffusion through a semipermeable membrane; crystalloids pass through readily, colloids very slowly or not at all.

diameter: Distance from any point on the periphery of a surface, body, or space to the opposite point such as measurements of the pelvic inlet and fetal head; **biparietal diameter:** the largest transverse diameter of the fetal skull at term.

diaphoresis: Perspiration, especially profuse perspiration.

diaphragmatic breathing: The use of the diaphragm to draw air into the bases of the lungs.

diaphragmatic hernia: Congenital malformation of the diaphragm that allows abdominal contents to displace into the thoracic cavity.

diastasis recti abdominis: Separation of the rectus abdominal muscles at the midline seen in women with multiple gestations or repeated childbirths.

diastole: Period of time between contractions of the atria or the ventricles during which blood enters the relaxed chambers from the systemic circulation and lungs; significant in blood pressure readings.

dichotomous thinking: Good/bad; black/white thinking.

diffuse: Spread out or dispersed. Not concentrated.

diffusion: The process of becoming diffused or widely spread. Dialysis through a membrane.

digital: Discrete form of information (e.g., a clock that displays only digits at any given moment, as opposed to analog).

dignity: Importance of valuing the inherent worth and uniqueness of each person.

dilation (dilatation): The stretching and enlarging of the pupils or veins; cervical opening to 10 cm to allow birth of the infant.

dilation and curettage (D & C): Widening of the cervical canal with a dilator and the scraping of the uterine endometrium with a curette.

diminutive: Suffix added to a medical term to indicate a smaller size, number, or quantity of that term.

diplegia: Involvement of two extremities.

diplopia: Double vision.

disability: The inability to engage in age-specific, gender-related, and sex-specific roles in a particular social context and physical environment. Any restriction or lack (resulting from an injury) of ability to perform an activity in a manner or within the range considered normal for a human being.

disability behavior: Ways in which people respond to bodily indications and conditions that they come to view as abnormal; how people monitor themselves, define and interpret symptoms, take remedial action, and use sources of help.

disablement: Used as an umbrella term to cover all the negative dimensions of disability together or separately.

discharge: The process of discontinuing interventions included in a single episode of care, occurring when the anticipated goals and desired outcomes have been met. Other indicators for discharge: the patient/client declines to continue care; the patient/client is unable to continue to progress toward goals because of medical or psychosocial complications. Also the flow of secretion or the excretion of pus, lochia, etc.

discharge planning: Plans made to prepare the client for moving from one setting to another, usually a multidisciplinary process.

disclosure: Informing the client of what he or she is going to do for a study in which he or she participates.

discontinue: Cease the treatment, medication, or action previously provided.

discordance: Discrepancy between twins in size; also discordant twins.

disc prolapse: Displacement of intervertebral disc tissue from its normal position between vertebral bodies; also referred to as slipped, herniated, or protruded disc.

discrimination: The act of making distinctions between two (or more) groups or things. Also refers to treating people differently based on such differences as culture, race, gender, or religion.

disease: Deviation from the norm of measurable biological variables as defined by the biomedical system; refers to abnormalities of structure and function in body organs and systems.

disease management program: A comprehensive approach directed toward specific outcomes of a specific disease.

disengagement theory of aging: Psychosocial theory of aging suggesting that successful aging occurs when both the elderly individual and society gradually withdraw from one another, ultimately leading to death.

disinhibition: The inability to suppress a lower brain center or motor behavior, such as a reflex, indicative of damage to higher structures of the brain.

dislocation: Displacement of bone from a joint with tearing of ligaments, tendons, and articular capsules. Symptoms include loss of joint motion, pain, swelling, temporary paralysis, and occasional shock.

disorder: Disruption or interference with normal functions or established systems.

disorganized: Schizophrenia type characterized by inability to speak appropriately, to conduct ADL, and to react appropriately. Characterized by sequence of steps being disorganized.

disorientation: Inability to make accurate judgments about people, places, and things.

displacement: Transfer of feeling from one target to another that is less threatening.

disruption: To disrupt or interrupt the orderly course of events.

disseminated intravascular coagulation (DIC): Pathological coagulation of clotting factors so that generalized bleeding occurs; seen in placenta abruption, eclampsia, amniotic fluid embolism, hemorrhage, sepsis, trauma, pancreatitis, and surgical procedures.

distal: In terms of anatomical position, located further from the trunk.

distractibility: Level at which competing sensory input can draw attention away from tasks at hand.

distress: The state of being in pain, discomfort, or suffering. Any affliction that is distressing.

distribution: Refers to manner through which a drug is transported by the circulating body fluids to the sites of action.

disuse atrophy: The wasting degeneration of muscle tissue that occurs as a result of inactivity or immobility.

diuresis: Increased secretion of urine.

divergence: The brain's ability to send information from one source to many parts of the central nervous system simultaneously.

diversity: Quality of being different or having variety.

diverticulosis: Pouches or sacs in the organ's wall, especially of the large intestine.

dizygotic: Related to two zygotes or fertilized ova.

documentation: Process of recording and reporting the information gathered and intervention performed on a client. It ensures that the client receives adequate services and that the provider is reimbursed for them.

doll's eyes: When the head is turned in one direction, the eyes look in the opposite direction; this indicates damage to the higher brain centers.

domain: Specific occupational performance area of work (including education), self-care and self-maintenance, and play and leisure.

dominant trait: One gene suppresses the expression of another (e.g., brown eyes are dominant over blue).

Doppler blood flow analysis: Device for noninvasive measure of blood flow in the placenta and fetus that detects restricted growth.

dormant: Time period when a disease remains inactive.

dorsal: In terms of anatomical position, located toward the back.

dorsosacral position: *See* lithotomy position.

dorsum: The back or analogous to the back.

double-blind study: Strategy used in research that attempts to reduce one form of experimental error. Neither the recipient nor the researcher knows which element is which.

Down's syndrome: Chromosomal abnormality involving an extra chromosome characterized by mental retardation and altered physical appearance including sloping forehead, low-set ears, and short broad hands with a single "simian" crease.

drug half-life: The time required for half the drug remaining in the body to be eliminated.

dual diagnosis: Presence of more than one diagnosis at the same time, most often a combination of a substance use disorder and some other condition, but may include any situation in which comorbidity exists.

ductus arteriosus: The channel between the pulmonary artery and aorta in the fetus, usually closing over soon after birth.

durable medical equipment (DME): Equipment typically covered by insurance.

durable power of attorney: Legal instrument authorizing one to act as another's agent for specific purposes and/or length of time. May also reference that related only to health care.

dyad: Relationship between two individuals in which interaction is significant.

dyadic activity: Activity involving another person.

dycem: A nonslip plastic material that is used in food trays and mats. Enables a person to eat without the plate slipping away. Also used to prevent any object from sliding on a surface.

dynametry: Measurement of the degree of muscle power.

dynamic equilibrium: The ability to make adjustments to the center of gravity with a changing base of support.

dynamic flexibility: Amount of resistance of a joint(s) to motion.

dynamics: Study of objects in motion.

dynamic systems theory: Theory concerning movement organization that was derived from the study of chaotic systems. Theorizes that the order and the pattern of movement performed to accomplish a goal come from the interaction of multiple, nonhierarchical subsystems.

dysarthria: Group of speech disorders resulting from disturbances in muscular control.

dyscalculia: Learning disability in which there is a problem mastering the basic arithmetic skills (e.g., addition, subtraction, multiplication, and division), and their application to daily living.

dysdiadochokinesia: The inability to perform rapid alternating movements.

dysesthesia: Sensation of "pins and needles" such as that experienced when one's extremity "goes to sleep." Manifested by unpleasant or painful touch perception.

dysfunction: Complete or partial impairment of function.

dysfunctional hierarchy: Levels of dysfunction including impairment, disability, and handicap.

dysfunctional labor: Abnormal uterine contractions that prevent normal labor progress (both dilatation and effacement).

dysfunctional uterine bleeding (DUB): Abnormal uterine bleeding with no apparent cause.

dysgraphia: Imperfect ability to process and produce written language.

dyskinesia: Impairment of voluntary motion.

dyslexia: Impairment of the brain's ability to translate images received from the eyes into understandable language.

dysmetria: Condition seen in cerebellar disorders in which the patient is unable with a finger to control movements such as touching specific objects.

dysmenorrhea: Painful menstruation related to ovulation (primary) and (secondary) related to organic disease such as endometriosis, pelvic inflammatory disease, or uterine neoplasm.

dyspareunia: Painful sexual intercourse (either gender).

dyspepsia: Poor digestion.

dysphagia: The inability to swallow.

dysplasia: Abnormal development in number, size, or organization of cells or tissue.

dyspnea: The inability to breathe; difficulty breathing.

dyspraxia: Difficulty or inability to perform a planned motor activity when the muscles used in this activity are not paralyzed.

dysreflexia: A life-threatening, uninhibited, sympathetic response of the nervous system to a noxious stimulus that is experienced by an individual with a spinal cord injury at T7 or above.

dysrhythmia: Disturbance in rhythm in speech, brain waves, or cardiac irregularity.

dyssomnia: Sleep disorder.

dysthmic disorder: Depressive neurosis without loss of contact with reality.

dystocia: Prolonged difficult birth due to mechanical factors related to the passenger (malpresentation of the fetus), the passage (inadequate size of the pelvis), or the powers (inadequate uterine muscle activity).

dystonia/dystonic: Distorted positioning of the limbs, neck, or trunk that is held for a few seconds and then released.

early intervention: Multidisciplinary, comprehensive, coordinated, community-based system for young children with developmental vulnerability or delay from birth to age 3 years and their families. Services are designed to enhance child development, minimize potential delays, remediate existing problems, prevent further deterioration, and promote adaptive family functioning.

ecchymosis: Bruise; caused by superficial bleeding under the skin due to trauma or infection.

echo densities: Ultrasound changes that can be evidence of brain tissue damage.

echolalia: Uncontrollable repetitive verbalization of words spoken by another person that does not fit the situation.

echopraxia: Repetitive movement that does not fit the situation.

eclampsia (also called toxemia): An acute toxic condition of pregnancy and puerperal women with symptoms of coma, seizures, high blood pressure, renal dysfunction, and proteinuria.

ecologic theory: Developmental theory that focuses on the process of development with all of the relevant variables (e.g., individual, contextual, mixed, cultural) of an individual's environment considered.

ectoderm: Layer of cells that develop from the inner cell mass of the blastocyst. This layer eventually develops into the outer surface of the skin, nails, part of teeth, lens of the eye, the inner ear, and central nervous system.

ectopia: Displacement or malposition; **ectopic pregnancy:** Implantation of the fertilized ova outside of the uterus in the abdomen, fallopian tubes, or ovaries.

ectropion: Eversion of the edge of the eyelid.

eczema: An inflammatory skin disease characterized by lesions varying greatly in character, with vesiculation, infiltration, watery discharge, and the development of scales and crusts.

edema: Accumulation of large amounts of fluid in the tissues of the body; **dependent edema:** Accumulation of fluid in lower or dependent parts of the body; **pitting edema:** Accumulation of fluid that leaves a small depression or pit when pressure is applied.

edentulous: Having no natural teeth.

effacement: Thinning and shortening of the cervix, occurring before or during dilation and expressed in percentages of 0% to 100%.

effectiveness: Degree to which the desired result is produced.

efferent: Conducting away from a structure, such as a nerve or a blood vessel.

efferent neuron: Includes motor neurons.

efficacy: Having the desired influence or outcome.

effleurage: Gentle stroking along the long axis of limbs or muscles; **abdominal effleurage:** Light stroking in a circular pattern over the abdomen used in the Lamaze technique of childbirth in the first stage of labor.

effusion: Escape of fluid into a joint or cavity.

ego: In psychoanalytic theory, one of three personality structures. Controls and directs one's actions after evaluating reality, monitoring one's impulses, and taking into consideration one's values and moral and ethical code. The executive structure of the personality.

ego defense mechanism: Strategies to protect the ego in view of threats to integrity.

ego differentiation: One of the three psychological developmental tasks in aging (Peck). Focus is on valued activities to replace work.

ego integrity: Eighth stage of Erikson's model of development. Self-acceptance.

egoistic suicide: Condition of individual who feels separated from society.

egophony: A bleating quality of voice observed in auscultation in certain cases of lung consolidation.

ejaculation: Ejection of semen from the male urethra.

ejection fraction: Percentage of blood emptied from the ventricles at the end of a contraction of the heart muscle.

elective abortion: *See* abortion.

electrical potential: The amount of electrical energy residing in specific tissues.

electrical stimulation: Intervention through the application of electricity.

electrocardiogram (EKG): A graphic recording of the electrical activity of the heart.

electrocautery: Cauterization by means of a wire loop or needle heated by direct current.

electroconvulsive therapy (ECT): Treatment consisting of electrical current through the brain to create grand mal seizure. Used to disrupt treatment-resistant depression.

electroencephalogram (EEG): Electrical activity of the brain.

electrolytes: Mineral salts that conduct electricity in the body when in solution.

electromyography (EMG): The examining and recording of the electrical activity of a muscle.

electronic fetal monitoring (EFM): The monitoring of the fetal heart rate and uterine contractions through internal electrodes and pressure catheter or external pressure and sound transducers during labor.

electrophysiologic testing: The process of examining and recording the electrical responses of the body.

electrophoresis: The movement of charged particles through a medium as a result of changes in electrical potential.

electrotherapeutic modalities: A broad group of agents that use electricity to produce a therapeutic effect.

electrotherapy: The use of electrical stimulation modalities in treatment.

elder: Term used to refer to individuals in the later years of the life span, arbitrarily set between the age 65 to 70 and beyond.

elder abuse: Intentional physical or psychological injury inflicted upon older adults by caretakers.

elopement: Client leaving a care facility without the knowledge of staff.

emaciated: State of physical wasting or excessive thinness.

embolism: Sudden blocking of an artery by a clot of foreign material (i.e., blood clot) brought to the site of lodging via the bloodstream.

embryo: The fetus from conception to 8 weeks of gestation.

embryo transfer (ET): Transfer of the fertilized ova (still in the embryonic stage) from medium to the uterus.

embryonic period: Prenatal period of development that occurs from 2 to 8 weeks after conception. During this period, cell differentiation intensifies, support systems for the cells form, and organs appear.

embryotomy: Extraction of a dead fetus by dismemberment.

emergency response system (ERS): Devices used to signify the need for help. Used typically by elderly who live alone.

emetic: Type of medication that promotes vomiting.

emotional lability: Rapid mood changes; often seen in early pregnancy.

empathy: While maintaining one's sense of self, the ability to recognize and share the emotions and state of mind of another person.

emphysema: An abnormal swelling of the lung tissue due to the permanent loss of elasticity or the destruction of the alveoli, which seriously impairs respiration.

empirical base: Knowledge based upon the observations and experience of master clinicians.

empowerment: To enable.

empty calories: Foods lacking vitamins, minerals, and fiber.

enablement: Assisting clients to locate needed resources.

encephalitis: Disease characterized by inflammation of the parenchyma of the brain and its surrounding meninges; usually caused by a virus.

encephalocele: Protrusion of the brain through a defect in the skull.

encephalopathy: Any disease that affects the tissues of the brain and its surrounding meninges.

encoding (cognitive): Processes or strategies used to initially store information in memory.

endarterectomy: The surgical removal of endarterium and atheromatous material from an arterial segment that has become stenosed.

endarterium: The innermost layer of the arterial wall; also called the intima.

end-diastolic volume: The amount of filling of the ventricles of the heart during diastole.

endocarditis: Inflammation of the endocardium; a disease generally associated with acute febrile or rheumatic diseases and marked by dyspnea, rapid heart action, and peculiar systolic murmurs.

endocardium: The thin endothelial membrane lining the cavities of the heart.

endocervical: Pertaining to the lining of the cervix.

endocrine: Any gland producing internal secretion (e.g., thyroid gland).

end-of-life care: Care that is culturally sensitive and appropriate to the individual during the final stages of dying.

endogenous: Growing from within. Developing or originating within the organism.

endometrial cancer: Malignant neoplasm of lining of the uterus.

endometriosis: Abnormal proliferation of the uterine mucous membrane into the pelvic cavity.

endometrium: Lining of the uterus which is shed monthly during menstruation.

endothelial: Pertaining to the epithelial cells that line the heart cavities, blood vessels, lymph vessels, and serous cavities of the body.

end-systolic volume: The amount of blood remaining in each ventricle after each heartbeat.

endurance: The ability of a muscle to sustain forces or to repeatedly generate forces.

endurance testing: Used to determine the capacity of an individual to sustain the energy output needed to fulfill a task.

endorphins: Polypeptides secreted in the brain that act as an opiate and increase the perceived pain threshold.

endotracheal: Within or through the trachea. Performed by passage through the lumen of the trachea (e.g., endotracheal tube).

energy conservation techniques: Applying procedures that save energy; may include activity restriction, work simplification, time management, and organizing the environment to simplify tasks.

en face positioning: Parent and infant facial alignment (eyes, mouth, etc.) when looking at each other face to face.

engagement: Signifies that the fetus has firm presenting part within the mother's pelvis; active involvement in activities.

engorgement: Vascular congestion and swelling, especially of the breast tissue following birth and prior to lactation.

engrossment: Total focus on something or someone; in obstetrics—the focus of parents on the newborn.

enmeshment: Exaggerated connectedness of group members exemplified by lack of differentiation among or between members of the group.

enteral: Administration of a pharmacologic agent directly into the gastrointestinal tract by oral, rectal, or nasogastric routes.

enteric: Pertaining to the intestines.

enterocele: Herniation of the intestine below the cervix associated with congenital weakness or obstetric trauma.

enterostomal therapist: Person designated to care for ostomies such as ileostomies or colostomies, frequently assumed by a registered nurse.

enterovirus: A group of viruses that infect the GI tract and include coxsackievirus, ECHO virus, and poliovirus.

enthesopathy: Any inflammation of a joint.

entrainment: Phenomenon observed between parent and infant in which the infant moves (parts of the body) in rhythm to the parents words. Is not observed with random sound. Believed to be an essential aspect in parent–infant bonding.

entropion: Inversion of the edge of the eyelid.

enucleation: Removal of an organ or other mass from its supporting tissues, e.g., removal of an eye.

enuresis: The inability to control urine, bedwetting.

environment: Social and physical conditions or factors that have the potential to influence an individual.

environmental approaches: Interventions based on changing the environment (e.g., changing support systems; modifying job, home).

environmental assessment: Process of identifying, describing, and measuring factors external to the individual that can influence performance or the outcome of treatment. Can include space and associated objects, cultural influences, social relationships, and system available resources.

environmental barrier: Any type of obstacle that interferes with a person's ability to achieve optimal occupational performance.

environmental factors: The background of a person's life and living, composed of elements of the natural environment (e.g., weather or terrain), the human-made environment (e.g., tools, furnishing, the built environment), social attitudes, customs, rules, practices, institutions, and other individuals.

enzyme: A protein functioning as a biochemical catalyst, necessary for most major body functions. Biochemical substances that are capable of breaking down necrotic tissue.

epicardium: The layer of the pericardium that is in contact with the heart.

epicritic sensation: The ability to localize and discern fine differences in touch, pain, and temperature.

epidemiology: A study of the relationships of the various factors determining the frequency and distribution of diseases in a human environment. Science concerned with factors, causes, and remediation as related to the distribution of disease, injury, and other health-related events.

epidermis: The outer cellular layer of skin.

epidural (block): Anesthesia injected into the epidural space of the spine, which can produce loss of sensation from the abdomen to the toes.

epigastric: Region of abdomen in upper center portion.

epigenesis: Elements of each developmental stage represented in all developmental stages.

epilepsy: Group of disorders caused by temporary sudden changes in the electrical activity of the brain that results in convulsive seizures or changes in the level of consciousness or motor activity.

epinephrine: A hormone secreted by the adrenal medulla in response to splanchnic stimulation and stored in the chromaffin granules, being released predominantly in response to hypoglycemia. Increases blood pressure, stimulates heart muscle, accelerates the heart rate, and increases cardiac output.

episiotomy: Refers to an incision through the perineum that allows for less pressure on the fetal head during delivery and prevents lacerations of the perineum.

episodic memory: Memory for personal episodes or events that have some temporal reference.

epispadias: Congenital opening of the urethra on the dorsum of the penis, or opening by separation of the labia minora and a fissure of the clitoris.

epistaxis: Nosebleed.

epistemology: Dimension of philosophy that is concerned with the questions of truth by investigating the origin, nature, methods, and limits of human knowledge.

epithelialization: Regeneration of the epidermis across a wound surface.

Epstein-Barr virus (EBV): The virus that causes infectious mononucleosis. It is spread by respiratory tract secretions (e.g., saliva, mucus).

equilibrium reaction: Reaction that occurs when the body adapts and posture is maintained, and when there is a change of the supporting surface; any of several reflexes that enables the body to recover balance.

equinovarus: Deformity of the foot in which the foot is pointing downward and inward; clubfoot.

ergometer: Device that can measure work done.

ergometry: Measurement of work.

ergonomics: Field of study that examines and optimizes the interaction between the human worker and the nonhuman work environment. The relationship among the worker, the work that is done, the tasks and activities inherent in that work, and the environment in which the work is performed. Scientific and engineering principles to improve the safety, efficiency, and quality of movement involved in work.

ergot: Drug which causes the uterus to contract by stimulating smooth muscle.

eructation: Producing gas from the stomach, often with a characteristic sound; belching.

erythema: First-degree reddening of the skin due to a burn or injury.

erythema chronicum migrans (ECM): Annular lesion at the site of a tick bite; an early symptom of Lyme disease.

erythroblastosis fetalis: Destruction of fetal blood cells by maternal antibodies resulting in severe fetal/newborn anemia requiring transfusion.

erythrocyte: Red blood cell that contains hemoglobin, an oxygen-carrying pigment responsible for the red color of blood.

eschar: Thick, leathery necrotic tissue; devitalized tissue; a slough produced by burning or by a corrosive application.

Escherichia coli (*E. coli*): A species of organisms constituting the greater part of the intestinal flora. In excess, it causes urinary tract infections and epidemic diarrheal disease.

esophageal atresia: Condition in which the esophagus is not connected to the stomach, either ending in a blind pouch or a thin cord.

esophageal varices: A tortuous dilatation of a vein; a result of excessive pressure from cirrhotic liver.

essential fat: Stored body fat that is necessary for normal physiologic function and found in bone marrow, the nervous system, and all body organs.

essential hypertension: High blood pressure that is idiopathic, self-existing, and has no obvious external cause. Intrinsic hypertension.

estimated date of birth (EDB): Estimate calculated using Nägele's rule.

estrogen: The female hormone that is responsible for maintenance of female sex characteristics and is formed in the ovary, placenta, testis, and adrenal cortex.

estrogen deficiency vulvovaginitis: Vaginal burning often with sexual intercourse caused by the decrease in estrogen.

estrogen replacement therapy (ERT): Hormone therapy used after menopause.

ethical dilemma: Conflict of choices with no clear solution that is often caused by attempting to balance two or more options with no over-riding principle to tell an individual what to do.

ethical relativism: View that each person's values should be considered equally valid.

ethics: System of principles or standards that govern personal and professional conduct.

ethnic: Member of, or pertaining to, groups of people with a common racial, national, linguistic, religious, or cultural history.

ethnicity: Component of culture that is derived from membership in a racial, religious, national, or linguistic group or subgroup, usually through birth.

ethnocentrism: Process of judging different cultures or ethnic groups only on the basis of one's own culture or experiences.

ethnogerontology: Study of ethnicity in an aging context.

ethologic theory: Branch of developmental theory that emphasizes innate, instinctual qualities of behavior that predispose individuals to behave in certain patterns.

ethology: The systemic study of the formation of the core characteristics of being human.

etiology: Dealing with the causes of disease.

euthanasia: The deliberate ending of life of a person suffering from an incurable disease; has been broadened to include the withholding of extraordinary measures to sustain life, allowing a person to die.

evaluation: Process of obtaining and interpreting data necessary for treatment; a dynamic process in which the practitioner makes clinical judgments based on data gathered during the examination.

eversion: Turning outward.

evidence-based practice: Practice founded on research that supports its effectiveness.

evisceration: Removal of the contents of a cavity.

exacerbation: Increase in the severity of a disease or any of its symptoms.

examination: The process of obtaining a history, performing relevant systems reviews, and selecting and administering specific tests and measures.

exchange transfusion: Replacement of 75% to 85% of a newborn's circulating blood volume due to excessive accumulation of bilirubin or other by-products of hemolysis and to correct for anemia and acidosis.

excitement phase: Physical and emotional changes that take place during human sexual response that increases the interest in sexual intercourse.

excoriation: Abrasions or scratches on the skin, frequently linear.

excretion: Process through which metabolites of medications (and the active medication itself) are eliminated from the body through urine and feces, evaporation from skin, exhalation from lungs, and secretion into saliva.

exertional angina: Paroxysmal thoracic pain due most often to anoxia of the myocardium precipitated by physical exertion. Synonym: angina.

exhaustion: Depletion of energy with the consequent inability to respond to stimuli.

exhibitionism: Attention-getting behavior, disorder evidenced in recurring urge to expose one's genitals to a stranger.

exocrine: Secreting outwardly (the opposite of endocrine).

exogenous: Growing by additions to the outside. Developed or originating outside the organism.

exophthalmos: Abnormal protrusion of the eyeball, which results in a marked stare.

expected outcomes: The intended results of patient/client management, with the changes in impairments, functional limitations, and disabilities and the changes in health, wellness, and fitness needs that are expected as the result of implementing the plan of care.

expectorate: To expel mucus or phlegm from the lungs; to spit.

exploratory laparotomy: Incision into the abdominal cavity to view the condition of abdominal organs.

expressive aphasia: The inability to verbalize one's own needs.

exstrophy of the bladder: Bladder lies open on the abdomen due to physical anomaly in which the anterior wall of the bladder and the lower abdominal wall are absent.

extended care facility (ECF): Facility that is an extension of hospital care; derived from Medicare legislation.

extension (EXT): Straightening a body part.

external stimulation: Factors in the area where the activity is being performed, which may enhance or impede performance.

external validity: The degree to which an experimental finding is predictable to the population at large.

exteroceptive: Receptors activated by stimuli outside of the body.

extinction: Behavioral approach to discouraging a particular behavior by ignoring it and reinforcing other more acceptable behaviors.

extracorporeal membrane oxygenation (ECMO): Oxygenation of the blood (primarily newborns with meconium aspiration syndrome) externally using cardiopulmonary bypass.

extracranial: Anatomic structures outside the cranial vault (skull).

extrahepatic biliary atresia: Closure/absence of major bile duct.

extrapyramidal: Outside of the pyramidal tracts or the compact bundle of nerve fibers in the medulla oblongata.

extrapyramidal signs: Motor symptoms that mimic Parkinson's disease, dyskinesia, and other lesions in the extrapyramidal tract.

extrauterine pregnancy: Pregnancy outside the uterus (usually some-place in the abdomen).

extrinsic: Coming from or originating outside.

extrinsic motivation: Stimulation to achieve or perform that initiates from the environment.

extrusion reflex: When the infant automatically extrudes the tongue when stimulated. This is a normal reflex.

exudate: Material, such as fluid, cells, or cellular debris, that has escaped from blood vessels and been deposited in tissues or on tissue surfaces, usually as a result of inflammation. In contrast to a transudate, is characterized by a high content of protein, cells, or solid materials derived from cells; accumulation of fluids in wound. May contain serum, cellular debris, bacteria, and leukocytes.

face validity: Dimension of a test by which it appears to test what it purports to test.

fact: Truth or reality.

factor analysis: Statistical test that examines relationships of many variables and their contribution to the total set of variables.

failure to thrive: Syndrome of malnutrition in neonates and children with growth patterns below the norm for the specific age; in the elderly, can be combined with a lack of will to live.

fallopian tubes: Tubes through which the ovum travels to the uterus.

false imprisonment: Charge related to deliberate and unauthorized confinement by use of threat or force. May result in cases involving the use of restraints.

false labor: Uterine contractions that fail to produce dilatation or effacement of the cervix; often irregular and are not usually progressive to a normal labor pattern.

false negative: Statistical research term indicating the rate of negative results on a diagnostic test when disease was actually present.

false positive: Statistical research term indicating the rate of positive results on a diagnostic test when no disease was actually present.

family structure: Set of unwritten principles by which a family operates as a unit and interacts with one another.

family therapy: Intervention that focuses on the context of the entire family system.

family violence: Violence (both physical and emotional) within the family that can be directed toward children, elders, siblings, or spouse.

farsightedness: An error in refraction in which a person can see distant objects clearly but has difficulty seeing objects which are close.

fascia: A thin layer of connective tissue covering, supporting, or connecting the muscles or inner organs of the body.

fasciculation: A small local contraction of muscles, visible through the skin, representing a spontaneous discharge of a number of fibers innervated by a single motor nerve filament.

fasciitis: Inflammation of a fascia.

fat emboli: Embolus formed by an ester of glycerol with fatty acids that causes a clot in the circulatory system and can result in vessel obstruction.

fatigue: State of exhaustion or loss of strength and endurance; decreased ability to maintain a contraction at a given force.

feces: Body waste material excreted from the bowels by way of the anus.

feedback: Information provided to an individual based on the individual's performance that influences the subsequent behavior in a positive or negative way.

festinating gait: Patient walks on his or her toes when pushed. Starts slowly, increases, and may continue until the patient grasps an object in order to stop (e.g., in Parkinson's disease).

fetal alcohol syndrome (FAS): Low birth weight, developmental delays, and physical defects in infants caused by mothers consuming alcohol during pregnancy.

fetal distress: Decrease in fetal heart rate and the possibility of meconium-stained amniotic fluid related to jeopardized fetal oxygen supply.

fetal growth retardation: Condition of babies who are especially small for their gestational age at birth.

fetal heart rate (FHR): The rate (beats per min) of the fetal heart; **acceleration:** Increase in FHR seen as reassuring; **baseline:** FHR average between contractions; **bradycardia:** When the baseline FHR is below 110; **deceleration:** A slowing of the FHR assessed in relationship to contractions; **early deceleration:** Begins at the same time as the contraction and is related to head compression; **late deceleration:** Begins after the peak of the contraction and continues after the contraction subsides and is related to uteroplacental insufficiency; **prolonged deceleration:** Decrease in FHR for at least two minutes; **variable deceleration:** Begins at times unrelated to contractions, thought to be related to cord compression.

fetal scalp electrode: Electrode placed in the fetal scalp which electronically monitors the FHR.

fetal tachycardia: When the baseline FHR exceeds 160 often related to maternal fever or anomalies.

fetishism: Disorder characterized by recurring sexual urges and fantasies involving use of inanimate objects.

fetotoxic: Poisonous to the fetus.

fetus: Describes the baby from the 8th week after conception until birth.

FEV1: The percentage of the vital capacity that can be expired in 1 minute.

fibrillation: Small, local involuntary muscle contraction.

fibrin: A whitish, insoluble protein formed from fibrinogen by the action of thrombin, as in the clotting of blood. Fibrin forms the essential portion of a blood clot.

fibroblast: Chief cell of connective tissue responsible for forming the fibrous tissues of the body, such as tendons and ligaments.

fibroid: Fibrous encapsulated tumor, frequently found in the uterus.

fibromyalgia: Myofascial syndrome with systemic symptoms.

fibrosis: Formation of fibrous tissue, fibroid degeneration.

fidelity: Duty to be faithful to the client and the client's best interest; includes the mandate to keep all client information confidential.

field dependence/independence: Extent to which a person is influenced by cues from the environment in making judgments.

fight or flight: Syndrome resulting from one's perception that harm or danger is imminent.

fimbria: Fringelike structure found at the end of the fallopian tubes.

fine motor coordination: Motor behaviors involving manipulative, discreet finger movements and eye–hand coordination. Dexterity.

first stage of labor: Initial part of labor when the cervix effaces and dilates to 10 cm; includes the early, active, and transition phases.

fiscal management: Method of controlling the economics of problems at hand. It is concerned with discovering, developing, defining, and evaluating the financial goals of a department.

fissure: Any cleft or groove.

fistula: Abnormal tubelike duct or passage from a normal cavity or tube to a free surface or another cavity.

flaccidity: State of low tone in the muscle that produces weak and floppy limbs.

flashes: Sudden flashes of light in the eyes.

flexibility: The characteristic of bending without breaking. Adaptability.

flexion/flex: Act of bending a body part.

floaters: Particles free floating in the vitreous humor of the eye. Can be seen by the individual.

floating: Refers to the fetus floating within the uterus in the abdomen above the bony pelvis.

flooding/implosion therapy: Bombardment usually consisting of mental imagery to desensitize individuals to phobic stimuli.

flow: Optimal experience.

fluid intelligence: The ability to use new information.

fluidotherapy: Dry whirlpool (i.e., the application of dry heat through a fluidotherapy machine).

focal epilepsy: Jerking or stiffening of many muscles on the same side of the body that crosses over to the opposite side and then continues. Person does not fully lose consciousness but consciousness is altered.

folkways: Social customs to which people generally conform; traditional patterns of life common to a people.

focal stimulus: Event or situation of immediate concern that threatens self-esteem.

Focus Charting: *See* documentation section in Part 2.

folk medicine: Health care provided by nonprofessional persons and based on tradition of a culture.

follicle stimulating hormone (FSH): One of the gonadotropic hormones of the anterior pituitary which stimulates the growth and maturation of graafian follicles in the ovary and stimulates spermatogenesis in the male.

fomites: Material/structures upon which living organisms may be conveyed (e.g., bed linens).

fontanel: "Soft spot" on head of newborn composed of connective tissue contiguous with cranial bones at their junctions; **anterior fontanel:** Diamond-shaped area above the baby's forehead between the frontal and two parietal bones; **mastoid fontanel:** Posterior fontanel usually not palpable; **posterior fontanel:** Small triangular area at the junction of the occipital and parietal bones at the lambdoidal and sagittal sutures; **sagittal fontanel:** Soft area between the anterior and posterior fontanels along the sagittal suture; **sphenoid fontanel:** Anterolateral fontanel, usually not palpable.

footling breech: *See* breech.

foramen ovale: Septal opening between the right and left atria of the fetal heart which normally closes shortly after birth. Surgery required to close, if it remains open.

force: Product of mass and acceleration; a kinematic measurement that encompasses the amount of matter, velocity, and its rate of change of velocity; also strength, energy, and power.

forceps: Locked tonglike obstetrical instruments used to aid in the delivery of the fetal presenting part.

forensic: Pertaining to law, legal aspect.

foreskin: Loose fold of skin covering the glans penis.

formative: Evaluation conducted during the course of a program to modify the remaining elements.

foremilk: Thin watery breast milk substance secreted at the beginning of a feeding.

formulary: List of specific medications available for prescription; for example, what might be used within a given organization.

fornix: Structure with an arched shape; **fornix of the vagina:** The upper vagina is divided into anterior and posterior spaces by the protrusion of the cervix into the vagina.

fourth stage of labor: First 1 to 2 hours after delivery of the placenta, the recovery period.

fourth trimester: The 3-month period after birthing including the return of the reproductive organs to their nonpregnant state; also called the puerperium, a period of psychosocial adaptation to becoming a parent.

fracture (Fx): Pertaining to broken bone(s).

frame of reference: Organization of interrelated, theoretical concepts used in practice.

frank breech: *See* breech.

Frank-Starling mechanism: The intrinsic ability of the heart to adapt to changing volumes of inflowing blood.

fraternal twins: Twins who come from two separate ova; nonidentical.

free association: A technique of having one verbalize whatever comes to mind when presented with a stimulus. Used in repression.

free radicals: Any molecule that contains one or more unpaired electrons. Changes in cells that result from the presence of free radicals are thought to result in aging.

free-standing birthing center: A center that provides obstetrical services, prenatal care, labor, birth, and postpartum care, outside of a traditional institution (e.g., hospital).

freedom: Allows the individual to exercise choice and to demonstrate independence, initiative, and self-direction.

fremitus: A thrill or vibration, especially one that is perceptible on palpation.

frenulum: Ridge of tissue in the midline under the tongue; varies as to where it attaches from the tip of the tongue.

Fresnel prism: Prism applied to a person's glasses that shifts images toward the center of the visual field.

friability: Refers to a fragile condition of tissue.

friction: A rubbing against another surface, especially skin.

Friedman's curve: A graph of the progress of labor represented by descent of the presenting part, dilatation, and effacement of the cervix. Created by Emmanuel Friedman based on his research on the progress of labor.

frontal plane: Runs side to side, dividing the body into front and back portions.

frostbite: Injury to the tissues of the body by exposure to intense cold.

frotteurism: Disorder characterized by sexual urge to touch or rub against another person without his or her consent.

fugue: Response to extreme psychological stress resulting in leaving normal places with the intent of establishing a new identity or not remembering one's past identity.

fulcrum: The intermediate point of force application of a 3- or 4-point bending construction; entity on which a lever moves.

fulminant: Sudden; severe; occurring suddenly and with great intensity.

full-thickness skin loss: Third-degree burn or wound in which skin is completely destroyed and underlying structures (e.g., muscles, vessels) can be visualized.

function: Those activities identified by an individual as essential to support physical, social, and psychological well-being and to create a personal sense of meaningful living. Performance; action.

functional assessment: Determining the ability to perform physical activities of daily living.

functional mobility: Moving from one position or place to another, such as in-bed mobility, wheelchair mobility, and transfers, performing functional ambulation, and transporting objects. The ability to perform functional activities and tasks without restriction.

fundoscopy: Procedure for viewing the base of an organ, such as a fundoscopic examination of the eye.

fundus: The larger part of a hollow organ.

funis: A cordlike structure, as in the umbilical cord.

furuncle: A painful nodule formed in the skin by circumscribed inflammation of the corium and subcutaneous tissue, enclosing a central slough or "core." Caused by bacteria that enter through the hair follicles or sudoriparous glands.

gag reflex: Involuntary contraction of the pharynx and elevation of the soft palate elicited in most normal individuals by touching the pharyngeal wall or back of the tongue.

gains: Reinforcements for exhibiting physical symptoms; **primary:** Added attention and nurturing; **secondary:** Avoiding difficult situations due to symptoms; **tertiary:** Focus of family/others to the individual rather than on the issue at hand.

gait: The manner in which a person walks, characterized by rhythm, cadence, step, stride, and speed.

galactorrhea: A symptom of a pituitary tumor; breast milk produced without pregnancy or breast feeding.

galactosemia: Recessive, inherited metabolic disorder that prevents an individual from converting galactose to glucose, which results in serious physical and mental challenges.

galvanic skin response (GSR): Change in the electrical resistance of the skin as a response to different stimuli.

Gamblers Anonymous: Support group for those addicted to gambling.

gamete: The mature sperm or ovum.

ganglion: A mass of nerve cells serving as a center from which impulses are transmitted. A cystic tumor on a tendon sheath.

gangrene: Decay of tissue in a part of the body when the blood supply is obstructed by disease or injury.

gastric intubation: Forced feeding, usually through a nasogastric tube.

gastric lavage: Washing out the stomach with repeated flushing of water.

gastroesophageal reflux disease (GERD): "Heart burn" or return of stomach contents.

gastroschisis: Anomalies of the abdominal wall usually near the umbilical cord that allows abdominal contents to extrude.

gastrostomy: A surgically created opening to the stomach through which patients can be fed when it is not possible to take oral feedings.

gate-control theory: The pain modulation theory developed by Melzak and Wall that proposes that presynaptic inhibition in the dorsal gray matter of the spinal cord results in blocking of pain impulses from the periphery.

gatekeeper: A primary care provider responsible for coordinating all services.

gavage: Oral feeding via a tube passed through the nose or mouth into the stomach.

gender identity: Awareness of what sex/gender one is and that there is a difference between males and females. Process begins in infancy and is reinforced throughout childhood and into adulthood by families and society at large.

general systems theory: Conceptualizes the individual as an open system that evolves and undergoes different forms of growth, development, and change through an ongoing interaction with the external environment.

generalization: Applying previously learned concepts and behaviors to a variety of new situations; skills and performance in applying specific concepts to a variety of related solutions.

generalized anxiety disorder: Excessive and unrealistic worry lasting more than 6 months.

Generation X: The generation of people born between 1961 and 1981.

Generation Y: The generation of people born between 1979 and 1994.

general anesthesia: Intravenous or inhalation anesthetic agents producing loss of consciousness and thus loss of all body sensation.

generic: Nonspecific, as in medication: non-brand-name product.

genes: Biologic unit that contains the hereditary blueprints for the development of an individual from one generation to the next.

genetic: Pertaining to reproduction or to birth of origin; hereditary traits.

genetic counseling: Counseling done with families regarding genetic disorders, their occurrences and risks. Information provided regarding alternatives for actions in pregnancy termination, sterilization, or care of an already affected child.

genetic disorder: Inherited anomaly or defect transmitted through a family, one generation to the next.

geniculostriate system: Visual system pathways that transmit information for identifying the nature of objects in the environment.

genital prolapse: The falling out or slipping out of place of an internal organ, such as the uterus, rectum, vagina, or bladder.

genitalia: External organs of reproduction.

genogram: Graphic portrayal of the family system.

genome: Complete copy of genetic material in an organism.

genotype: The genetic constitution of an organism or group. In humans, hereditary combinations determining physical characteristics.

geophagia: Eating nonfood substances, e.g., dirt or clay. Observed in pregnancy.

geriatric day care: Ambulatory health care facility for older adults.

geriatrics: Area of study concerned with health care of individuals in old age. Branch of medicine that treats all problems unique to old age and aging, including the clinical problems associated with senescence and senility.

germinal period: Stage or interval of time from conception to implantation of the blastocyte to the uterus, approximately 8 to 10 days.

gerontological tripartite: Approach to the study of aging that collectively combines three phenomena of the aging process: the biological capacity for survival, the psychological capacity for adaptation, and the sociological capacity for the fulfillment of social roles.

gerontology: Area of study concerned with the care, health issues, and special problems of the elderly.

gerontophobia: Fear of aging.

gerophsychiatric: Care of older adults with mental health issues.

gestation: Total period of time the baby is carried in the uterus, approximately 40 weeks in humans.

gestational age: The number of completed weeks of development for the fetus, beginning with the first day of the last normal menstrual period.

gestational diabetes: Hyperglycemia first diagnosed in pregnancy, usually in the second or third trimester.

GIFT: Gamete intrafallopian transfer, a procedure in which the ova are retrieved via laparoscopy and are transferred with sperm into the fallopian tube.

gingivitis: Gum disease characterized by inflammation (redness and swelling) and a tendency to bleed.

glaucoma: Eye disease with increased intraocular pressure. Without treatment, can lead to blindness.

globin: The protein constituent of hemoglobin; also any member of a group of proteins similar to the typical globin.

glomerulonephritis: Infection of the kidney primarily involving the glomeruli and occurring frequently after an upper respiratory infection involving strains of streptococci.

glomerulus: A tuft or cluster; used in anatomical nomenclature as a general term to designate such a structure, as one composed of blood vessels or nerve fibers.

glottis: The vocal apparatus of the larynx, consisting of the true vocal cords and the opening between them (i.e., rima glottidis).

glucagon: A hyperglycemic-glycogenolytic factor thought to be secreted by the pancreas in response to hypoglycemia or stimulation by the growth hormone of the anterior pituitary gland.

glucocorticoid: Hormone from the adrenal cortex that raises blood sugar and reduces inflammation.

glucose: A thick, syrupy, sweet liquid generally made by incomplete hydrolysis of starch.

glucose tolerance test: Screening test used to diagnose diabetes.

glucosuria: Presence of glucose in the urine; often a sign of diabetes mellitus.

glycogenesis: The formation or synthesis of glycogen.

glycogenolysis: The splitting up of glycogen in the body tissue.

glycoprotein: A substance produced metabolically that creates osmotic force.

Golgi tendon organ (GTO): Sensory receptors in the tendons of muscles that monitor tension of muscles.

gonad: A sex gland; either the ovary or testis.

gonadotropic hormone: Hormone that stimulates the sex glands.

gonadotropin-releasing hormone (GnRH): Stimulation of the pituitary gland by a hormone from the hypothalamus producing follicle-stimulating hormone (FSH) and luteinizing hormone (LH).

goniometry: Measurement of the angle of the joint or a series of joints.

gonorrhea: Sexually transmitted bacterial disease (*N. gonorrhea*).

Goodell's sign: Softening of the cervix indicating possible pregnancy and occurring in the second or third month.

gout: Painful metabolic disease that is a form of acute arthritis; characterized by inflammation of the joints, especially of those in the foot or knee.

graafian follicle (vesicle): A small secretory sac containing the ripe ovum. Secretes estrogens and later estrogen and progesterone after the rupture of the sac.

grading: A scheme or categorization of treatments, movements, disease stages, and wound stages.

graft: The replacement of a defect in the body with a portion of suitable material, either organic or inorganic. Also, the material used for such replacement.

grand mal: Type of seizure in which there is a sudden loss of consciousness immediately followed by a generalized convulsion.

grand multipara: A woman who has given birth seven or more times.

granulation: The formation of a mass of tiny red granules of newly formed capillaries, as on the surface of a wound that is healing.

granulocyte: Any cell containing granules, especially a granular leukocyte. A heterogeneous class of leukocytes characterized by a multilobed nucleus and intracellular granules. Include neutrophils, eosinophils, basophils, and mast cells.

granulocytosis: Increase in circulating granulocyte number.

graphesthesia: The ability to identify letters or designs on the basis of tactile input to the skin.

graphomotor: Pertains to movement involved in writing.

gratification: The ability to receive pleasure, either immediate (immediately upon engaging in an activity) or delayed (after completion of the activity).

gravida: A pregnant woman.

gravidity: The number of times a woman has been pregnant.

gravity: Constant force that affects almost every motor act characterized by heaviness or weight. The tendency toward the center of the earth.

gray matter: Area of the central nervous system that contains the cell bodies.

grief: Response to real or perceived loss of someone or something valuable.

grieving process: The somatic and psychologic symptoms associated with extreme sorrow, usually a death.

gross motor coordination: Using large muscle groups for controlled, goal-directed movements. Motor behaviors concerned with posture and locomotion.

group: Plurality of individuals (three or more) who are in contact with one another, who take each other into account, and who are aware of some common goal.

group dynamics: Forces that influence the interrelationships of members and ultimately affect group outcome.

group process: Interpersonal relationship among participants in a group.

group therapy: Any intervention directed toward groups of individuals rather than an individual alone.

growth spurts: Times of increased growth, e.g., in neonates occurs at approximately 6–10 days, 6 weeks, 3 months, and 4–5 months. Frequent feedings required to increase the needed caloric intake. In puberty, the rapid increase in growth—height—requires marked caloric intake.

guardian: Individual appointed by court to exercise financial decisions.

Guillain-Barré syndrome: Peripheral polyneuritic syndrome that ascends the body and can cause paresis or paralysis.

gustatory: Pertaining to the sense of taste.

gynecoid pelvis: Typical female pelvis, rounded as opposed to oval or blunt.

gynecology: The study of female diseases such as genital, urinary, and rectal organs of the female.

gynecomastia: Enlargement of breasts in men.

gyral atrophy: Decreases in the gray or white matter of the brain or both.

habilitation: Process of giving a person the resources, including specialized treatment and training, to promote improvement in activities of daily living, thereby encouraging maximum independence.

habit: Performed on an automatic, preconscious level.

habitual (recurrent) abortion: *See* abortion.

habituate: Process of accommodating to a stimulus through repeated diminishing exposure. In newborns, the ability to decrease and then eliminate any response to a given repeated stimulus.

half-life: Measure of the amount of time required for 50% of a drug to be eliminated from the body. The time in which the radioactivity originally associated with an isotope will be reduced by one half through radioactive decay.

hallucinate: Sense (e.g., see, hear, smell, or touch) of something that does not exist externally.

halo effect: Error based on the fact that if a person is believed to possess one positive trait, he or she may possess others as well.

handicap: Disadvantage, resulting from an impairment or disability, that limits or prevents the fulfillment of a role that is normal (depending on age, sex, and social and cultural factors) for that individual. The social disadvantage of a disability.

haploid number: A cell which has half the normal number of chromosomes; e.g., germ cells which have half each of the 23 chromosomes found in humans.

harlequin sign: Rare color change in neonates in which the dependent half of the infant's body is noticeably more pink than the superior half. Has no pathologic implications.

Hawthorne effect: Research error due to response differences paid to the participant by the researcher.

Hayflick's limit: Biologic limit to the number of times a cell is able to reproduce before it dies. A finite capacity for cellular division.

hazard: State that could potentially harm a person or do damage to property.

head injury (HI): Caused by direct impact to the head, most commonly from traffic accidents, falls, industrial accidents, wounds, or direct blows; known also as traumatic brain injury.

healing: To make whole including the physical, psychological, social, spiritual, and environmental aspects of a human being and does not necessarily imply curing.

healing touch: A combination of techniques utilizing the energy fields of the body. Can relieve areas of pain and can be used for identification of physical problems areas. Sometimes relieves pain and creates a sense of well-being and harmony.

health: Physical and mental well-being with freedom from disease, pain, or defect and normalcy of physical, mental, and psychological functions.

health assessment: Comprehensive inventory of current status and needs related to health.

health education: A combination of educational, organizational, economic, and environmental supports for behavior conducive to health.

Health Insurance Portability and Accountability Act (HIPAA): Legislation passed in 1996 that provides certain protections that limit exclusions for preexisting conditions, prohibits discrimination in health care coverage, guarantees renewability and availability of health care coverage to certain groups, protects some workers who lose coverage, and increases requirements for disclosure.

health maintenance: Screening and intervention for potential health risks to prevent disease and promote health and well-being.

health promotion: Programs put in place to promote the physical, mental, and social well-being of the person. Includes a focus on the individual's ability to function optimally in her or his environment and a balance in mind and body across all of an individual's life experiences.

health care: The encompassing term for medical, nursing, therapeutic, and pharmaceutic practice.

Healthy People 2010: Report related to US needs in health promotion and education by 2010; typically revised every 10 years.

heart disease: Any of the diseases of the heart.

heart failure: The inability of the heart to pump enough blood to maintain an adequate flow to and from the body tissues.

heart–lung machine: Performs functions of the heart and lungs during open-heart surgery so these organs may undergo surgical procedures.

heat therapy: Application of heat on a body part; used to relieve the symptoms of musculoskeletal disorders.

heavy work: Exerting up to 50 to 100 pounds of force occasionally, or 25 to 50 pounds of force frequently, or 10 to 20 pounds of force constantly to move objects.

Hegar's sign: The softening of the lower uterine segment of the uterus which is present in the second or third month of pregnancy. Can be a diagnostic sign of pregnancy.

HELLP: A condition of severe preeclampsia of pregnancy that is diagnosed with laboratory findings of **h**emolytic anemia, **e**levated **l**iver function, and **l**ow **p**latelet levels; can be life threatening.

helplessness: Psychological state characterized by a sense of powerlessness or the belief that one is not capable of meeting an environmental demand competently.

hemangioma: Benign tumor composed of newly formed blood vessels clustered together.

hemangiosarcoma: A malignant tumor formed of endothelial and fibroblastic tissue.

hematocrit: The volume percentage of erythrocytes in whole blood.

hematoma: Localized collection of blood in an organ or within a tissue.

hematopoiesis: Production of blood cells.

hemianesthesia: Total loss of sensation to either the left or right side of the body.

hemianopsia: Blindness in one half of the field of vision in one or both eyes.

hemiparesis: Weakness of the left or right side of the body.

hemiplegia (hemi): Condition in which half of the body is paralyzed due to anoxia during birth or as a result of an aneurysm or cerebral vascular accident.

hemoconcentration: A decrease in plasma volume or an increase in production of red blood cells resulting in an increase in number of red cells in proportion to the total volume.

hemodilution: An increase in total volume of blood resulting in a decrease of the proportion of red blood cells.

hemodynamics: The study of the interrelationship of blood pressure, blood flow, vascular volumes, physical properties of the blood, heart rate, and ventricular function.

hemoglobin: The oxygen-carrying pigment of the erythrocytes formed by the developing erythrocyte in bone marrow.

hemoglobin electrophoresis: Test (most often from cord blood) used to diagnose sickle-cell disease in newborns.

hemolysis: The liberation of hemoglobin. The separation of the hemoglobin from the corpuscles and its appearance in the fluid in which the corpuscles are suspended.

hemolytic: Pertaining to, characterized by, or producing hemolysis.

hemolytic disease of the newborn: Usually found in cases of Rh incompatibility between mother and infant resulting in the breakdown of fetal red blood cells by maternal antibodies.

hemophilia: Lack of clotting factors that results in a hemorrhage.

hemoptysis: Expectoration of blood due to hemorrhage in the respiratory system.

hemorrhage: The escape of large quantities of blood from a blood vessel; heavy bleeding.

hemorrhagic disease of the newborn: A deficiency of vitamin K creating a bleeding disorder during the first few days of life.

hemothorax: A collection of blood in the pleural cavity.

hepatic encephalopathy: Condition resulting from cirrhosis where conversion of ammonia to urea is not possible, which results in impaired mental acuity, sleep disturbances, and confusion.

hepatitis: Inflammation of the liver.

hereditary: The genetic transmission of a particular quality or trait from parent to offspring.

hermaphrodite: Having genital and sexual characteristic of both sexes.

hernia: The protrusion of all or part of an organ through a tear in the wall of the surrounding structure such as the protrusion of part of the intestine through the abdominal muscles.

herniated vertebral disc: Weakness in annulus allowing nucleus pulposus to protrude; sometimes presses against the nerve root and spinal cord, causing radicular symptoms.

heroin: Highly addictive narcotic from the opium family.

HET model (Human-Environment-Technology Model): Conceptual framework designed to convey the relationship between human performance deficits and the use of technologies to address these deficits.

hiatal hernia: Protrusion of part of stomach into chest through esophageal hiatus of diaphragm.

heterozygous: Having two dissimilar genes at the same site, e.g., at the site for eye color, one gene for blue and one gene for brown create eyes of different colors.

heuristic: Clinical reasoning strategies, or shortcuts, that simplify complex cognitive tasks.

hidrosis: Formation and excretion of sweat.

hierarchy: A ranking system having a series of levels running from lowest to highest.

hierarchy of needs: Model developed by Abraham Maslow to explain people's needs in life in a specific order.

high-density lipoproteins (HDL): The "good" cholesterol. Helps to eliminate low-density lipoproteins.

high-risk pregnancy: A pregnancy in which the mother or fetus is in danger of a compromised outcome.

hilus: A depression or pit at that part of an organ where the vessels and nerves enter.

hindmilk: Thick, high fat content breast milk present at the end of breast feeding session.

hippocampus: A nuclear complex forming the medial margin of the cortical mantle of the cerebral hemisphere forming part of the limbic system.

hirsutism: Excessive growth of hair in unusual places, especially in women.

histogram: Bar graph.

histrionics: Overly dramatic behaviors designed to draw personal attention.

History (Hx): An account of past and present health status that includes the identification of complaints and provides the initial source of information about the patient/client.

HIV: *See* human immunodeficiency virus.

holism: View of the human mind and body as being one entity.

holistic: A concept in which understanding is gained by examination of all parts working as a whole; a model or approach to health care that takes into account all internal and external influences during the process.

holographic will: Document written by the individual, usually handwritten.

holophrase: Infants' one word utterances.

Homans' sign: Pain in the calf of the leg when the foot is flexed serving as a diagnostic sign for thrombophlebitis of deep veins.

home birth: Delivery of an infant in the home, frequently supervised by a lay or nurse midwife.

home health program: Health or rehabilitation services provided in a client's home.

homeostasis: Physiological system used to maintain internal processes and constancy of the internal metabolic balance despite changes in the environment.

homogamy: Notion that similar interests and values are important in forming strong, lasting personal relationships.

homogeneity of variance: Assumption that the variability within each of the sample groups should be fairly similar.

homologous: Corresponding in structure, position, and origin. Derived from an animal of the same species but of different genotype.

homologous insemination: Insemination where the semen is provided by the husband, not through intercourse.

homonymous hemianopsia: Loss of the same side of the field of vision in both eyes, usually due to optic nerve damage.

homosexual family: Family in which the parents are homosexual partners.

homosexuality: Sexual preference for individuals of the same gender.

homozygous: Having two similar genes at the same site.

horizontal plane: Runs transversely across, dividing the body into upper and lower parts. Parallel to the ground.

hormone: A chemical substance, produced in the body, that has a specific effect on the activity of a certain organ; applied to substances secreted by endocrine glands and transported in the bloodstream to the target organ on which their effect is produced.

hormone replacement therapy (HRT): Replacement of estrogen or progestin to restore desired levels after menopause.

hospice programs: Care for terminally ill clients and emotional support for them and their families.

hot flash: In women, a common sign of declining ovarian function and the onset of menopause as exemplified by sudden brief episodes of heat and sweating during which the face and chest are flushed.

human: An organism that maintains and balances itself in the world of reality and actuality by being in active life and active use.

human chorionic gonadotrophin (HCG): A growth hormone that influences the gonads.

human development: Ongoing changes in the structure, thought, or behavior of a person that occur as a function of both biologic and environmental influences.

human genome project: Mapping of genetic structure. Designed to be able to predict and treat diseases more effectively.

human immunodeficiency virus (HIV): The virus that causes AIDS, which is contracted through exposure to contaminated blood or bodily fluid (e.g., blood, semen, or vaginal secretions).

human papillomavirus (HPV): Viruses that cause warts.

humerus: Long bone of the upper arm.

hyaline membrane disease (HMD): *See* respiratory distress syndrome (RDS).

humoral: Pertaining to any fluid or semifluid in the body.

humoral immunity: Immune function via soluble factors found in blood and other body fluids.

hyaluronic acid: Substance that under compressive forces lubricates cells.

hydatidiform mole: Anomaly of the placenta, which forms a nonmalignant mass from cystic swelling of the chorionic villi; no embryo is present.

hydramnios (polyhydramnios): An excessive amount of amniotic fluid; usually more than 1.5 liters; often indicative of fetal anomaly; seen in insulin-dependent diabetic pregnant women.

hydration: Providing adequate water.

hydrocele: Accumulation of serous fluid in a saclike cavity, especially in the testes.

hydrocephalus: Enlargement of the head due to an increase in cerebrospinal fluid within the brain.

hydrocephaly: Condition characterized by abnormal accumulation of cerebrospinal fluid within the ventricles of the brain, which leads to enlargement of the head.

hydrophilic: Attracting moisture.

hydrophobic: Repelling moisture.

hydrops fetalis: Severe fetal hemolytic disorder, sometimes as a result of maternal Rh isoimmunization; the infant exhibits gross edema, cardiac decompensation, and profound anemic pallor; often fatal.

hydrostatic pressure: A pressure created in a fluid system, such as the circulatory system.

hydrotherapy: Intervention using water.

hydroureter: Abnormal distention of the ureter with urine due to an obstruction.

hymen: Fold of membranous tissue partially covering the vaginal opening, often present in females who have not experienced sexual intercourse.

hymenal tag: A redundant piece of hymen tissue found in newborn females which disappears spontaneously shortly after birth.

hyperalimentation: The ingestion or administration of a greater than optimal amount of nutrients.

hyperbaric oxygen: Oxygen under greater pressure than normal atmospheric pressure.

hyperbilirubinemia: Excessive amount of bilirubin in the blood.

hypercalcemia: Excessive amount of calcium in the blood.

hypercapnia: Excessive amount of carbon dioxide in the blood.

hypercholesterolemia: Excessive amount of cholesterol in the blood.

hyperemesis gravidarum: Extreme vomiting in pregnancy.

hyperemia: Presence of excess blood in the vessels; engorgement.

hyperesthesia: Increased sensitivity, often unpleasant, to cutaneous stimulation.

hyperglycemia: Abnormally increased content of sugar in the blood.

hyperkalemia: Excessive amount of potassium in the blood.

hyperlipidemia: An abnormally high concentration of lipids in the blood.

hypermobility: Condition of excessive motion.

hypernatremia: Excessive amount of sodium in the blood.

hyperopia: Farsightedness; a defect in vision in which the light rays focus behind the retina.

hyperpathia: Severely exaggerated, subjective, painful response to stimuli.

hyperplasia: Increased number of cells.

hyperpnea: Abnormal increase in the depth and rate of the respiratory movements.

hyperreflexia: Increased action in the reflexes.

hypersomnia: Excessive sleeping.

hyperesthesia: Abnormally increased sensitivity to stimulation.

hyperglycemia: Increased amount of glucose (above normal) in the blood.

hypertensive crisis: Life-threatening syndrome typically resulting from consumption of foods high in tyramine when taking MAO inhibitor medications.

hypertonus: Muscular state wherein muscle tension is greater than desired, spasticity; hypertonus increases resistance to passive stretch.

hypertonic uterine dysfunction: Uncoordinated frequent uterine contractions without dilatation or effacement of the cervix.

hypertrophic cardiomyopathy: Enlargement and loss of elasticity of the left ventricle resulting in decreased cardiac output.

hypertrophic scarring: Excessive markings left by the healing process in the skin or an internal organ.

hypertrophy: Increased cell size leading to increased tissue size. The morbid enlargement or overgrowth of an organ or part due to an increase in size of its constituent cells (e.g., hypertrophic cardiomyopathy).

hyperuricemia: Excess of uric acid in the blood.

hyperventilation: Increased expiration and inspiration potentially caused by anxiety.

hyperventilation of pregnancy: Increase in the respiratory minute volume, which makes the mother feel like she is hyperventilating, because of an increase in respiratory tidal volume during normal respiration.

hypnosis: Act of inducing a state of subconsciousness in order to recall memories not capable of being expressed when conscious.

hypnotic: Medications or conditions that produce drowsiness or sleep.

hypocalcemia: Calcium deficiency seen in preterm infants or as a result of a long stressful labor or in infants of diabetic mothers.

hypochondria: In the absence of medical evidence, a sustained conviction that one is ill or about to become ill; abnormal concern about one's health.

hypoesthesia: Diminished ability to recognize stimuli.

hypofibrinogenemia: Significantly decreased levels of fibrinogen (clotting factor) in the blood.

hypoglycemia: Decreased amount of glucose in the blood (below normal), as a result of excessive insulin production in the pancreas or administration of an excessive amount of insulin in relation to caloric intake.

hypokalemia: Low serum potassium level.

hyponatremia: Low sodium level in blood.

hypotension: Low blood pressure.

hypoxia: Low level of oxygen in arterial blood.

hypoxia-ischemic (H/I): Decreased oxygen and decreased blood flow to organs or tissues or both.

hypoxic-ischemic encephalopathy: Neurological damage from decreased oxygen and decreased blood flow to the brain.

hypokinetic disease: Complications arising from inactivity. Synonym: disuse syndrome.

hypometria: Distortion of target-directed voluntary movement in which the limb falls short of reaching its target.

hypomobile: When motion is less than that which would normally be permitted by the structures.

hyponatremia: Decreased amount of sodium in the blood.

hypoplasia: Defective or incomplete development (e.g., osteogenesis imperfecta).

hypospadias: Abnormal congenital opening of the male urethra on the undersurface of the penis.

hypotension: Abnormally low blood pressure.

hypothermia: Body temperature that falls below normal range (98.6° F) often caused by exposure to cold. Known as cold stress in neonates.

hypothesis: Conclusion drawn before all the facts are known; working assumption that serves as a basis for further investigation; a plausible explanation or best guess about a situation.

hypothetico-deductive reasoning: Form of problem solving in which several possible ideas are tested in order of probability to reach a solution.

hypotonicity: Decrease in the muscle tone and stretch reflex of a muscle resulting in decreased resistance to passive stretch and hyporesponsiveness to sensory stimulation.

hypotonic uterine dysfunction: Ineffective uterine contractions occurring during the active phase of labor; can be related to cephalopelvic disproportion or malposition of the fetus.

hypotonus: Muscular state wherein muscle tension is lower than desired; flaccidity; hypotonus decreases resistance to passive stretch.

hypovolemia: Abnormally decreased volume of circulating fluid (i.e., plasma) in the body.

hypoxia: Any state in which an inadequate amount of oxygen is available to the tissues, without respect to cause or degree. Deficiency of oxygen in the blood. *See* anoxia.

hysterectomy: Surgical removal of the uterus; **total abdominal hysterectomy and bilateral salpingo-oophorectomy (TAH-BSO):** Removal of uterus, both tubes, and ovaries; **vaginal hysterectomy (VH):** Removal of the uterus by vaginal approach.

hysteria: Disorder with multiple complaints presented in a dramatic manner.

hysterical conversion: Somatoform disorder characterized by the loss of functioning of some part of the body not due to any physical disorder, but apparently due to psychological conflicts.

hysterosalpingography: Radiographic evaluation of the uterus and fallopian tubes after injection with radiopaque dye.

hysterotomy: Surgical incision into the uterus.

iatrogenic: Complication caused by medical intervention and health care providers.

ICD Code: International Classification of Diseases codes used for billing and reimbursement purposes.

icing: Ice is applied in small, overlapping circles for 5 to 10 minutes until skin flushing and numbness occur.

iconic representation: Memory of the stimuli in terms of pictorial images or graphics that stand for a concept without defining it fully.

icterus neonatorum: Jaundice in the newborn.

id: In psychoanalytic theory, the unconscious part of the psyche that is the source of primitive, instinctual drives and strives for self-preservation and pleasure. The primary process element of personality.

ideation: An internal process in which the nervous system gathers information from stimuli in the environment or recruits information from memory stores to formulate an idea about what to do.

ideational apraxia: The inability to formulate a plan to complete a request or command.

identity: Gradually emerging and continually changing sense of self; used in Erik Erikson's theory of development.

identity diffusion: Eriksonian psychosocial crisis in which integration of childhood skills, goals, and roles does not occur.

ideomotor apraxia: Interference with the transmission of the appropriate impulses from the brain to the motor center; results in the inability to translate an idea into motion.

idiopathic: Designating a disease whose cause is unknown or uncertain.

IDM: Infant of a diabetic mother.

illness: Experience of devalued changes in being and in social function. It primarily encompasses personal, interpersonal, and cultural reactions to sickness.

illusion: Misperception of real external stimuli.

imaginative play: Activities that include make-believe games.

imbalance: Lack of balance, as in proportion, force, and functioning.

immediate recall: The ability to recall information within a short time after the information has been received.

immersion: To plunge, dip, or drop into a liquid; to involve deeply.

immunity: Protection from microorganisms; **acquired immunity:** Protection from microorganisms as a result of exposure to the organism or from passive injection of immunoglobulins; **active immunity:** Protection from specific microorganisms in response to infection from that organism or from inoculation against that organism; **natural immunity:** The first line of defense by the body including skin and phagocytic cells or simple incompatibility of environment to the organism (e.g., the measles virus cannot reproduce in canine cells; thus dogs have natural immunity to measles); **passive immunity:** Acquired through transfer of antibodies or lymphocytes from an immune donor.

immunocompetent: The body's immune system responding to foreign antigens and developing antigen-specific antibodies.

immunoglobulin (Ig): Glycoprotein found in blood and other body fluids that may exert antibody activity. All antibodies are Ig molecules, but not all Ig exhibits antibody activity. **IgA:** The immunoglobulin in colostrums; **IgG:** Passive immunity to the fetus acquired transplacentally from the mother's immunities to specific infections; **IgM:** Immunoglobulin that is manufactured by the infant shortly after birth (e.g., the fetus manufactures IgM when amnionitis is present).

immunology: The study of the body's immune system; its recognition of foreign antigens as a significant part of the body's defenses.

immunosuppression: A decrease in responsiveness of the immune system with an imbalance of the antigen-antibody relationship.

impairment: A loss or abnormality of psychological, physiological, or anatomical structure or function; **secondary:** Impairments that originate from other, preexisting impairments.

impedance: Resistance to flow or movement.

imperforate anus: Physical anomalies of the rectum and anus, usually diagnosed because the anus has no opening into the rectum.

impingement: To trap and compress.

implantation: The fertilized ovum embeds in the uterine mucosa.

implosion therapy: *See* flooding.

impotence: Weakness, especially the inability of the male to achieve or maintain erection.

impulsive: To act without planning or reflection.

in situ: Localized site, confined to one place (e.g., cancer that has not invaded neighboring tissues).

incapacitated: Legal designation for loss of thought processes including memory and judgment; limitation of any function.

incest: Sexual exploitation of a minor by a relative.

incidence: During a specified time period, the number of new cases of a certain illness or injury in a population. Demonstrated as the number of new cases divided by the total number of people at risk.

incidence report: *See* unusual occurrence report.

incompetence: Failing to meet requirements; incapable; unskillful. Lacking strength and sufficient flexibility to transmit pressure, thus breaking or flowing under stress.

incompetent cervix: Cervix that prematurely dilates as pregnancy progresses.

incomplete abortion: *See* abortion.

incontinence: Inability to control excretory functions.

incubator: An apparatus for maintaining a premature infant in an environment of proper temperature and humidity.

independence: Lack of requirement or reliance on another; adequate resources to accomplish everyday tasks.

indirect hemagglutination: The clumping of red blood cells.

indirect services: Those activities, strategies, and interventions provided to agencies and others to assist them in providing direct care services.

individual habilitation plan (IHP): A written multidisciplinary plan of care for a developmentally disabled adult that identifies needs, strategies for meeting those needs, and the individuals involved in providing the program.

induction: Artificial stimulation of labor through use of drugs (usually Pitocin) to create contractions.

inductive fallacy: Overgeneralizing on the basis of too few observations.

inductive reasoning: Generation and testing of a hypothesis on the basis of evidence to indicate its validity.

induration: Abnormal firmness of tissue with a definite margin.

industry: According to Erik Erikson and his theory of development, this is when children in elementary school focus on applying themselves in doing certain activities that are reflective of being successful in the adult world.

infancy: Time of development of a child from 28 days after birth until the second year of life.

infant of a diabetic mother (IDM): Infant born to a mother who has diabetes mellitus.

infantile myoclonic: Sudden, brief, involuntary muscle contractions producing head drops and flexion of extremities.

infarct: An area of coagulation necrosis in a tissue due to local anemia resulting from obstruction of circulation to the area.

infection: The state of being infected, especially by the presence in the body of bacteria, protozoa, viruses, or other parasites.

infective: To cause infection; infectious.

inference: Possible result or conclusion that could be deduced from evaluation data.

inferential (predictive) statistics: Utilizing the measurements from the sample to anticipate characteristics of the population.

inferior: In terms of anatomical position, located below the head.

infertility: Inability to conceive a pregnancy throughout a year of unprotected sexual intercourse.

inflammation: The condition into which tissues enter as a reaction to injury, including signs of pain, heat, redness, and swelling.

inflammatory: Pertaining to or characterized by inflammation.

informal social network: People who provide support but who are not connected with any formal social service agency.

informant interview: Interview in which a therapist gathers information about the client or environment from significant others.

informational support: A type of social support that informs, thereby reducing anxiety over uncertainty.

informed consent: Requirement that the person must be given adequate information about the benefits and risks of planned treatments or research before he or she agrees to the procedures.

inguinal: Pertaining to the groin.

inhibition: Arrest or restraint of a process.

injury: Physical harm or damage to a person.

inlet: Passage leading into a cavity; **pelvic inlet:** Upper brim of the pelvic cavity.

innate goodness: View presented by Swiss-born French philosopher Jean-Jacques Rosseau that emphasized that children are inherently good.

inpatient: Services delivered to the patient during the hospitalization.

inquiry: An investigation or examination.

insertion: Distal attachment of a muscle that exhibits most of the movement during muscular contraction.

insight: Self-understanding. Understanding of consequences or ramifications of a situation or an action.

insemination: Fertilization of the ovum through discharge of semen from the penis into the vagina; **artificial insemination:** Introduction of semen into the vagina or uterus mechanically.

insomnia: Inability to begin or sustain sleep.

instability: Description of a joint that has lost its structural integrity and is overtly hypermobile.

instinctual drives: Aspect of the psychodynamic theory in which Freud believes that there are two primary instinctual impulses that demand gratification: sex and aggression.

institution: Any public or private entity or agency.

institutionalization: Effects of dehumanizing and depersonalizing characteristics of the environment that result in apathy, a significant decrease in motivation and activity, and increased passivity of an individual. Also refers to confinement.

instrumental activities of daily living (IADL): Essential activities that are used to measure independent living capability and are not considered basic daily living activities or self-care tasks. Activities include shopping, cooking, home chores, heavy household chores, managing money, and structured play for infants and children. Activities that are important components of maintaining independent living.

insufficiency: Deficiency or inadequacy. The failure or inability of an organ or tissue to perform its normal function.

intake interview: Interview in which the therapist identifies the client's needs and his or her suitability for treatment.

integration: Unifying or bringing together; in children, the developmental ability to link successive actions instead of viewing each action as a separate, unrelated event; usually acquired by 2 years of age.

integumentary: Pertaining to or composed of skin.

intellectualization: Using logic and reason to avoid expressing emotions in a stressful situation.

intelligence: Potential or ability to acquire, retain, and use experience and knowledge to reason and problem solve.

intention tremor: Rhythmical, oscillatory movement initiated with an arm or hand.

interactive reasoning: Process involving individualizing treatment for the specific needs of the patient/client.

interdependence: A concept that recognizes the mutual dependencies of individuals within social groups.

interdisciplinary: Integration of members from numerous disciplines working toward a common goal.

interferon (IFN): A class of unrelated cytokine proteins formed when cells are exposed to viruses. It is an antiviral chemical, secreted by an infected cell, that strengthens the defenses of nearby cells not yet infected.

intermediate care facilities (ICF): Facilities designed to give personal care, simple medical care, and intermittent nursing care.

intermittent positive-pressure breathing (IPPB): Mechanical device that uses air pressure to inflate and deflate the lungs for breathing.

internal: Having to do with the inner nature of a thing.

internal os: Inside opening of a cavity (e.g., of the cervix).

internal validity: The cause and effect relationship that can be identified by the results of an experiment.

International Classification of Diseases (ICD): Disease classification system developed by the World Health Organization.

international unit (IU): Measure for labeling certain medications: $1 \text{ IU} = 0.30 \text{ } \mu$.

interneuron: Nerve cell that links motor and sensory nerves.

internodal: The space between two nodes; the segment of a nerve fiber connecting two nodes (often called internodal bundles or pathways).

interoceptive: Receptors activated by stimuli from within visceral tissues and blood tissues.

interpolar: Situated between two poles.

intertuberous diameter: Distance between ischial tuberosities. Measurement to determine capacity of the pelvic outlet.

interval data: Measurements that are assigned values so the order and intervals between numbers are recognized noncontinuous data.

intervention: The purposeful and skilled interaction of the caregiver with the patient/client, and when appropriate, with other individuals involved in care, using various methods and techniques to produce changes in the condition. The interactions and procedures used in treating and instructing patients/clients. The confronting process of defining a substance abuse situation with the abuser.

intervertebral disks: Pads of fibrous elastic cartilage found between the vertebrae. They cushion the vertebrae and absorb shock.

intervillous space: Spaces between the villi on the maternal side of the placenta filled with blood which serves as the site of maternal-fetal exchange of gases, nutrient, and waste products.

intima: Refers to the innermost surface of a vessel, especially an artery.

intracranial: Occurring within the cranium.

intracranial hemorrhage: Bleeding within the cranium.

intrafusal muscle: Striated muscle tissue found within the muscle spindle.

intrapartum: Period during labor and birth.

intrathecal: Within the subarachnoid space.

intrauterine device (IUD): A plastic or metal device placed in the uterus to interfere with conception or implantation of the fertilized ovum.

intrauterine growth restriction (IUGR): A decreased rate of fetal growth (usually below 10th percentile for gestational age) due to inadequate placental perfusion, infection, congenital anomalies, placental abnormalities, or maternal medical disorders. Cause is unknown in 50% of cases.

intrauterine hypoxia: Stopping of the pulse and loss of consciousness as a result of too little oxygen and too much carbon dioxide in the blood leading to suffocation during the birthing process.

intrauterine pressure catheter (IUPC): Catheter inserted in the uterus to determine uterine activity including the strength of contractions by electronic means.

intrauterine resuscitation: Interventions to improve uterine blood flow when a nonreassuring fetal heart rate exists.

intravascular: Directly into a vessel.

intrinsic motivation: Concept in human development that proposes that people develop in response to an inherent need for exploration and activity.

introitus: Entrance to a canal or cavity such as the vagina.

introjection: Incorporation of beliefs and values of another so that it is difficult to feel separate or distinct from the other person.

intubation: The insertion of a tube; especially the introduction of a tube into the trachea through the glottis, performed for the introduction of an external source of oxygen.

intussusception: Telescoping of the bowel within itself.

in utero: Inside the uterus.

inventory: Assessment composed of a list of items to which the person gives responses.

inversion: Turning inward or inside out.

inversion of the uterus: When the uterus is turned inside out and the fundus intrudes out of the cervix or vagina; can be caused by too aggressive approach to removal of the placenta rather than allowing the natural process to occur.

in vitro fertilization: Fertilization of the ovum in a culture dish.

involuntary movement: Movement that is not done of one's own free will; not done by choice. Unintentional, accidental, not consciously controlled movement.

involution: A rolling or turning inward over a rim, such as a toenail growing back into the soft tissue of the toe. Also a term used to describe the return of the uterus to the nonpregnant size and position following delivery of a baby.

iodine: Element important for the development and functioning of the thyroid gland.

iontophoresis: Introduction of ions into tissues by means of electric current.

ipsilateral: Situated on or affecting the same side.

ischemia: Reduced oxygen supply to a body organ or part. Deficiency of blood in a part due to functional constriction or actual obstruction of a blood vessel.

ischemic heart disease: Lack of blood supply to the heart.

Islets of Langerhans: Irregular structures in the pancreas composed of cells smaller than the ordinary secreting cells. Produces an internal secretion, insulin, which is connected with the metabolism of carbohydrates. Their degeneration is one cause of diabetes.

isoenzyme: One of the multiple forms in which a protein catalyst may exist in a single species, the various forms differing chemically, physically, and/or immunologically.

isoimmunization: Development of antibodies with antigens from the same species (e.g., development of anti-Rh antibodies in an Rh negative mother).

isokinetic strength: Force generated by a muscle contracting through a range of motion at a constant speed.

isolation: Separation of physical or mental self from environmental or emotional contacts.

isthmus: Narrow structure connecting two larger parts.

itinerant: Traveling from place to place.

ITP: Idiopathic thrombocytopenic purpura. Hemorrhagic disease often following a viral infection where destruction of circulating platelets occurs.

IVF-ET: In vitro fertilization and embryo transfer. Eggs are aspirated from ovarian follicles and are fertilized in the laboratory and a growing embryo is introduced into the uterus.

jaundice: A condition in which the eyeballs, the skin, and the urine become abnormally yellow as a result of increased amounts of bile pigments in the blood. Usually secondary to conditions such as hepatitis or liver failure; **breast milk jaundice:** Late-onset jaundice (more than 5 days) in the breast-fed infant, cause unknown; **pathologic jaundice:** First noticeable within 24 hours of birth and caused by some abnormal condition such as Rh or ABO incompatibility. This toxicity can cause brain damage or death in newborns; **physiologic jaundice:** Increased serum levels of unconjugated bilirubin that create a yellow tinge to the skin and mucous membranes.

joint capsule: Any sac or membrane enclosing the junction of the bones.

joint mobility: Functional joint play and flexibility allowing for freedom of joint movement. The capacity of the joint to be moved passively, taking into account the structure and shape of the joint surface in addition to the characteristics of the tissue surrounding the joint.

joints: Junctures in the body where bones articulate. The classifications are synarthrosis (i.e., nonmoving), amphiarthrosis (i.e., slightly moving), or diarthrosis (i.e., freely moving).

judgment: The ability to use data or information to make a decision.

jump sign: A test that screens for binocular vision, which is when both eyes cannot focus on a single point or target. The patient/client focuses on an object with one eye covered and uncovered eye "jumps" to refocus on the object (positive jump sign).

junctional rhythm: Rapid heart rate with a characteristically inverted P wave often preceding, following, or falling within the QRS complex on an EKG. Causes are usually digitalis toxicity, acute inferior myocardial infarction, or heart failure.

justice: Notion that all people should be treated alike and fairly in accord with general standards of right and wrong.

juvenile: Pertaining to youth or childhood diseases, such as juvenile diabetes or juvenile arthritis.

juvenile ankylosing spondylitis: A chronic inflammatory process in juveniles affecting mainly joints and vertebrae similar to rheumatoid arthritis.

kalemia: The presence of potassium in the blood.

kangaroo care: Naked infant is placed against skin of the mother or father and covered with a warm blanket. Skin-to-skin source of warmth for the infant used in normal and preterm infants.

Kantianism: Ethical principle related to sense of duty.

Kaposi's sarcoma: Malignant cell proliferation typically associated with AIDS.

karyotype: Arrangement of the chromosomes within a cell to demonstrate their numbers and morphology.

Kawasaki disease: An acute or chronic febrile disease of children of unknown etiology.

Kegel exercises: Pelvic floor strengthening exercises developed by Dr. Arnold Kegel.

keratin: A scleroprotein that is the principal constituent of epidermis, hair, nails, and the organic matrix of the enamel of the teeth.

keratitis: Inflammation of the cornea.

keratosis: Any horny growth, such as a wart or callosity.

kernicterus: Deposit of unconjugated bilirubin in brain cells resulting in damaged intellectual, perceptive, or motor function, or even death.

ketoacidosis: Hyperglycemia which creates an accumulation of ketone bodies in the blood leading to metabolic acidosis.

ketone: Any compound containing a carbonyl group; CO.

ketosis: A condition characterized by an abnormally elevated concentration of ketone (acetone) bodies in the body tissues and fluids, causing an acidosis. Also referred to as ketoacidosis.

kinesics: The study of body movements, gestures, and postures as a means of communication. Synonym: body language.

kinesiology: The study and science of motion.

kinesthetic: Sense derived from end organs located in muscles, tendons, and joints and stimulated by movement. Also called proprioception.

kinetics: Area of kinesiology that is concerned with cause, as well as the forces that produce, modify, or stop a motion.

kleptomania: Repetitive stealing of objects not needed for personal or monetary value.

Kohn's pores: Openings in the interalveolar septa of the lungs.

Korsakoff's psychosis: Alcoholic syndrome due to deficient thiamin levels that results in confusion, memory loss, and distortion of truth.

Krebs cycle: Tricarboxylic acid cycle that results in the energy production of adenosine triphosphate.

Kurzweil reading machine: Computerized device that converts print into speech. User places printed material over a scanner that "reads" the material aloud by means of an electronic voice.

Kussmaul's respiration: Air hunger (as seen in patients with chronic obstructive pulmonary disease).

kyphoscoliosis: Backward and lateral curvature of the spinal column, such as that seen in vertebral osteochondrosis (Scheuermann's disease).

kyphosis: Abnormal anteroposterior curving of the spine; hunchback or roundback.

labia: The external folds surrounding the vagina and urethra; **labia majora:** Two folds of skin, fat tissue, and hair on either side of the labia minora and vaginal opening that form either side of the vulva; **labia minora:** The two thin folds of skin that lie inside the labia majora and anteriorly enclose the clitoris.

labile: Changeable.

labor: Refers to the uterine contractions that produce dilation and effacement of the cervix, assisting in descent of the fetus and delivery of the fetus and products of conception through the vaginal opening; **active phase of labor:** Phase in the first stage of labor from

4 cm to 7 cm dilatation; **arrested labor:** Failure of labor to progress through the normal stages due to uterine inertia, pelvic obstruction, or maternal disease; **artificial labor:** Induction of labor through use of drugs; **augmented labor:** Strength of contractions increase through use of drugs; **back labor:** Experience of severe back pain during labor due to the position of the fetal head to the mother's sacrum; **dysfunctional labor:** Lack of progress in labor either in dilatation or descent; **false labor:** Uterine contractions that do not result in dilatation or effacement of the cervix; **first stage of labor:** From the onset of regular contractions to full dilatation of the cervix (10 cm); **induction of labor:** (*see* induction); **latent phase of labor:** Beginning of the first stage of labor from 0 cm to 3 cm dilatation; **precipitate labor:** Onset of contractions to delivery in less than 3 hours; **preterm (premature) labor:** Labor that begins prior to 38 weeks of gestation and affects 7–10% of all live births; it is the primary cause of preterm birth, which is the primary cause of neonatal mortality; **prodromal labor:** Changes which precede actual labor, usually 24–48 hours, such as an energy surge, excessive vaginal discharge, scant bloody show, and diarrhea; **prolonged labor:** Abnormally slow labor usually more than 20 hours; **second stage of labor:** From full dilatation of the cervix to birth of the infant(s); **spontaneous labor:** Labor with no drugs, mechanical, or operative intervention; **third stage of labor:** From birth of the baby to expulsion of the placenta; **transition phase of labor:** Phase in first stage from 8 cm to 10 cm dilatation; **trial of labor:** Labor that progresses long enough to ascertain if normal vaginal birth is possible.

labor, delivery, recovery (LDR): A single room where the mother labors, delivers, and recovers before being moved to a postpartum unit.

labor, delivery, recovery, postpartum (LDRP): A single homelike room where all aspects of care from admission to discharge take place with continuity of nursing staff.

labyrinthine righting reflexes: Begin at birth and continue through life. Head orients to a vertical position with the mouth horizontal when the body is tipped or tilted. Tested with the eyes closed.

laceration: Irregular tear of tissue.

lactation: Refers to the process by which milk is made in the breasts and secreted for nourishment of the infant; **lactation consultant:** A specially educated health care professional whose focus is lactation and breast feeding; **lactation suppression:** Stopping the production of breast milk through either pharmaceutical or nonpharmaceutical methods.

lactiferous: Secreting milk.

lactogen: Pharmaceutical or other substance that enhances milk production and secretion.

lactogenesis stage I: Initial breast milk components that appear during pregnancy and the first few days after birth, also called colostrums.

lactogenesis stage II: Beginning of breast milk production, usually 2–5 days after birth.

lactose intolerance: Difficulty digesting milk and some milk products; can cause abdominal bloating, cramping, and diarrhea.

lactosuria: The presence of lactose in the urine, can occur during pregnancy or during breast feeding and must be differentiated from glycosuria.

laissez-faire style: A management style in which managers have low involvement with staff.

La Leche League: International organization that promotes breast-feeding.

Lamaze (psychoprophylaxis) method: Method of childbirth preparation developed to minimize fear and the perception of pain and to support positive family relationships. Gained popularity in the 1960s and requires practice during pregnancy and coaching during labor and birth.

Laminaria digitata: Dried seaweed that expands as it absorbs moisture; used to dilate the cervix and prepare it for induction of labor or for abortion.

laminectomy: Surgical excision of the posterior arch of the vertebra.

Landau reflex: Seen with infants at 3 months to 2 years. When lifting under thorax in a prone position, first head and then back and legs extend. If head is put into a flexed position, extensor tone disappears.

lanugo: Fine hair on the body of the fetus after the fourth month in utero.

laparoscopy: A type of endoscope (a device consisting of a tube and electrical optical system) is used to explore the interior abdominal cavity.

large for gestational age (LGA): Newborn birth weight that exceeds 90th percentile for the weeks of gestation.

laryngospasm: Spasmodic closure of the larynx.

last menstrual period (LMP): First day of the last normal menstrual period.

latch on: Ability of the newborn to obtain an appropriate sucking response on the breast.

latent period: Time during which a disease is in existence but does not manifest itself.

latent phase: *See* labor.

latent stage (latency): Fourth of Freud's stages of psychosexual development, characterized by the development of the superego (i.e., conscience) and by the loss of interest in sexual gratification; typically occurs from the age of 6 to 11 years in Western cultural groups. Also, latency in the duration of effectiveness following cessation of treatment or intervention.

lateral: In terms of anatomical position, located away from the midline of the body.

lateral corticospinal tract (LCST): Contralateral descending motor tract. Upper motor neurons influencing lower motor neurons either directly or indirectly.

laterality: Tendency toward one side or the other (e.g., right-handedness, left-handedness). Dominant side for skilled activities.

lateralization: The tendency for certain processes to be more highly developed on one side of the brain than the other. In most people, the right hemisphere develops processes of spatial and musical thoughts, and the left hemisphere develops areas for verbal and logical processes.

lateral shift: Apparent translatoric displacement of the trunk on the lower lumbopelvic region.

lateral trunk flexion: The ability to move the trunk from side to side without moving the legs, which is essential for maintaining balance.

launching: Process in which youths move into adulthood and leave their family of origin.

learned helplessness: Process in which the person attributes his or her lack of performance to external factors rather than lack of effort.

learned nonuse: A process that occurs after an injury such as a cerebrovascular accident.

learning: Acquiring new concepts and behaviors. Enduring ability of an individual to comprehend and/or competently respond to changes in information from the environment and/or from within the self.

learning disability: Learning problem that is not due to environmental causes, mental retardation, or emotional disturbances; often associated with problems in listening, thinking, reading, writing, spelling, and mathematics.

learning theory: Theoretical base behind the behavioral frame of reference in which behavior is best learned when environmental influences are introduced.

left ventricular hypertrophy (LVH): Left ventricle (of heart) enlargement.

lecithin: A phospholipid that decreases surface tension; surfactant.

lecithin/sphingomyelin ratio: Ratio of lecithin to sphingomyelin found in the amniotic fluid and used to assess fetal lung maturity.

leiomyoma: Benign smooth muscle tumor.

leisure: Category of activities for which freedom of choice and enjoyment are the primary motives.

length of stay (LOS): The duration of hospitalization, usually expressed in days.

Leopold's maneuvers: Use to determine the position of the fetus through four different abdominal palpation maneuvers of the mother.

lesbian: Female homosexual.

lesion: Injury to the central or peripheral nervous system that may prevent the expression of some functions and/or may allow the inappropriate, uncoordinated, or uncontrolled expression of other functions.

letdown reflex: The involuntary release of milk through the nipples that occurs at the beginning of breastfeeding.

lethargy: Sluggishness or inactivity.

letting-go phase: The last phase in maternal role attainment occurring during the postpartum period and includes letting go of the pregnancy and becoming a mother; this requires multiple relationship adjustments.

leukocyte: White cell; colorless blood corpuscles that function to protect the body against microorganisms causing disease.

leukocytosis: An increase in circulating lymphocyte number.

leukopenia: Decreased white blood cell count.

leukorrhea: A mucous discharge, white or yellow in color, from the vagina or cervical canal that can be either normal or pathological resulting from abnormal conditions of the genital tract.

levator syndrome: Spasm of the muscles surrounding the anus, causing severe rectal pain.

level: Even; no slope.

level of arousal: An individual's responsiveness and alertness to stimuli in the environment.

levels of processing: Durability of the memory trace; a function of the level to which the information was encoded.

libel: Sharing with a person in a written form information that is detrimental to another.

libido: Freud's term for the psychic element to fulfill basic needs.

licensure: Legal authority to practice a specific role, typically based on specific education and testing, although other credentials may be required.

lie of the fetus: Relationship of the long axis of the fetus to the long axis of the mother.

life cycle: From conception to death of an organism.

life expectancy: Number of years in the life span of an individual in a particular cultural group.

life review: Process in which one looks back at one's life experiences, evaluating, interpreting, and reinterpreting them.

life roles: Daily life experiences that occupy one's time, including roles of student, homemaker, worker (active or retired), sibling, parent, mate, child, and peer.

life span perspective: Makes seven basic contentions about development: it is lifelong, multidimensional, multidirectional, plastic, historically embedded, multidisciplinary, and contextual.

lifestyle: Pattern of daily activities over time that is stable and predictable, through which an individual expresses his or her self-identity.

ligament: Inelastic fibrous thickening of an articular capsule that joins one bone to its articular mate, allowing movement at the joint.

ligation: Application of a ligature (a ligature being any material used for tying a vessel or to constrict a part).

lightening: Occurs when the fetal head drops into the pelvic inlet, allowing the uterus to descend to a lower level, relieving pressure on the diaphragm and making breathing easier during the last few weeks of pregnancy.

light work: Exerting up to 20 pounds of force occasionally, up to 10 lbs of force frequently, or a negligible amount of force constantly to move objects.

Likert scale: Point system that is used to rate a particular level of skill, function, or attitude.

limbic system: Primitive central nervous system associated with emotional and visceral functions in the body. A group of brain structures that include amygdala, hippocampus, dentate gyrus, cingulate gyrus, and their interconnections with the hypothalamus, septal areas, and brainstem.

limitation: Act of being restrained or confined.

limits of stability: The boundary or range that is the farthest distance in any direction a person can lean away from vertical (midline) without changing the original base of support (e.g., stepping, reaching, etc.) or falling.

linear processing: Learning or solving a problem using a step-by-step process in which each step is dependent on what occurred before.

linea nigra: Pigmented line appearing on the abdomen, from the pubis to the umbilicus, in pregnant women.

lingula: A small tonguelike structure. In the cerebellum, part of the vermis of the cerebellum on the ventral surface where superior medullary velum attaches (lingula cerebelli). In the lung, projection from lower portion of upper lobe of left lung, just beneath the cardiac notch, between cardiac impression and inferior margin (lingula of left lung). In lower jaw, sharp medial boundary of mandibular foramen to which is attached the sphenomandibular ligament (lingula mandibulae); **Lingula sphenoidalis:** A ridge of bone on the lateral margin of the carotid sulcus projecting backward between the body and great wing of the sphenoid bone.

lipofuscin: A dark, pigmented lipid found in the cytoplasm of aging neurons.

lithotomy position: Position in which the client lies on his or her back with thighs flexed upon the abdomen and the lower legs on the thighs, which are abducted.

live birth: When the newborn, regardless of gestational age demonstrates a heartbeat, breath, or voluntary movement.

living ligature: The smooth muscle fibers of the uterus that gives the uterus the ability to ligate blood vessels or stop bleeding after childbirth, miscarriage, or abortion.

living will: Legal instrument to authorize certain activities at the end of life.

lobectomy: Excision of a lobe, as of the lung, thyroid, brain, or liver.

localized inflammation: Swelling, redness, and increased temperature that are isolated to the injured or infected part of the body.

lochia: Discharge of blood, mucus, and tissue from the vagina after delivery, often lasting up to 6 weeks after birth; **rubra lochia:** Referring to the bright red discharge of the first 2 weeks postpartum; **alba lochia:** Thin yellowish discharge that follows serous lochia and lasts 2–6 weeks; **serous lochia:** Serous, pinkish brown, watery vaginal discharge that follows rubra lochia.

locomotion: The ability to move from place to place.

locus of control: Psychological term referring to one's orientation to the world of events. In most simplistic form, internal locus of control reflects belief in self-control. External locus of control, conversely, relates to outcomes of events largely as a matter of fate or chance (i.e., that one cannot have influence over the outcome of events).

logical classification: The ability to sort objects by their defining properties occurs at the age of 5 or 6 years.

longevity: Long life or life expectancy.

longitudinal research: Study in which subjects are measured over the course of time to gather data on potential trends.

long-term care (LTC): Array of services needed by individuals who have lost some capacity for independence because of a chronic illness or condition.

long-term memory: Permanent memory storage for long-term information.

long-term support system: Ensuring that individuals have access to the services that are needed to support independent living.

loose associations: Thoughts shift with little or no apparent logic, and the individual is unaware of the illogical flow.

lordosis: Abnormal forward curvature of the lumbar spine; swayback.

low birth weight (LBW): Infant born weighing less than 2500 gm.

low-density lipoproteins (LDL): The "bad" cholesterol associated with heart and vascular disease.

lower motor neuron (LMN): Sensory neuron found in the anterior horn cell, nerve root, or peripheral nervous system.

L/S ratio: *See* lecithin/sphingomyelin.

lumbar puncture: Diagnostic test involving insertion of needle into spinal column.

lumpectomy: Excision of a small primary breast tumor, leaving the rest of the breast intact.

lunar month: Four weeks or 28 days.

lung: The organ of respiration.

lupus erythematosus: A chronic multiorgan, autoimmune, inflammatory disease.

luteinizing hormone (LH): A gonadotrophic hormone of the anterior pituitary that acts with the follicle-stimulating hormone to cause ovulation of mature follicles and secretion of estrogen by specific cells. Also concerned with corpus luteum formation and, in the male, stimulates the development and functional activity of interstitial cells.

luteotropin hormone (LTH): Lactogenic hormone; prolactin, which is partially responsible for breast development and for stimulating breast milk.

lymphadenitis: Inflammation of the breast tissue causing enlargement.

lymphadenopathy: Disease of the lymph nodes, characterized by malaise and general enlargement of the nodes.

lymphatic system: The system containing or conveying lymph.

lymphedema: Swelling of an extremity caused by obstruction of the lymphatic vessels.

lymphoblast: T lymphocytes that have been altered during a viral attack to release a variety of chemicals that encourage greater defensive activity by the immune system.

lymphocyte: A particular type of white blood cell that is involved in the immune response and produced by lymphoid tissue.

lymphoidectomy: Excision of lymphoid tissue.

lymphoma: Any of the various forms of cancers of the lymphoid tissue.

lysozyme: Enzyme present in saliva, sweat, tears, and breast milk that has antiseptic qualities that destroy foreign organisms.

maceration: Softening of tissue by soaking in fluids; breaking down of fetal skin as seen in postterm infant or in fetal death.

macroglossia: A tongue which is large for the oral cavity; present in neonates with Down's syndrome and in some preterm infants.

macrosomia: Large for gestational age infants; often seen in infants of diabetic mothers.

macular degeneration: Common eye condition in which the macula is effected by edema, the pigment is dispersed, and the macular area of the retina degenerates. It is the leading cause of visual impairment in persons older than 50.

macrophage: A phagocyte cell residing in tissues and derived from the monocyte.

magnetic resonance imaging (MRI): A scanning technique using magnetic fields and radio frequencies to produce a precise image of the body tissue; used for diagnosis and monitoring of disease.

magical thinking: Process of thinking will make it true.

magnification: Thinking in which the negative is exaggerated.

main effects: The action of two or more independent variables each working separately.

mainstreamed: Concept in education that a child with a disability be put into a typical classroom for a portion or all of the school day.

maintenance: Programs for the maintenance of functional capabilities.

maladaptation: Failure to return to homeostasis after a stressful event.

malaise: A vague feeling of bodily discomfort or uneasiness, as in an early illness.

malnutrition: Inadequate amount and or quality of food to maintain wellness.

malposition: Faulty or abnormal position.

malpractice: Failure to exercise prudent judgment and actions based on community standards of acceptable practices.

mammary gland: Gland of the female breast composed of lobes and lobules that secrete milk for the young; glands also exist in males in a rudimentary state.

mammogram: X-ray of breast tissue to determine presence of abnormalities.

managed care: Delivery of care based on balancing cost with quality.

mania: Elevated mood in bipolar disorder characterized by high energy.

manipulation: A passive therapeutic movement, usually of small amplitude and high velocity, at the end of the available range.

Mann-Whitney U-Test: Test on rank-ordered data of the hypothesis of difference between two independent random samples. The independent t-test is its ordinal likeness.

Marfan syndrome: An inherited disorder characterized by elongation of the bones causing musculoskeletal abnormalities and associated with cardiovascular and eye anomalies.

mask of pregnancy: *See* chloasma.

masochism: Sexual stimulation resulting from demeaning behavior of another.

mass: A quantity, such as cells; a measure of amount, usually in kilograms or pounds.

massage: Manipulation of the soft tissues of the body for the purpose of affecting the nervous, muscular, respiratory, and circulatory systems.

mastectomy: Removal of the breast (mammary gland); **radical mastectomy:** Removal of breast, involved skin, pectoral muscle, axillary lymph nodes, and subcutaneous fat; **simple mastectomy:** The breast, nipple areola, and involved skin are removed; **prophylactic (preventive) mastectomy:** In an effort to prevent breast cancer, the removal of one or both breasts.

master care plan: Treatment plan that includes the list of client problems and identifies the treatment team's intervention strategies and responsibilities.

mastery: Achievement of skill to a criterion level of success.

mastication: Chewing; tearing and grinding food with the teeth while it becomes mixed with saliva.

mastitis: An infection of the breast; symptoms include fever, redness, and tenderness in the breast, usually confined to a milk duct.

maternal adaptation: Adaptive process for a woman adjusting the maternal role first identified by Reva Rubin and including: taking in, taking hold, and letting go.

maternal mortality: Death of a woman directly related to childbearing.

maternal sensitization: Process by which the maternal immunologic system forms antibodies against fetal blood cells.

maternal serum a-fetoprotein (MS-AFP): Screen of maternal blood for the presence and amount of AFP.

maternal-infant bonding: Forming of an emotional attachment between the mother and the infant.

maturation: Sequential unfolding of behavioral and physiological characteristics during development.

maturational crisis: Crisis arising from a transition between phases of normal growth and development.

maturational theory: Developmental theory that views development as a function of innate factors, which proceed according to a maturational and developmental timetable.

mature group: Members take on all necessary roles, including leadership. To balance task accomplishment with need satisfaction of all group members. A therapist is equal member of this group.

mature milk: Breast milk that contains the appropriate calories and nutrients for energy and growth in the infant.

maximal oxygen consumption (max VO_2, maximal oxygen uptake, aerobic capacity): The greatest volume of oxygen used by the cells of the body per unit time.

maximal voluntary ventilation (MVV): The greatest volume of air that can be exhaled in 15 seconds.

maximum heart rate (age predicted): Highest possible heart rate usually achieved during maximal exercise. Maximum heart rate decreases with age and can be estimated as $220 -$ the age.

McBurney's point: Anatomical location of appendix.

mean (x): Arithmetic average. Measure of central tendency.

meaning: To make sense out of a situation using everything a person brings to it, including perception, attitudes, feelings, and social and cultural values.

meaningfulness: Amount of significance or value an individual associates with an experience after encountering it.

mean arterial pressure (MAP): Calculated value of blood pressure.

meatus: Passage or opening within the body.

mechanical ventilation: The use of a respirator for external support of breathing and the use of an Ambu bag to mechanically inflate the lungs.

mechanics: The study of physical forces.

mechanism of labor: Describes the five positions that the fetal head assumes through the pelvis: descent, flexion, internal rotation, extension, and external restitution.

mechanistic view (reductionism): Belief that a person is passive and that his or her behavior must be controlled or shaped by the society or environment in which he or she functions. Supports that the mind and body should be viewed separately and that the human being, like a machine, can be taken apart and reassembled if its structure and function are sufficiently well understood.

meconium: Fetal bowel movements of an infant; sticky, dark greenish brown, or nearly black; it is also sterile and odorless; **meconium aspiration syndrome (MAS):** Occurs in fetal hypoxia which creates relaxation of the sphincter, meconium is released into the amniotic fluid; reflex gasping during respiratory distress, rales, and chemical pneumonia; **meconium ileus:** Lower intestinal obstruction by dried meconium that may occur with cystic fibrosis; **meconium-stained fluid:** Release of meconium in utero which creates a greenish color to the fluid.

medial: In terms of anatomical position, located closer to the midline of the body.

medial longitudinal fasciculus (MLF): Pathway in the brainstem that connects the vestibular system with the cranial nerves that serve the eye muscles (III, IV, VI).

median (Mdn): The value or score that most closely represents the middle of a range of scores.

mediastinum: The mass of tissues and organs separating the two lungs, between the sternum in front and the vertebral column behind, and from the thoracic inlet above to the diaphragm below. Contains heart and its large vessels, trachea, esophagus, thymus, lymph nodes, and other structures and tissues.

medical neglect: Lack of needed health care.

medicine: The profession practiced by physicians.

medicolegal: Legal issues related to health care.

meditation: Method of relaxation involving focusing on object or thought.

medium work: Exerting up to 20 to 50 pounds of force occasionally, 10 to 25 lbs of force frequently, or greater than negligible up to 10 pounds of force constantly to move objects.

meiosis: Sperm and ova are produced by the reduction division process, each having only half of the parent cell's original complement of chromosomes (23 in humans).

melancholia: A major depressive episode with extreme symptoms and loss of interest in any activity.

melatonin: Hormone produced by the pineal gland and secreted into the bloodstream.

membrane(s): Thin pliable tissue that lines a cavity or separates structures or covers an organ; the amnion and chorion surrounding the fetus; **artificial rupture of membranes (AROM):** Rupture of membranes using a plastic amnio hook or a surgical clamp; **premature rupture of membranes (PROM):** Rupture of membranes with leaking from the amniotic sac prior to the onset of labor at any time during pregnancy; **preterm premature rupture of membranes (PPROM):** Rupture of membranes occurring prior to 37 weeks gestation; **spontaneous rupture of membranes (SROM):** Natural rupture of membranes or no medical intervention.

memory: Recalling information after brief or long periods of time; the mental process that involves registration and encoding, consolidation and storage, and recall and retrieval of information; **immediate:** Events of a few minutes ago; **recent:** Events of no more than a few days ago; **remote:** Events of many years ago.

memory processes: Strategies for dealing with information that is under the individual's control.

memory structure: Unvarying physical or structural components of memory.

menarche: First menstrual period of a female; usually occurs between 9 and 17 years of age.

meningomyelocele: A congenital defect of the spinal column through which a saclike protrusion appears usually containing some portion of the spinal cord.

menopause: Period of life in women marking the end of the reproductive cycle; accompanied by cessation of menstruation, decreases in hormonal levels, and alteration of the reproductive organs.

menorrhagia: Excessive menstrual flow or bleeding.

menstruation (menses): Periodic discharge of a bloody fluid from the uterus through the vagina occurring at more or less regular intervals from puberty to menopause.

mental health: Personal wellness, satisfaction.

mental illness: Condition exhibiting behaviors, feelings, and thoughts that are culturally inconsistent with the norms and that produce inabilities to function adequately in society.

mental imagery: Visualization of some place or event that is particularly relaxing.

mental retardation: Significantly subaverage general intellectual functioning concurrent with deficits in adaptive behavior and manifested during the developmental period.

mental status exam: Any diagnostic procedure used to evaluate intellectual, emotional, psychological, and personality functions.

mentum: Chin; used as a reference point when designating the position of the presenting fetal part, in relation to the maternal pelvis, during labor.

meridians: Pathways in body in Chinese medicine in which Chi (healing energy) flows.

mesoderm: Middle layer of cells that develops from the inner cell mass of the blastocyst, eventually becoming the muscles, the bones, the circulatory system, and the inner layer of the skin.

mesothelioma: A tumor developed from mesothelial tissue.

meta-analysis: Type of research in which previous research studies are examined to determine outcome trends.

metabolic acidosis: Metabolic environment of acidity. A pathologic condition resulting from accumulation of acid or loss of base in the body and characterized by an increase in hydrogen ion concentration (decrease in pH).

metabolic alkalosis: A pathologic condition resulting from the accumulation of base or loss of acid in the body and characterized by a decrease in hydrogen ion concentration (increase in pH).

metabolic equivalent level (MET): Method used to measure endurance levels; represents the energy requirements needed to maintain metabolic functioning as well as perform varying activities. An abbreviation for oxygen consumption during activities; the greater the exertion, the greater the METs required for an activity.

metabolism: The sum of all physical and chemical processes by which living organized substance is produced and maintained, and also the transformation by which energy is made available for the uses of the organism. The process by which the body inactivates drugs. Synonym: biotransformation.

metaethics: Branch of philosophy that examines similarities in ways decisions between right and wrong are made.

metastasis: When tumor cells spread from site of origin to other parts of the body.

metrorrhagia: Abnormal uterine bleeding occurring outside of the normal menstrual period.

microbacteria: A genus of microorganism made up of gram-positive rods found in dairy products and characterized by relatively high resistance to heat.

microcephaly: Condition in which an atypically small infant skull results in brain damage and mental retardation.

micturition: The act of urinating.

midwives: Attendants who assist women during labor and delivery; **certified nurse midwife:** Registered nurse with advanced education in midwifery, usually a master's degree; **lay midwife:** A person who is not a professional nurse and may have some advanced education and who has learned most skills experientially.

migraine: Headache associated with periodic instability of the cranial arteries; may be accompanied by nausea.

milia: Closed sebaceous glands appearing on the neonatal forehead, nose, cheeks, and chin as tiny white papules which disappear spontaneously in a few days or weeks after birth.

milieu: The environment.

milieu therapy: Treatment in which the environment is designed to provide specific levels of feedback.

milk ejection reflex (MER): Release of milk from the milk glands (breasts) in response to hormonal stimulus (oxytocin); also called letdown.

milk leg: Femoral thrombosis resulting in painful swelling of the leg.

millenial generation: The generation born between 1982 and 2000.

mind–body relationship: The effect of the mind (and mental disorders) on the body and the effect of the body (and physical disorders) on the mind.

minimal brain damage (MBD): Superficial damage to the brain that cannot be detected using objective instruments. Such damage is usually assessed from deviations in behavior.

minimal risk: The probability and magnitude that harm and discomfort anticipated in research are not greater in and of themselves than those ordinarily encountered in daily life or during the performance of routine physical or psychological examinations or tests.

minimization: Undervaluing positive aspects of an event.

minimum data set (MDS): Required data to be completed by a registered nurse within the first 14 days of admission.

minority group: Group differing, especially in race, religion, or ethnic background, from the majority of a population.

minute ventilation: The volume of air inspired and exhaled in 1 minute. The highest minute ventilation achieved during exercise is also called the maximum breathing capacity.

miscarriage: Spontaneous delivery or abortion of a fetus.

mission statement: Statement of purpose of an agency or organization.

mitleiden: Psychosomatic symptoms of fathers-to-be.

mitogen: A substance that stimulates cell division (i.e., mitosis) in lymphocytes.

mitosis: Cell duplication and division that generates all of an individual's cells except for the sperm and ova.

mitral valve prolapse (MVP): Incomplete closure of the mitral valve due to one or both of the mitral valves protruding backward into the left atrium during systole.

mitral valve stenosis: An obstruction of the blood flow from the atrium to the ventricle caused by narrowing of the opening and the stiffening of the leaflets of the mitral valve.

mittleschmerz: Pain associated with ovulation.

mnemonics: Memory-enhancing, learning techniques that link a new concept to an established one.

mobilization: The condition in which a fixed part is moveable.

modality: A broad group of agents that may include thermal, acoustic, radiant, mechanical, or electrical energy to produce physiologic changes in tissues for therapeutic purposes.

mode: Value or score in a set of scores that occurs most frequently.

model: An approach, framework, or structure that organizes knowledge to guide reasonable decision making.

modeling: Process by which a behavior is learned through observation and imitation of others.

modernization theory: Theory that looks at how a society is organized as a basis for how older adults are treated.

modulation: A variation in levels of excitation and inhibition over sensory and motor neural pools.

molecular pharmacology: The study of interaction of drugs and subcellular entities.

molding: The shaping of the fetal head by the overlapping fetal skull bones to adjust to the size and shape of the birth canal.

mongolian spot: Dark nonelevated pigmented area found over the buttocks after birth; usually fades by age 5 or 6.

mongolism: See Down's syndrome.

monitrice: A person who supports a woman during labor and has extensive knowledge of psychoprophylactic childbirth methods.

monitoring: Determining a client's status on a periodic or ongoing basis.

monoamine oxidase inhibitor (MAOI): Class of antidepressants to block MAO.

monochorionic: A single chorion as in the case of identical twins.

monocular: Pertaining to one eye.

monocyte: A circulating phagocytic leukocyte that can differentiate into a macrophage upon migration into tissue.

monosomy: Chromosomal anomaly characterized by one missing chromosome from the normal diploid complement.

monozygotic: Coming from a single fertilized ovum as in identical twins.

mons veneris: Pad of fatty tissue, coarse skin and hair that overlies the symphysis pubis in women.

Montgomery's glands: Small nodules on the areolas around the nipples of the breast; enlarge during pregnancy.

mood: Pervasive and sustained emotion that, when extreme, can color one's whole view of life; generally refers to either elation or depression.

morbidity: Illness or abnormal condition.

mores: Very strong norms; often laws.

morning sickness: Nausea and vomiting occurring in the first trimester of pregnancy which can occur at any time of the day.

Moro's reflex: Normal generalized startle reflex in an infant caused by a sudden loud noise.

morphogenesis: The morphological transformation, including growth, alterations of germinal layers, and differentiation of cells and tissues, during development.

mortality: Being subject to death; number of deaths in relation to a specific population; **fetal mortality:** Number of fetal deaths per 1,000 live births; **infant mortality:** Number of deaths per 1,000 children 1 year or younger; **maternal mortality:** Number of maternal deaths per 100,000 births; **neonatal mortality:** Number of neonatal deaths per 1,000 live births; **perinatal mortality:** Combined fetal and neonatal deaths per 1,000 live births.

motivation: An individual's drive toward the mastery of certain goals and skills; may be intrinsic or involve inducements and incentives.

motivational theory: Theory in which motivation is described as an arousal to action, initiating, molding, and sustaining specific action patterns. Certain reinforcers may be used to increase or decrease motivation. Internal rewards appear to be better motivators than extrinsic ones.

motor control: Using the body in functional and versatile movement patterns. The ability of the central nervous system to control or direct the neuromotor system in purposeful movement and postural adjustment.

motor deficit: Lack or deficiency of normal motor function that may be the result of pathology or other disorder. Weakness, paralysis, abnormal movement patterns, abnormal timing, coordination, clumsiness, involuntary movements, or abnormal postures may be manifestations of impaired motor function (motor control and motor learning).

motor development: Growth and change in the ability to do physical activities, such as walking, running, or riding a bike.

motor function: The ability to learn or demonstrate the skillful and efficient assumption, maintenance, modification, and control of voluntary postures and movement patterns.

motor neuron: A nerve cell that sends signals from the brain to the muscles throughout the body.

motor skill: The ability to execute coordinated motor actions with proficiency.

mourning: Experiencing the emotional response to the loss of a significant loved person until there is acceptance of the loss and an ability to continue with life.

mucous plug: An accumulation of mucus in lung diseases. A plug produced by the endocervical glands to seal the cervical canal and extruded from the vagina in early labor.

multicultural counseling: Process in which a therapist from one ethnic or racial background interacts with a person of a different background to assist in the psychological and interpersonal development and adjustment to the dominant culture.

multiculturalism: Awareness and knowledge about human diversity in ways that are translated into more respectful human interactions and effective interconnections.

multidisciplinary care: Different disciplines providing specific services to the patient/client.

multigenerational model: Model of family therapy that focuses on reciprocal role relationships over a period of time and thus takes a longitudinal approach.

multigravida: A woman who has completed two or more pregnancies to the stage of viability.

multi-infarct dementia: Form of organic brain disease characterized by the rapid deterioration of intellectual functioning and caused by vascular disease.

multilingual: Speaking many languages fluently.

multiparity: Refers to a condition of having two or more children.

multiparous: Refers to having given birth to two or more offspring in separate pregnancies, regardless of whether they ended in live births.

multiple melanoma: Multiple malignant tumors on the skin often beginning in moles that can metastasize widely.

multiple myeloma: Primary malignant tumor of the plasma cells usually arising in bone marrow.

multiple regression: Making predictions of one variable (using the multiple R) based on measures of two or more others.

Munchausen syndrome by proxy: The fabrication of the disease symptoms of another's illness to gain attention from caregivers.

murmur: A gentle blowing auscultatory sound caused by friction between parts, a prolapse of a valve, or an aneurysm.

muscle tone: Demonstrating a degree of tension or resistance in a muscle at rest and in response to stretch; amount of tension or contractibility among the motor units of a muscle; often defined as the resistance of a muscle to stretch or elongation.

muscle weakness: Lack of the full tension-producing capability of a muscle needed to maintain posture and create movement.

muscular atrophies: Diseases of unknown etiology that are caused by the breakdown of cells in the anterior horn of the spinal cord.

muscular system: Framework of voluntarily controlled skeletal muscles in the body.

musculoskeletal: System in the human body that is associated with the muscles and the bones to which they attach.

mutation: An error in gene replication that results in a change in the molecular structure of genetic material.

mutual support group: Type of group in which members organize to solve their own problems, usually led by the group members themselves who share a common goal and use their own strengths to gain control over their lives.

mutuality: In parent–infant attachment, the corresponding parent behaviors and characteristics to the infant behaviors and characteristics.

myalgia: Pain in a muscle or muscles.

myelin: A fatlike substance forming the principal component of the sheath of nerve fibers in the central nervous system.

myelination: The process of forming the "white" lipid covering of nerve cell axons; myelin increases the conduction velocity of the neuronal impulse and forms the "white matter" of the brain and spinal cord.

myelitis: Inflammation of the spinal cord with associated motor and sensory dysfunction.

myelography: Radiograph process used to view spinal lesions in the subarachnoid space after injection with dye or air.

myelomeningocele: A defect in the vertebral column through which a sac containing meninges, spinal fluid, and nerves extrudes.

myelopathy: A general term denoting functional disturbances and/or pathological changes in the brain.

myoclonus: Sudden, quick spasms of a muscle or group of muscles.

myokymia: Continual irregular twitching of a muscle often seen around the eye in the facial region.

myoma: Benign tumor consisting of muscle tissue.

myometrium: Fixed, smooth muscle forming the middle layer of the uterine wall.

myopathy: Abnormal muscle function.

myopia: Seeing distinctly at close range; light rays focus in front of the retina.

myorrhaphy: Suture of a muscle.

myosin: A protein in muscles.

myotasis: Stretching of muscle.

myringoplasty: Reconstruction of the eardrum.

myringotomy: Puncture of the eardrum with evacuation of fluids from the middle ear.

myxoma: A tumor composed of mucous tissue.

Nägele's (Naegele's) rule: Method for calculating a pregnant woman's estimated date of confinement or due date; the formula is the date of the last menstrual period minus 3 months, plus 7 days.

narcissism: Egocentricity; dominant interest in one's self.

narcolepsy: Chronic sleep disorder manifested by excessive and overwhelming daytime sleepiness.

narcotic antagonist: A compound that reverses the effects of narcotics, such as Narcan, which counteracts the effects of Demerol.

narrative: The interpretation of events through stories.

narrative documentation: System of documentation that uses summary paragraphs to describe evaluation data and treatment progress.

natal: Pertaining to birth.

natriuresis: The excretion of sodium in the urine.

navel: The depression in the abdomen where the umbilical cord attaches to the fetus.

nebulizer: An atomizer; a device for throwing a spray or mist.

necrosis: Death of tissue usually resulting in gangrene.

necrotic: Dead; avascular.

necrotizing enterocolitis (NEC): Acute inflammation of the bowel that occurs in preterm or low birth weight infants; characterized by ischemic necrosis or death of the mucosa of the bowel and may lead to perforation of the bowel and peritonitis; formula-fed infants are at a higher risk for the disease than breast-fed infants.

needs assessment: Systematic gathering of information about strengths, problems, resources, and barriers in a given population or community. Results of needs assessment are the basis of program planning.

negative reinforcement: Removing an aversive stimulus following an inappropriate response.

negligence: Commission of an act that a prudent person would not have done or the omission of a duty that a prudent person would have fulfilled resulting in injury or harm to another person. May be basis for a malpractice suit.

neocerebellum: Those parts of the cerebellum that receive input via the corticopontocerebellar pathway.

neologism: A new, meaningless word, often spoken by fluent aphasic clients.

neonatal abstinence syndrome: Symptomatology associated with drug withdrawal in the neonate.

neonatal mortality: *See* mortality.

neonatal narcosis: Newborn central nervous system depression caused by narcotic; symptoms include respiratory depression, hypertonia, lethargy, and problems with temperature regulation.

neonate: Represents the first 4 weeks of an infant's life.

neonatology: A branch of medicine that focuses on research about and care for neonates.

nephrotoxicity: The quality of being toxic or destructive to kidney cells.

neoplasia: The development of new and abnormal tissue such as a tumor which can be benign or malignant.

nervous system: The network of neural tissues in the body comprising the central and peripheral divisions, which are responsible for the processing of impulses.

neural tube: The tube from which the brain and spinal cord develop in the embryo; **neural tube defect:** Improper development of the tube that causes malformations of the brain or spinal cord.

neuralgia: Attacks of pain along the entire course or branch of a peripheral sensory nerve.

neurapraxia: Interruption of nerve conduction without loss of continuity of the axon.

neuritic plaque: Normative age-related change in the brain involving the collection of amyloid protein on dying or dead neurons. A discrete structure found outside the neuron that is composed of degenerating small axons, some dendrites, astrocytes, and amyloid. Also known as senile plaque.

neuritis: Condition causing a dysfunction of a cranial or spinal nerve; in sensory nerves, paresthesia is present.

neuroanatomy: Structures within the central, peripheral, and autonomic nervous systems.

neurobehavioral approach: Analysis of tactile, kinesthetic, visual, auditory, and olfactory sensations and their required motor, visual, and verbal responses for each activity. Neurological integration of the input from the senses and muscular responses are included.

neuroblastoma: A malignant tumor of the nervous system composed chiefly of neuroblasts.

neurodevelopment: The progressive growth and development of the nervous system.

neuroendocrinology: Study of hormones in the neurological system.

neurofibrillary tangle (NFT): A darkly stained, thick, and twisted band of material found in the cytoplasm of aging neurons. Associated with dementias of the Alzheimer's type.

neurofibromatosis: Growth of multiple tumors from the nerve sheath (i.e., von Recklinghausen's disease).

neurogenic pain: Pain in the limbs caused by neurologic lesions.

neurography: The study of the action potentials of nerves.

neurohypophysis: The posterior lobe of the pituitary gland.

neuroleptic: Drug or agent that modifies psychotic behavior, antipsychotic.

neurologic impairment: Any disability caused by damage to the central nervous system (brain, spinal cord, ganglia, and nerves).

neurolysis: Destruction of nerve tissue or loosening of adhesions surrounding a nerve.

neuroma: Tumor or growth along the course of a nerve or at the end of a lacerated nerve, which is often very painful.

neuromechanism: A neurologic system whose component parts work together to produce central nervous system function.

neuromuscular: Pertaining to the nerves and the muscles.

neuron: Nerve cell.

neuronal sprouting: The process of regrowing a neuronal process (e.g., an axon, in an injured neuron, attempting to reestablish innervation with a target structure).

neuropathy: Any disease or dysfunction of the nerves.

neuropharmacology: The study of the effects of medications on the brain.

neuroplasty: Surgical repair of nerves.

neurosis: Mental disorder in which reality testing is not seriously disturbed, but the individual is fearful or overly anxious about various elements of his or her life.

neurosyphilis: Syphilis of the central nervous system.

neurotic: Analytic concept that reflects psychodynamic conflicts that cause difficulty for an individual to remain in contact with reality.

neurotransmitters: Chemical substances that are released from presynaptic cells and travel across the synapse to stimulate or inhibit postsynaptic cells, thereby facilitating or inhibiting neural transmission.

neurotrophic: Nutrition and maintenance of tissues as regulated by nervous influence.

neutrophil: A phagocytic leukocyte characterized by a multilobed nucleus and many intracellular granules.

nevus: A congenital pigmentation of the skin such as a mole, mark, or natural blemish; **nevus flammeus:** A port wine stain usually reddish in color, flat, and found on the neck or face. Due to its size and color, it is considered a serious deformity; **nevus vasculosus (strawberry hemangioma):** A lesion which is elevated and composed of immature capillaries and endothelial cells that fades over the years.

nipple confusion: Difficulty establishing successful breast feeding after an infant has been given a pacifier or a bottle; the confusion seems to arise over the texture of the artificial nipple versus the mother's nipple.

nipple cup: A plastic cup which fits over the nipple and is used to make an inverted nipple erectile.

nociceptor: A peripheral nerve ending that appreciates and transmits painful or injurious stimuli.

nominal (or categorical) data: Numbers are utilized to name mutually exclusive categories.

nominal scales: Measurement scales that contain information that is categorical and mutually exclusive (i.e., it can only be contained in one category).

nonfenestrated trach: The inability to create an opening through the trachea.

nonjudgmental acceptance: Therapist or group therapist lets the client know that his or her ideas and thoughts will be valued and not rejected.

nonmaleficence: Obligation to avoid doing harm to another individual or creating a circumstance in which harm could occur.

nonnutritive sucking: Infant use of a pacifier.

nonparametrics: Statistical tests that do not predict the population parameter or normality of the underlying population distribution.

nonrapid eye movement (NREM): Sleep state in which brain waves become slower and less regular.

nonreassuring fetal heart rate pattern: A pattern that indicates the fetus is not well oxygenated and requires intervention.

nonshivering thermogenesis: When an infant produces heat from brown fat through increasing the metabolic rate.

nonstress test (NST): The fetal response, as demonstrated by the fetal heart rate, to natural contractions or to an increase in fetal activity.

norepinephrine: A hormone secreted by the adrenal medulla in response to splanchnic stimulation and stored in the chromaffin granules, being released predominantly in response to hypotension. Stimulates the sympathetic nervous system.

normal curve: When scores and frequency of occurrence are plotted on the x and y axis, respectively, this frequency distribution curve ensues.

normality: Range of behavior considered acceptable by a social group or culture.

normative ethics: Examination of daily debates between group members about what is right and what is wrong.

normoglycemia: Normal blood glucose level that indicates good glycemic control.

norm-referenced test: Any instrument that uses the typical scores of members of a comparison group as a standard for determining individual performance.

norms: Standards of comparison derived from measuring an attribute across many individuals to determine typical score ranges.

nosocomial: Diseases originating in hospitals.

noticing: Act of knowing; awareness of critical issues.

novitiate: Beginning stages or apprenticeship within a professional career.

noxious: Harmful to health; injurious (e.g., noxious gas, noxious stimuli).

nuchal cord: One or more loops of umbilical cord encircling the fetal neck.

nuchal rigidity: Reflex spasm of the neck extensor muscles resulting in resistance to cervical flexion.

nuclear family: Family unit consisting of parents and their dependent children.

null hypothesis: In research, a hypothesis that predicts that no difference or relationship exists among the variables studied that could not have occurred by chance alone.

nulligravida: Woman who has never been pregnant.

nullipara: Woman who has yet to carry a pregnancy to viability.

nurse practitioner: A registered nurse with advanced education and experience capable of legal recognition within a geographic area.

nurses: A broad term referring to the people who perform nursing, frequently including licensed practical nurses along with registered nurses. Also used to refer to registered nurses only.

nursing: The profession nurses practice. As stated in the American Nurses Association social policy statement: "Protection, promotion, and optimization of health and abilities, prevention of illness and injury, alleviation of suffering through the diagnosis and treatment of human response, and advocacy in the care of individuals, families, communities, and populations."

nursing diagnosis: The clinical judgments about responses to actual or potential health problems; the basis for subsequent actions to achieved desired outcomes.

nursing process: *See* nursing process section.

nutrition: The balance of nutrients needed to sustain life.

nyctalopia: The inability to see well in faint light or at night.

nystagmus: Rhythmic, constant, and rapid involuntary movement of the eyeball. A series of automatic, back-and-forth eye movements. Different conditions produce this reflex. A common way of producing nystagmus is by an abrupt stop following a series of rotations of the body. The duration and regularity of postrotary nystagmus are some of the indicators of vestibular system efficiency.

obesity: Body mass index of 30 or more.

objective measure: Method of assessment that is not influenced by the emotions or personal option of the assessor.

observer bias: When the previous experiences of the individual influence his or her observations and interpretation of behaviors being assessed or evaluated.

obsession: Irresistible thought pattern, usually anxiety provoking, that intrudes on normal thought processes.

obsessive-compulsive disorder: Anxiety disorder characterized by recurrent uncontrollable thoughts, irresistible urges to engage repetitively in an act, or both, such that they cause significant anxiety or interfere with daily functioning.

occipitobregmatic: Pertaining to the occiput, which is the back part of the skull, and the bregma or anterior fontanel where the coronal and sagittal sutures meet.

occipitofrontal: A line from the root of the nose to the most prominent portion of the occipital bone of the fetus at term.

occipitomental: Diameter from the chin of the fetus to the most prominent portion of the occipital bone; the correct angle for the application of forceps during delivery.

occiput: The back part of the fetal head.

occiput anterior: Fetal occiput to the mother's symphysis pubis.

ocular dysmetria: The eyes are unable to fix on an object or follow a moving object with accuracy.

oculogyric crisis: Involuntary condition of fixation of eyeballs, usually in an upward position, associated with some antipsychotic medication side effects.

oculomotor: Pertains to movement of the eyeballs.

old age: Arbitrary or societally defined period of life; specifically, over 65 years of age in the United States.

older person: Term used to refer to individuals in the later years of the life span. Arbitrarily set between 65 and 70 years old in American society for the purpose of age-related entitlements.

oldest old: Persons over 85 years of age.

old old: Persons over 75 years of age.

olfactory: Interpreting odors; pertaining to the sense of smell.

oligoclonal banding: A process by which cerebrospinal fluid IgG is distributed, following electrophoresis, in discrete bands. Present in approximately 90% of clients with multiple sclerosis.

oligodendroglia: Myelin-producing cells in the central nervous system.

oligohydramnios: Abnormally small amount of amniotic fluid that can occur with a fetal urinary tract defect.

oligomenorrhea: Longer intervals between menstrual periods, from 38 days to 3 months.

oliguria: Diminished amount of urine formation and excretion, below 25–30 ml for 2 consecutive hours in adults.

ombudsman: An individual within an organization with accountability for advocacy.

omphalitis: Infection of the umbilical stump; symptoms include redness, edema, and purulent exudates.

omphalocele: Failure in the closure of the abdominal wall or muscles that allows the abdominal contents to herniate through the navel of the neonate.

one-tail (directional) test: A test of the null hypothesis in which only one tail of the distribution is utilized.

ontogeny: Course of development during an individual's lifetime.

onychia: Inflammation of the nail bed.

onychogryphosis: Ingrown nail, either finger or toe.

onychomycosis: Parasitic fungal condition between skin and nail, frequently seen in the great toe.

onychosis: Any disease of the nails.

oocyte: A primitive cell in the ovary that becomes an ovum after meiosis.

oogenesis: Formation and development of the ovum.

open-ended question: Question that may have multiple correct responses rather than a finite correct answer.

open system: System of structures that functions as a whole and maintains itself by means of input from the environment and organismic change occurring as needed.

operant conditioning: A form of conditioning in which positive or negative reinforcement is contingent upon the occurrence of the desired response.

operculum: Mucous plug that fills the cervical canal during pregnancy.

ophthalmia neonatorum: Infection in the eyes of a neonate contracted from the mother during passage through the birth canal; usually gonorrheal.

ophthalmoplegia: Paralysis of ocular muscles.

opioid: Terminology used to refer to synthetic drugs that have pharmacological properties similar to opium or morphine.

opisthotonos: Position of extreme hyperextension of the vertebral column caused by a tetanic spasm of the extensor musculature.

opportunistic infection: Infections, especially bacterial and fungal, occurring during an altered physiological state such as with AIDS.

opposition: The movement in which the thumb is brought across to meet the little finger.

Optacon: Camera that allows blind people to read by converting print to an image of letters, which are then produced onto the finger using vibrations.

optokinetic nystagmus: Nystagmus induced by watching stripes on a drum revolving around one's face.

oral defensiveness: Avoidance of certain textures of food and irritation with activities using the mouth.

oral-motor control: Coordinated ability of opening and closing the mouth and being able to manage chewing, swallowing, and speaking.

orchitis: Inflammation of one or both testes including edema and pain, can be caused by mumps, syphilis or tuberculosis.

order: The desired state of affairs, which is an absence of disease in medicine and competence in the performance of work, play, or self-care; **disorder:** A disease in medicine and/or performance dysfunction.

ordinal data: Rank-ordered data.

ordinal scales: Measurement scales that contain information that can be rank ordered.

ordinate: In the coordinate system, the ordinate is the vertical axis (also known as the y axis).

organismic view: Concept that an individual is active in determining and controlling his or her own behavior and can change that behavior if it is desirous to do so.

organization: Group of individuals organized for the attainment of a common goal.

orgasm: The apex and culmination of sexual excitement.

orientation: Identifying person, place, time, and situation; the initial stage of group development that includes a search for structure, goals, and dependency on the leader.

origin: Proximal attachment of a muscle that remains relatively fixed during normal muscular contraction.

orifice: Mouth or entrance to any aperture, cavity.

orthopedic: Branch of medical science that deals with the prevention or correction of disorders involving locomotor structures of the body.

orthopedic impairment: Any disability caused by disorders to the musculoskeletal system.

orthopnea: The inability to breathe except in an upright position.

orthosis/orthotic: Device added to a person's body to support, position, or immobilize a part; to correct deformities; to assist weak muscles and restore function; or to modify tone.

orthostatic hypotension: A dramatic fall in blood pressure when a patient assumes an upright position, usually caused by a disturbance of vasomotor control decreasing the blood supply returning to the heart.

orthotic: *See* orthosis.

os: mouth or opening; **external os:** External opening of the cervix; **internal os:** Internal opening of the cervix.

oscilloscope: Instrument that displays a visual representation of an electrical wave, such as that which causes a muscle contraction.

osmosis: The passage of pure solvent from the lesser to the greater concentration when two solutions are separated by a membrane, which selectively prevents the passage of solute molecules but is permeable to the solvent. An attempt to equalize concentrations on both sides of a membrane.

ossification: Mineralization of bone.

osteoarthritis: Joint degeneration due to stress of movement.

osteoblast: Any cell that develops into bone or secretes substances producing bony tissue.

osteochondrosis: A disease of one or more of the growth or ossification centers that begins as a degeneration or necrosis followed by regeneration or recalcification, especially in children.

osteoclast: Any of the large multinucleate cells in bone that absorb or break down bony tissue.

osteogenisis imperfecta: A genetic disorder of the connective tissue which manifests in short stature and extreme bone fragility occurring in childhood; no known cause.

osteoplasty: Plastic surgery of the bones; bone grafting.

osteoporosis: Weakened, thinned bones.

osteotomy: Operation to cut across a bone.

otitis media: Inflammation of the inner ear, which usually causes dizziness.

otosclerosis: Hardening of the bony tissue of the ear, resulting in conductive hearing loss.

outcome: The way something turns out; result; consequence. The result of patient/client management. Relate to remediation of functional limitation and disability, primary or secondary prevention, and optimization of patient/client satisfaction.

outcome measure: Instrument designed to gather information on the efficacy of service programs; a means for determining if goals or objectives have been met.

outlet: Opening by which something can leave; **pelvic outlet:** Lower opening of the true pelvis.

outpatient services: Ambulatory care.

ovary: The female glands that are found on either side of the pelvic cavity and produce the ovum or female egg for reproduction and the hormones, estrogen and progesterone.

overgeneralization: Broad conclusions based on limited events or data. Also known as absolutistic thinking.

overuse syndrome: Musculoskeletal disorder manifested from repetitive upper extremity movements occurring during activities. Symptoms include persistent pain in joints, muscles, tendons, or other soft tissues of the upper extremities. Synonyms: cumulative trauma disorder, repetitive strain disorder.

ovulation: The ripening and discharge of the ovum from the ovary, usually 14 days prior to the onset of menstrual flow.

ovum: Female reproductive cell or egg.

oximeter: A photoelectric device for determining the oxygen saturation of the blood.

oxygen consumption (VO_2): The amount of oxygen used by the tissues of the body, usually measured in oxygen uptake in the lung; normally about 250 ml/minute and it increases with increased metabolic rate.

oxygen saturation: The degree to which oxygen is present in a particular cell, tissue, organ, or system.

oxygen toxicity: Concentration of oxygen is so high that it produces tissue changes such as retinopathy of prematurity or bronchopulmonary dysplasia.

oxytocics: Drugs that stimulate uterine contractions, can stimulate labor and speed up childbirth, and stimulate the release of milk (letdown reflex) for breast feeding.

oxytocin: A hormone stored in the pituitary that causes contraction of the uterus.

oxytocin challenge test (OCT): Assessment of fetal response to uterine contractions stimulated by low doses of oxytocin.

pacemaker: Electrical device implanted to control the beating of the heart.

pachymeningitis: Acute inflammation of the dura mater.

pacing: Accommodating for time in a test or treatment session; the rate at which instruction is given or practice is provided.

pain: A sensation of hurting or strong discomfort in some part of the body caused by an injury, disease, or functional disorder and transmitted through the nervous system.

pain character measurements: Any of the tools used to define the character of a patient's/client's pain.

pain estimate: A pain intensity measurement in which a patient's/client's pain is rated on a scale, usually 0 to 10.

pain experience: Individual response of living with persistent pain, includes functioning, stress, helplessness.

pain intensity measurements: Any of the scales used to quantify pain intensity.

pain management: Use of treatment to control chronic pain, including the use of behavioral modification, relaxation training, physical modalities and agents, medication, and surgery.

pain modulation: Variation in the intensity and appreciation of pain secondary to CNS and ANS affects on the nociceptors and along the pain pathways, as well as secondary to external factors such as distraction and suggestion.

pain pathway: The route along which nerve impulses arising from painful stimuli are transmitted from the nociceptor to the brain, including transmission within the brain itself.

pain quality: A description of the nature, type, or character of pain (e.g., burning, dull, sharp, throbbing, etc.).

pain response: Interpreting noxious stimuli.

palilalia: Repetition of one's own words or sounds, such as the vocal tic associated with Tourette's syndrome.

pallesthesia: The ability to sense mechanical vibration.

palliative care: Care rendered to temporarily reduce or moderate the intensity of an otherwise chronic medical condition.

pallidotomy: Brain surgery (globus pallidus) used to decrease some conditions associated with Parkinson's disease.

pallor: Paleness; absence of skin coloration.

palmar: Palm of the hand.

palmar erythema: Rash of the palms sometimes seen in pregnancy.

palpate: To examine by touching or feeling.

palpation: Examination using the hands (e.g., palpation of muscle spasm, palpation of the thoracic cage, etc.).

palpitation: Rapid, violent, or throbbing pulsation in a body part.

palsy: The loss of movement or ability to control movement; **Bell's palsy:** Peripheral paralysis of the facial nerve (cranial nerve VII) so that the muscles of the unaffected side of the face pull it into a distorted position. **Erb's palsy (Erb-Duchenne paralysis):** Paralysis caused by injury to the upper brachial plexus, usually occurring in childbirth, symptoms include loss of feeling in the arm, paralysis and atrophy of the deltoid, biceps, and brachialis muscles.

pancreatitis: Inflammation of the pancreas, with pain and tenderness of the abdomen, tympanites (i.e., gaseous pockets), and vomiting.

panic attack: State of extreme anxiety, usually including sweating, shortness of breath, chest pains, and fear. May come on unpredictably or as a result of a particular stimulus.

Papanicolaou (Pap) smear: Test of cervical scrapings to determine abnormal conditions such as cervical cancer.

papilledema: Edema and hyperemia of the optic disc.

paracervical block: Anesthesia produced by injection of a local anesthetic into the lower uterine segment beneath the mucosa at 3 and 9 o'clock.

paracrine: The method of extracellular hormonal communication.

para (parity): Number of past viable pregnancies (greater than 20 weeks) regardless of whether the fetuses were stillborn or live born.

paracyesis: Pregnancy that develops outside the uterus in the abdominal cavity.

paradigm: Refers to the organization of knowledge, as well as the changes in scientific thought over time; an organizing framework.

paradox: A statement to the contrary of belief. A statement that is self-contradictory and, hence, false.

paraffin bath: A superficial thermal modality using paraffin wax and mineral oil.

parallel processing: Learning or solving a problem through a global approach integrating data into a whole experience.

paralysis: Condition in which one loses voluntary motor control over a section of the body due to trauma or injury.

paranoia: Thought pattern that reflects a belief that others are persecuting or attempting to harm one, in the absence of a realistic basis for such fears.

paraphilias: Repetitive actions involving nonhuman objects, suffering, or nonconsenting people.

paraplegia (PARA): Paralysis of the spine affecting the lower portion of the trunk and legs. Impairment or loss of motor and/or sensory function in thoracic, lumbar, or sacral (but not cervical) segments of the spinal cord secondary to damage of neural elements within the spinal canal.

parasomnia: Abnormal sleep behavior, including sleepwalking and bruxism (i.e., grinding the teeth).

parasympathetic nervous system: Autonomic nervous system that serves to relax the body's responses and is the opposite of the sympathetic nervous system.

parasympatholytic: Producing the effects resembling those of interruption of the parasympathetic nerve supply to a part. An agent that opposes the effects of impulses conveyed by the parasympathetic nerves.

parasympathomimetic: Producing effects resembling those of stimulation of the parasympathetic nerve supply to a part. An agent that produces effects similar to those produced by stimulation of the parasympathetic nerves.

paraxial: Lying near the axis of the body.

parenchyma: Essential parts of an organ which are concerned with its function rather than its framework.

parenteral: Administration by subcutaneous, intramuscular, or intravenous injection, thereby bypassing the gastrointestinal tract.

paresis: Weakness in voluntary muscle with slight paralysis.

paresthesia: Abnormal sensation, such as burning, pricking, tickling, or tingling.

parietoalveolar: Pertaining to the cavities of the alveoli in the lungs.

parish/shull nursing: Nursing services through a church or synagogue to provide health education and counseling.

parity: A condition of having produced viable offspring. The state or condition of being the same in power, value, and rank. Equality.

Parkinson's disease: Neurological deficit of dopamine resulting in tremors, muscle rigidity, and slow movement.

paroxysm: Sudden, periodic attack or recurrence or intensification of symptoms of a disease (e.g., paroxysmal atrial tachycardia).

paroxysmal nocturnal dyspnea (PND): Severe respiratory difficulty occurring at night while sleeping flat and characteristic of left-sided heart failure.

partial thickness: Loss of epidermis and possible partial loss of dermis.

participant-observer: Descriptor that can be applied when a therapist observes and evaluates an individual's performance while engaged in an activity with the person.

parturient: Woman giving birth.

parturition: The act or process of giving birth.

passive-aggressive personality disorder: Disorder that is characterized by resistance to social and occupational performance demands through procrastination, dawdling, stubbornness, inefficiency, and forgetfulness that appears to border on the intentional.

passive range of motion (PROM): Amount of motion at a given joint when the joint is moved by the therapist.

paternalism: Acting or making decisions on behalf of others without their consent.

patent: Open.

patent ductus arteriosis: A connection in the newborn between the main pulmonary artery and the aorta which persists after birth; requires surgery if it fails to close.

pathogen: Any disease-producing agent or microorganism.

pathology: The study of the characteristics, causes, and effects of disease, as observed in the structure and function of the body.

pathophysiology: An interruption or interference of normal physiological and developmental processes or structures.

patient management interview: Interview used by multiple professionals to identify the type of intervention or treatment needed.

patient-related consultation: When the health professional shares information with other professionals regarding individuals who are presently receiving services.

patient/client: A person receiving care or treatment. Individual who is the recipient of therapy and direct intervention.

patient's rights: The right of a patient to be informed about his or her conditions and prognoses and to make decisions concerning his or her treatment.

patterned responses: The programs, either preprogrammed or created by the motor system, to succeed at the presented task in the most efficient and integrated response possible at that moment in time.

patterns of help-seeking: Culturally distinct ways in which people go about finding help at particular times in an illness. Refers to both range of options (often categorized as the biomedical, popular, and traditional health sectors) and decision-making process.

Pearson's r: Statistical technique that shows the degree of relationship between variables (also called the product-moment correlation).

peau d'orange: A skin condition that appears like orange peel due to cancerous lesions and most often seen in extremely edematous breasts.

pectus carinatum: Undue prominence of the sternum, called also chicken or pigeon chest/breast.

pectus excavatum: Undue depression of the sternum, called also funnel chest or breast.

pedagogy: The art and science of teaching children.

pedigree: A shorthand method of tracking a person's family heredity to determine genetically linked physical disorders.

pedophilia: Recurrent sexual urges or fantasies related to children.

peer culture: Stable set of activities or routines, artifacts, values, and concerns that a group of individuals produce or share.

peer review: Appraisal by professional coworkers of equal status of the way health practitioners conduct practice, education, or research.

pelvic: Related to the pelvis; **pelvic exenteration:** Surgical removal of all the reproductive organs and parts of the intestine and bladder; **pelvic inflammatory disease (PID):** Infection of the female reproductive organs usually as a result of sexually transmitted diseases; **pelvic inlet:** *See* inlet; **pelvic outlet:** *See* outlet; **pelvic relaxation:** The lengthening or weakening of the fascial tissues supporting the pelvic structures; **pelvic tilt (rock):** An exercise used to relieve low back pain associated with menstruation and pregnancy.

pelvic contraction: A condition in which one or more diameters of the pelvis is narrower than normal, not allowing for normal progression of labor.

pelvic floor: A sling arrangement of ligaments and muscles that supports the reproductive organs.

pelvimetry: A method of obtaining pelvic measurements by X-ray to determine adequacy for vaginal birth.

pelvis: Bony structure which supports the abdominal contents formed by the sacrum, coccyx, symphysis pubis, and the innominate bones and the uniting ligaments.

pendular knee jerk: Upon elicitation of the deep tendon reflex of the knee, the lower leg oscillates briefly like a pendulum after the jerk, instead of returning immediately to resting position.

penis: Male reproductive organ, also used for urination.

percent body fat: Percent of body weight that is fat, includes storage fat (expendable), essential fat, and sex-specific fat reserve.

perception: The ability to organize and interpret incoming sensory information.

perceptual-motor skill: The ability to integrate perceptual (sensory) input with motor output to accomplish purposeful activities.

percussion (diagnostic): A procedure in which the clinician taps a body part manually or with an instrument to estimate its density.

percussion: A procedure utilized with pulmonary postural drainage to loosen secretions from the bronchial walls.

percutaneous: Administration of a drug by inhalation, sublingual, or topical processes.

percutaneous transluminal coronary angioplasty (PTCA): Opening of coronary arteries by flattening plaque against vessel.

percutaneous umbilical blood sampling (PUBS): An operative procedure performed while the fetus is in utero in which the fetal umbilical cord is accessed and blood is withdrawn for testing or blood is transfused.

perfusion: The act of pouring over or through, especially the passage of a fluid through the vessels of a specific organ or body part.

periodontal disease: Condition of gums and alveolar bones of mouth, frequently associated with tooth loss in older adults.

perimenopause: The phase prior to menopause when periods become irregular or menstrual flow may decrease to almost nothing.

perinatal: Time period from 28 weeks gestation to 28 days of life.

perinatologist: A physician who specializes in the research and care for mothers, fetuses, and neonates.

perineum: The area bounded by the pubis, coccyx, and the thighs, which is between the external genitalia and the anus.

period of concrete operations: Stage in the child's cognitive development in which he or she is bound by immediate physical reality.

periodic breathing: Episodes in which respirations cease for 10 seconds or less without cyanosis; commonly seen in preterm infants.

peripartum heart failure: Inadequate cardiac output leading to heart failure during pregnancy.

peripheral nerve: Any nerve that supplies the peripheral parts and is a branch of the central nervous system (i.e., the spinal cord).

peripheral nerve injuries: Loss of precision pinch and grip due to crushing, severance, or inflammation/degeneration of the peripheral nerve fibers.

peripheral nervous system (PNS): Consists of all of the nerve cells outside the central nervous system, including motor and sensory nerves.

peripheral neuropathy: Any functional or organic disorder of the peripheral nervous system; degeneration of peripheral nerves supplying the extremities, causing loss of sensation, muscle weakness, and atrophy.

peripheral pain: Pain arising from injury to a peripheral structure.

peristalsis: Movement by which a tube in the body (primarily the alimentary canal) sends contents within it to another part of the body.

Accomplished through alternative contractions and relaxations, which resemble a wavelike or wormlike movement.

peritonitis: Inflammation of the peritoneum; a condition marked by exudations of serum, fibrin, cells, and pus in the peritoneum. Attended by abdominal pain and tenderness, constipation, vomiting, and moderate fever.

periventricular hemorrhage: Bleeding around a ventricle.

perseveration: The inability to shift from thought to thought; persistence of an idea even when the subject of conversation changes.

personal care services: Services performed by health care workers that assist patients in meeting the requirements of daily living.

personal distance/space: Culturally based space between two interacting individuals. U.S. culture distance is approximately 18–40 inches.

personal factors: The background of a person's life and living that is composed of features of him- or herself that are not parts of a health condition or disablement, including age, gender, educational background, experiences, personality, character style, aptitudes, other health conditions, fitness, lifestyle, habits, upbringing, coping styles, social background, profession, and past and current experience.

personality: Individual's unique, relatively consistent, and enduring methods of behaving in relation to others and the environment.

personality trait: Distinguishing feature that reflects one's characteristic way of thinking, feeling, and adapting.

personalization: Attributing responsibility to self without considering other potential factors.

pessary: A circular ring device used to hold a prolapsing organ in place when surgical repair is contraindicated.

petechiae: Pinpoint hemorrhagic areas.

petit mal: Type of seizure characterized by a momentary lapse of consciousness that starts and ends abruptly.

pH: Hydrogen ion concentration.

phacoemulsification: Method of treating cataracts by using ultrasonic waves to disintegrate the cataract, which is then aspirated.

phagocytosis: A process by which a leukocyte (monocyte, neutrophil) engulfs, ingests, and degrades a foreign particle or organism.

phalanges: Bones of the fingers and toes.

phantom limb pain: Paresthesia or severe pain felt in the amputated part of a limb.

pharmacodynamics: The study of how medications affect the body.

pharmacokinetics: The study of how the body handles medications, including absorption, distribution, and elimination.

pharmacotherapy: Treatment of a disease primarily using medications.

phenotype: Observable characteristics of an organism that result from the interaction of the genotype with the organism's environment.

phenylketonuria (PKU): Recessive hereditary disease resulting in a metabolic defect of the amino acid phenylalanine. If not treated, brain damage leading to mental retardation may occur.

phimosis: Tightness of the prepuce (foreskin) of the penis.

phlebitis: Inflammation of a vein resulting in pain, edema, and redness.

phlebothrombosis: A clot or thrombus in the vein which can become dislodged and travel in the circulatory system.

phlebotomy: Opening or piercing the vein.

phobia: Characterized by an extreme fear of a person, place, or thing when the situation is not hazardous; **specific:** Related to one type of situation, e.g., agoraphobia; **social:** Fear of social situations.

phocomelia: Developmental anomaly in which the limbs are irregularly shaped and resemble the fins of seals. Hands and feet attached to the trunk of the body.

phosphatidylglycerol: A component of pulmonary surfactant; its presence in amniotic fluid is a sign of lung maturity.

phototherapy: Intervention using the application of light.

physical: Pertaining to the body.

physical agent: A form of thermal, acoustic, or radiant energy that is applied to tissues in a systematic manner to achieve a therapeutic effect; a therapeutic modality used to treat physical impairments.

physical function: Fundamental component of health status describing the state of those sensory and motor skills necessary for mobility, work, and recreation.

physical therapy: Treatment of injury and disease by mechanical means, such as heat, light, exercise, massage, and mobilization.

physiology: Area of study concerned with the functions of the structures of the body.

pica: Compulsive eating of nonnutritive substances such as dirt. A bizarre appetite.

pinna: Cartilage structure of external ear.

pitocin: A synthetic oxytocic hormone administered through intravenous drip to induce or augment uterine contractions.

placebo: A substance with no physiologically active elements to substitute for such a true medication.

placenta: The organ that develops within the uterus from which the fetus derives its nourishment and oxygen; also serves as a filtering system; **abruptio placenta:** *See* abruptio placenta; **battledore placenta:** Umbilical cord insertion at the margin of the placenta; **circumvallate placenta:** The placenta has a white ring at the edge; **placenta accreta:** The placenta invades the uterine muscle making it extremely difficult to separate the placenta from the uterine muscle wall; **placenta increta:** Deep penetration in the myometrium by the placenta; **placenta previa:** Placenta that is implanted in the lower uterine segment causing the placenta to separate and bleed as the cervix dilates. Typed according to the closeness to the cervical os; **total previa:** When the placenta completely covers the os, **partial previa:** When it only partly occludes the os; **marginal previa:** When the placenta encroaches on the margin of the os; **placenta succenturiata:** An accessory placenta.

placental: Relating to the placenta; **placental infarct:** Ischemic hard area on the fetal or maternal side of the placenta; **placental soufflé:** *See* soufflé.

plan of care: Statements that specify the anticipated long-term and short-term goals and the desired outcomes, predicted level of optimal improvement, specific interventions to be used, duration, and frequency of the intervention required to reach the goals, outcomes, and criteria for discharge.

plaque: A lesion characterized by loss of myelin and hardening of tissue in diseases such as multiple sclerosis (peripherally) or Alzheimer's disease (in the brain).

plasma cell: Mature antibody-secreting cell derived from the B cell.

plasmapheresis: A process by which blood is removed from the patient/client; plasma is discarded and replaced by normal plasma or human albumin. Reconstituted blood is then returned to the patient/client. Process believed to rid blood of antibodies or substances that are damaging.

plasticity: In neuroscience, the ability of the central nervous system to adapt structurally or functionally in response to environmental demands. Anatomical and electrophysiological changes in the central nervous system. **biomechanics:** Defined as continued elongation of a tissue without an increase in resistance from within the tissue.

platypelloid pelvis: Broad pelvis with a flattened, oval, transverse shape and a shortened anteroposterior diameter.

play or leisure activities: Intrinsically motivating activities for amusement, relaxation, spontaneous enjoyment, or self-expression.

plethora: Polycythemia of the newborn, or a deep-red skin color caused by an increased number of red blood cells.

pleura: The serous membrane investing the lungs and lining the thoracic cavity, completely enclosing a potential space known as the pleural cavity. Two pleurae, right and left, entirely distinct from each other.

pleurisy: Inflammation of the pleural membrane surrounding the lungs. Synonym: pleuritis.

plugged ducts: Breast milk ducts blocked by dried milk curds that are hard and can be palpated.

pneumoencephalogram: Radiographic examination of ventricles and subarachnoid spaces of the brain following withdrawal of cerebrospinal fluid and injection of air or gas via lumbar puncture.

pneumonectomy: The excision of lung tissue.

pneumopathology: Any disease involving the respiratory system.

pneumothorax: An accumulation of air or gas in the pleural cavity, which may occur spontaneously or as a result of trauma or a pathological process. Prevents the lung from expanding.

podalic version: Manipulation of a breech fetus presentation internally or externally so that the feet are at the pelvic outlet.

podiatrist: A health care provider licensed to treat conditions of the foot.

point stimulation: The stimulation of sensitive areas of skin using electricity, pressure, laser, or ice for the purpose of relieving pain.

poliomyelitis: Viral infection of the motor cells in the spinal cord.

polycythemia: Excessive number of red corpuscles in the blood.

polydactyly: Extra digits, either fingers or toes.

polydrug abuse: Abuse of several psychoactive drugs (e.g., alcohol and cocaine).

polyhydramnios: *See* hydramnios.

polymyositis: Systemic connective tissue disease characterized by inflammatory and degenerative changes in the muscles. Leads to symmetric weakness and some degree of muscle atrophy; unknown etiology.

polyneuritis: Inflammation of many nerves at once.

polyneuropathy: A disease involving several nerves such as that seen in diabetes mellitus.

polyp: Tumor with a stem (pedicle) that projects from a mucous membrane surface.

polypharmacy: The excessive and unnecessary use of medications.

polyradiculopathy: Inflammation of multiple nerve roots.

polysomnography: The study of sleep.

polyuria: Excessive urine secretion by the kidneys.

population at-risk: Group of people who share a characteristic that causes each member to be vulnerable to a particular event (e.g., non-immunized children exposed to the polio virus).

position: Relationship of the fetal presenting part to the maternal pelvis (i.e., the fetal occiput is at the anterior of the maternal pelvis, the position is OA or occiput anterior). *See* diagrams.

positive reinforcement: Providing a desired reinforcer following an appropriate response.

positive signs of pregnancy: These signs include audible fetal heart tones, visualization and palpation of fetal movement, or sonogram visualization.

positron emission tomography (PET): Dynamic brain-imaging technique that produces a very detailed image of the brain that reflects changes in brain activity.

posterior: Toward the back of the body.

posterior fontanel: *See* fontanel.

postmature infant: Infant born after the beginning of the 43rd week of gestation and exhibiting physical signs of dysmaturity including desquamation, an absence of lanugo, vernix caseosa, and decrease in subcutaneous fat.

postnatal: Happening after birth of the newborn.

postpartum: The period following birth; **postpartum blues:** Maternal feelings of let down, sadness, anxiety or irritability occurring from 3 days to 2 weeks after the birth and resolves spontaneously; **postpartum depression:** Clinical depression occurring within 6 months of birth and characterized by symptoms that interfere with activities of daily living and maternal responsibilities. Condition thought to be related to hormonal changes or membrane transport; **postpartum hemorrhage:** Excessive bleeding after childbirth, usually more than

500 ml; **postpartum psychosis:** Symptoms may begin as postpartum blues or depression but progress to delusions, hallucinations, confusion, delirium, or panic.

postpolio syndrome: Collection of impairments occurring in persons who have had poliomyelitis many years ago; related to chronic mechanical strain of weakened musculature and ligaments.

postrotary nystagmus: Reflexive movement of the eyes that occurs after quick rotational movements have ceased; used to indicate the level of processing of vestibular information.

postterm pregnancy: Pregnancy extending beyond 42 weeks gestation (also called postdates).

post-traumatic amnesia: The time elapsed between a brain injury and the point at which the functions concerned with memory are determined to have been restored.

post-traumatic stress disorder (PTSD): Characterized by intense negative feelings or terror in reexperiencing a traumatic or disastrous event either in thoughts, nightmares, or dreams experienced over time. May also include physiological responses such as excessive alertness, the inability to concentrate or follow through on tasks, or difficulty sleeping.

postural alignment: The relationship of all the body parts around the center of gravity. Relationship of one body segment to another in standing or sitting or any other position. Maintaining biomechanical integrity among body parts; *see also* posture.

postural drainage: Positioning a person so that gravity aids in the drainage of secretions from the respiratory system.

postural hypotension: *See* orthostatic hypotension.

posture: The attitude of the body.

posturing: Voluntary positioning that is inappropriate or bizarre.

power of attorney: Document authorizing one person to take legal action on behalf of another who acts as an agent for the grantor.

pragmatics: The study of language as it is used in context.

pragmatism: Practical way of solving problems.

praxis: Conceiving and planning a new motor act in response to an environmental demand; the ability to conceive and organize a new motor act.

preassaultive tension state: Behaviors, such as tense body position, clenched teeth, argumentative statements, that are predictive of possible violence.

precipitous delivery: An unexpected or sudden birth following a labor of less than 3 hours.

preconception care: Focus on health maintenance prior to pregnancy.

predictive validity: Positive correlation between test scores and future performance.

predisposing factors/conditions: Those elements that influence response or condition subsequently.

preeclampsia: Illness occurring after 20 weeks gestation to early postpartum, characterized by high blood pressure, swelling, and protein in the mother's urine. Synonym: toxemia.

preexisting condition: Medical problem experienced by person prior to acceptance into a health care plan.

prefix: Word element of one or more syllables placed in front of a combining form in order to change its meaning.

pregnancy: Condition of carrying a fertilized ovum (zygote) in the uterus from conception through birth of all products of conception; in humans, normal length is 280 days.

pregnancy-induced hypertension (PIH): Hypertension occurring during pregnancy, which includes transient hypertension, preeclampsia, and eclampsia.

prejudice: Unreasonable feelings, opinions, or attitudes directed against a race, religion, or other definable group.

preload: Conditions in the heart prior to beating (e.g., blood pressure, filling volume, etc.).

premature: Child born before the 37th week of gestation; birth of infant.

premature dilation of the cervix: *See* incompetent cervix.

premature rupture of the membranes (PROM): *See* membrane(s).

premenstrual syndrome (PMS): A set of symptoms that occurs monthly after ovulation and usually cease at menstruation or shortly thereafter.

premonitory: An early symptom or warning.

premorbid personality: Psychosocial factor referring to personality characteristics that are present before the development of a disease and have either a positive or negative effect on the rehabilitative process.

prenatal period: Time between conception and birth. Body does not change more during entire lifespan as in these 38 weeks.

prepartum: Before birth.

prepuce: Fold of skin that covers the glans penis of the male; **prepuce of the clitoris:** Fold of the labia minora that covers the clitoris.

presentation: The part of the fetus that first enters the pelvis; also called presenting part.

presbyastasis: Age-related disequilibrium in the absence of known pathology.

presbycusis: Age-related hearing loss in the absence of pathology.

presbyopia: Age-related farsightedness with the loss in the ability to focus on objects that are near.

presenile: Pertaining to a condition in which a person manifests signs of aging in early or midlife.

presenting part: The part of the fetus that is first engaged in the pelvis.

pressure edema: Edema of the lower extremities caused by the heavy pregnant uterus pressing against the large veins.

pressure point: Point over an artery where the pulse may be felt.

pressure sore: An area of localized tissue damage caused by ischemia due to pressure.

presumptive signs of pregnancy: Suggestive signs of pregnancy that are not absolutely positive including cessation of menses, Chadwick's sign, morning sickness, and quickening.

preterm birth: Birth occurring prior to 37 weeks gestation.

preterm premature rupture of membranes (PPROM): *See* membrane(s).

prevalence: The total number of persons with a disease in a given population at a given point in time. Usually expressed as the percentage of the population that has the disease.

prevention: The act of preventing. Decreasing the risk of disease or disability. **primary:** Prevention of the development of disease in a susceptible or potentially susceptible population through such specific measures as general health promotion efforts; **secondary:** Efforts to decrease the duration of illness, reduce severity of diseases, and limit sequelae through early diagnosis and prompt intervention; **tertiary:** Efforts to limit the degree of disability and promote rehabilitation and restoration of function in patients/clients with chronic and irreversible diseases.

priapism: Penile erection that is painful and prolonged.

primary care provider (PCP)/physician: The initial practitioner who is expected to coordinate care, the "gate keeper."

primary effect: Tendency to remember first items of a list.

primary prevention: Services to prevent illness or conditions from occurring.

primigravida: First pregnancy.

primipara: First pregnancy carried to viability whether it is live born or stillborn.

primordial: Existing first or in the simplest form.

principal: Person authorizing another to act on the person's behalf.

principle: Fundamental truth or belief.

probable signs of pregnancy: Evidence of the likelihood of pregnancy including enlarged abdomen, Goodell's sign, Hegar's sign, Braxton Hicks sign, and positive hormonal tests of pregnancy.

prodromal: An early sign or warning of a disease (e.g., rash).

progesterone: Hormone produced by corpus luteum and placenta to prepare the uterus for implantation of the fertilized egg, and maintain the pregnancy.

progressive relaxation: Strategy of relaxing groups of muscles by concentrating on specific areas at a time.

projection: Attributing one's own feeling to another.

prolactin: A pituitary hormone that stimulates milk production.

prolapsed cord: When the umbilical cord precedes the presenting part into the vagina.

prophylactic: Prevention of disease or condition; a condom or "rubber."

proscription: Forbidden or taboo.

prostaglandin (PG): Substance with a role in many reproductive tract functions, used to induce abortions and cervical ripening for labor induction.

prostate specific antigen (PSA): Blood test screen for abnormal prostate condition.

proteinuria: Presence of large amounts of protein in urine.

proximodistal: Process of developmental direction from the center outward.

pseudocyesis: Conversion reaction of appearing to be pregnant without actually being so.

psychoanalysis: Service provided by psychiatrist to explore the complexity of an individual's psychological construct.

psychomotor: Referring to motor skills (fine and gross) to perform a skill.

psychoneuroimmunology: Study of the relationship between the central nervous system, autonomic nervous system, the endocrine system, the immune system, and psychiatry.

psychoprophylaxis: Mental and physical preparation for childbirth to minimize fear and pain and to promote positive family relationships.

psychosomatic: Psychological influence on physical conditions.

ptyalism: Excessive salivation.

puberty: Period in human development when the reproductive organs mature and one is able to reproduce.

pubic: Pertaining to the pubis.

pubis: Pubis bone at the front of the pelvis.

pudendal block: Numbness of the genital and perianal region produced by injection of anesthetic agent into the pudendal nerve root.

puerperal infection: Infection of reproductive organs in association with childbirth; also known as childbed fever.

puerperium: Time period from just after birth to 6 weeks after birth or until involution of the uterus is complete.

pulmonary artery catheter (PAC): A flow-directed, balloon-tipped multilumen catheter that is inserted into the pulmonary artery and measures pulmonary artery pressure continuously; also called Swan-Ganz catheter.

pulmonary artery pressure (PAP): Systolic and diastolic pressures in the pulmonary artery that reflects right afterload.

pulmonary capillary wedge pressure (PCWP): Catheter positioned in the pulmonary artery so it floats into a wedge position; measurement reflects left atrial pressure and, if the mitral valve is competent, also indicates left ventricular end-diastolic pressure. Elevated pressures found in congestive heart failure or fluid overload.

pulmonary edema: Accumulation of fluid in lung associated with left-sided heart failure.

pulmonary emboli: Blockage of pulmonary artery by foreign substance.

pulmonary vascular resistance: A measure for the tension required to eject blood from the right ventricle into the circulatory system.

pulse oximetry: Noninvasive measure of oxygenation. Sensor typically is applied on one ear lobe or finger.

pursed-lip breathing: Exhaling through mostly closed lips in an effort to control respiratory distress typically associated with chronic obstructive pulmonary disease.

pyromania: Impulse to set fires.

pyrosis: A burning sensation (heartburn) in the epigastric and sternal region usually caused by stomach acid.

quadrigeminal: Fourfold, or in four parts, such as the heart.

quadrilateral: Having four sides.

quadriplegia (QUAD): Paralysis of all four extremities.

qualitative: Subjective elements; **qualitative research:** Methods that consider the unique properties of a natural setting without a reliance on quantitative data.

quality improvement (QI): Continuous improvement of performance; sometimes referred to as continuous quality improvement, or CQI.

quality of care: Providing the optimal care in any practice setting.

quality of life: The degree of satisfaction that an individual has regarding a particular style of life. Concept defined by an individual's perceptions of overall satisfaction with his or her living circumstances, including physical status and abilities, psychological well-being, social interactions, and economic conditions; the degree of satisfaction that an individual has regarding a particular style of life.

quantitative: Methods that concern measurements.

quantum: As in the quantum theory, a fixed elemental unit, as of energy, angular momentum, and other physical properties of physics.

quickening: The sensation of fetal movement, usually initially occurring between 16 and 20 weeks gestation.

race: Group of people united or classified together on the basis of common history, nationality, or geographical distribution.

rachitis: Inflammation of the spinal column due to vitamin D deficiency.

radical mastectomy: Removal of the entire breast and lymph nodes.

radicular: Pertaining to a radical or root. Commonly associated with a nerve root.

radiographic anatomy: The study of the structures of the body using X-rays.

radiography: Commonly referred to as an X-ray.

radioimmunoassay: A method of determining the concentration of a substance; for example, in pregnancy tests, human chorionic gonadotropin is identified using radioactively labeled markers.

rale: *See* crackle.

ramus: A branch; used in anatomical nomenclature as a general term to designate a smaller structure given off by a larger one, such as a blood vessel or a nerve.

randomization: Process of assigning participants or objects to a control or experimental group on a random basis.

random practice: Tasks practiced in a mixed order.

range of motion (ROM): Moving body parts through an arc; path of motion a joint can move in any one direction, measured in degrees.

rape: Power exerted through sexual violence; an act of aggression, not an act of passion.

rape–trauma syndrome: Characteristic symptoms seen in rape victims, not unlike those seen in post-traumatic stress disorder, such as horrifying memories, recurring fears, and feelings of helplessness.

rapid eye movement (REM): Sleep state in which brain waves show an active pattern; dreaming is occurring. Thought to be important for adequate rest, repair, immunity, and health.

rapport: Harmonious relationship between people.

rapid plasma reagin (RPR): A test for syphilis.

rationalization: Justifying unacceptable behaviors or feelings by making excuses or creating reasons for the behaviors or feelings.

raw score: Unadjusted score derived from observations of performance; frequently, the arithmetic sum of a subject's responses.

reaction formation: Exaggerating thoughts and behaviors opposite of the unacceptable or undesirable ones.

reaction time (RT): The interval between the application of a stimulus and the detection of a response. The time required to initiate a movement following stimulus presentation.

reactive hyperemia: Extra blood in vessels in response to a period of blocked blood flow.

reality orientation: Therapeutic technique often used with confused or disoriented clients. Includes group techniques to remind the client of facts, as well as a patterned environment, which provides memory cues.

reappraisal: In coping, reconsideration of a harm, threat, or loss episode after an initial appraisal has taken place. Thought that individuals constantly reassess the stressful episode and their resources and alternatives for dealing with it.

reasoning: The use of one's ability to think and draw conclusions, motives, causes, or justifications, which will form the basis of actions.

rebound phenomenon: Sudden withdrawal causing worsening of a condition or reflexive response.

recency effect: Tendency for an individual to remember the last items of a list better than those in the middle.

receptive aphasia: The inability to comprehend normal speech.

receptive field: Receptor area served by one neuron.

receptor: Specific site at which a drug acts through forming a chemical bond.

recessive trait: Genetically determined characteristic that comes from a recessive gene, one that is not dominant.

recidivism: Relapse to a former state. Noncompliance.

reciprocal: Present or existing on both sides expressing mutual, corresponding, or complementary action.

reciprocal inhibition/counterconditioning: Technique to decrease or eliminate behavior by substituting a more acceptable one.

recognition: A recognizing or being recognized as an object, person, accomplishment, or place. Identification of a person, place, or object.

recommended dietary allowances (RDA): National standards for levels of intake of specific vitamins and minerals on a daily basis.

reconditioning: Restoration to good physical and mental condition.

rectocele: Herniation of the rectum with protrusion into the vaginal canal, or prolapse of the rectum onto the perineum.

reduction: Realignment of a dislocated bone to its original position.

reductionistic: An approach to understanding in which the problem is broken into parts, and the parts are viewed and managed separately.

reexamination: The process by which patient/client status is updated following the initial examination (because of new clinical indications, failure to respond to interventions, or failure to establish progress from baseline data).

referral: A recommendation that a patient/client seek service from another health care provider or resource.

referred pain: Visceral pain felt in a somatic area away from the actual source of pain.

reflex: Eliciting an involuntary muscle response by sensory input; subconscious, involuntary reaction to an external stimulus.

reflex bradycardia: Slowing of the heart in response to a specific stimuli.

reflex incontinence: A form of incontinence caused by the inability to inhibit bladder stimulatory reflexes.

reflux: Backflow of any substance (e.g., urine from bladder to ureters or food returning to the esophagus from the stomach).

refractive error: Nearsightedness (i.e., myopia), farsightedness (i.e., hyperopia), astigmatism, or presbyopia. All improved with corrective lenses.

reframing: Changing the context or viewpoint of a situation by placing it in a different perspective to change its entire meaning so that the consequences of behavior are different.

regional anesthesia: The injection of local anesthetic to block a group of nerve fibers that innervate a certain area of the body.

regression: A retreat or backward movement in conditions, signs, and symptoms; **regression analysis:** Statistical method where mean of variable(s) is predicted conditioned on other variable(s).

regurgitate: Spitting up or vomiting of solids or liquids.

rehabilitation: Helping individuals regain skills and abilities that have been lost as a result of illness, injury, disease, disorder, or incarceration. The restoration of a disabled individual to maximum independence commensurate with his or her limitations.

reinforcement: Desired outcome of behavior. In behavior therapy, reinforcement provided to encourage specific activities; strengthened by fear of punishment or anticipation of reward.

relaxation: Techniques that decrease mental, physical, and emotional tension by quieting the mind and body.

relaxation techniques: A cognitive treatment technique that addresses muscle tension accompanying pain such as biofeedback; systematic relaxation exercises used in prepared childbirth.

relaxin: A polypeptide ovarian hormone secreted by the corpus luteum that possibly acts on the ligamentous structures of the body, slackening the ligaments to allow greater opening in the pelvic outlet.

release phenomenon: Ongoing action of one part of the central nervous system without modulation from a complementary functional component.

reliability: Predictability of an outcome regardless of observer. In diagnosis, refers to the probability that several therapists will apply the same label to a given individual.

religiosity: Intense focusing on religious behaviors and ideas, common to schizophrenia.

reminiscence effect: Tendency for the recall of an item to improve for a short period of time after initial learning before being forgotten.

reminiscence therapy: Strategy to help individuals celebrate past experiences to gain insight into the value of their life.

remission: Lessening in severity or abatement of symptoms of a disease.

renin: An enzyme secreted by the kidneys that converts angiotensinogen into angiotensin.

repression: Involuntary blocking of uncomfortable feelings from one's level of awareness.

reprimand: Expression of disapproval of conduct.

research: Systematic investigation, including development, testing, and evaluation design.

residual urine: The urine remaining in the bladder after normal urination (patients may be catheterized to determine residual urine).

resistance: Amount of weight to be moved.

resistance exercise training: Exercise that applies sufficient force to muscle groups to improve muscle strength.

resonance: The prolongation and intensification of sound produced by the transmission of its vibrations to a cavity, especially a sound elicited by percussion. Decrease in resonance is dullness; absence of resonance is flatness.

respiration: The act or process of breathing; inhaling and exhaling air. The process by which a living organism or cell takes in oxygen from the air or water, distributes and utilizes it in oxidation, and gives off products of oxidation, especially carbon dioxide.

respiratory distress syndrome (RDS): Condition resulting from decreased pulmonary gas exchange, retention of carbon dioxide and increase in PCO_2, commonly seen in premature infants with immature lungs/hyaline membrane disease (HMD).

respiratory exchange ratio (CO_2/VO_2): The ratio of the volume of carbon dioxide expired and the oxygen consumed.

respiratory failure: Failure of the pulmonary system in which inadequate exchange of carbon dioxide and oxygen occurs between an organism and its environment.

respite care: Short-term health services to the dependent adult, either at home or in an institutional setting.

restitution: The turning of the fetal head after it emerges from the introitus and assumes a normal alignment with the shoulders (*see* diagrams). Also a return to a prior state.

restraints: Devices used to aid in immobilization of patients.

rest/relaxation: Performance during time not devoted to other activity and during time devoted to sleep.

resuscitation: Restoration of consciousness or life in one whose respirations or cardiac function (or both) have ceased.

retained placenta: Retention in the uterus of parts or all of the placenta after birth of the infant.

retardation: Slowed, especially as in mental capacity.

retention: Keeping in the body materials or fluids which are normally excreted such as urine or feces; also keeping information cognitively.

reticulospinal tract: Pathway that supports action of the flexors and extensors of the neck for postural control.

retinal detachment: Condition of retina separating from the choroids of the eye. Without immediate treatment may result in blindness.

retinopathy of prematurity (ROP): Eye injury or blindness in premature infants associated with too intense a concentration of oxygen.

retraction: The process by which muscle remains slightly shortened after a contraction of the muscle; the drawing in of soft tissues of the chest or a straining indicative of an obstruction someplace in the respiratory tract.

retrograde amnesia: The inability to recall events that have occurred during the period immediately preceding a brain injury.

retrolental fibroplasia (RLF): *See* retinopathy of prematurity.

retrospective memory: Remembering information that occurred in the past.

retroversion of the uterus: The body of the uterus is tipped back while the cervix is pointing forward toward the symphysis pubis.

retroviruses: A group of ribonucleic acid (RNA) viruses causing a variety of diseases in humans and which have RNA as their genetic code and are capable of copying RNA and deoxyribonucleic acid and incorporating them into an infected cell.

Rh factor: Hereditary blood factor found in red blood cells determined by specialized blood tests; when present, a person is Rh positive; when absent, a person is Rh negative.

Rh immune globulin (RhG): Gamma globulin containing Rh antibodies; administration of this immune globulin to Rh negative mothers prevents sensitization by exposure to any Rh positive blood cells, usually from the fetus.

rheumatic heart disease: Damage to the heart muscle and valves as a result of rheumatic fever.

rheumatoid arthritis (RA): Chronic disease resulting in inflammation, swelling, and joint deformity.

rhizotomy: A neurosurgical intervention at the level of the caudal equinus, or the lumbar level of the spine, to interrupt abnormal sensory feedback that appears to maintain hypertonus.

rhonchus: A snoring sound; a rattling in the throat; also a dry, coarse rale in the bronchial tubes due to a partial obstruction.

rhythm method: A method of preventing pregnancy involving abstinence from sexual intercourse during the ovulatory phase of the menstrual cycle; commonly known as the calendar method.

ribonucleic acid (RNA): Basic genetic material in which a nucleic acid is associated with the control of chemical activities within a cell.

riboflavin: B vitamin that breaks down carbohydrates, fats, and proteins.

right: That to which an individual is entitled.

right to die: A person's right to die on his or her terms.

rigidity: Hypertonicity of agonist and antagonist that offers a constant, uniform resistance to passive movement. The affected muscles seem unable to relax and are in a state of contraction even at rest.

risk factors: Factors that cause a person or group of people to be particularly vulnerable to an unwanted, unpleasant, or unhealthy event.

rite of passage: Significant life event and celebration as a person moves from one developmental level to the next.

Ritgen maneuver: Procedure used to control the birth of the fetal head and avoid lacerations of the mother's birth canal.

ritualistic behavior: Repetitive, purposeless activities, usually associated with desire to decrease anxiety, as in obsession-compulsion behaviors.

robotics: Science of mechanical devices that work automatically or by remote control.

roentgenogram: An X-ray. A film produced by roentgenography.

Rolfing: Technique of massage and deep muscular manipulation designed to realign the body with gravity; structured integration.

Romberg's sign: The inability to maintain body balance when the eyes open and then close with the feet close together; unsteadiness when eyes are closed indicates a loss of proprioceptive control.

rooming-in unit: Postpartum area designed so that the mother and baby remain together, as opposed to mother's room and the baby in a nursery down the hall.

rooting reflex: This normal reflex in infants up to 4 months of age consists of head turning in the direction of the stimulus when the cheek is stroked gently.

rotation: Movement around the long axis of a limb; in obstetrics, the turning of the fetal head as it moves through the birth canal.

rotator cuff: The muscle complex of the shoulder that provides stability of the glenohumeral joint inclusive of the supraspinatus, infraspinatus, teres minor, and subscapularis muscles.

rotavirus: A group of viruses that cause dehydrating diarrhea in children.

rote: Habit performance without meaning.

round ligament: A pair of ligaments that hold the uterus in place, extending laterally from the fundus between the folds of the broad ligaments to the lateral pelvic wall, terminating in the labia majora.

rubella vaccine: Live attenuated rubella virus given to form antibodies and produce active immunity. Rubella infections in pregnant women produce defects in the developing fetus.

rugae: Skin folds in the vaginal mucosa or the scrotum.

rumination: Repetitive chewing of food; regurgitated after ingestion.

rupture: A bursting or the state of being broken apart.

saccadic eye movement: Extremely fast voluntary movement of the eyes, allowing the eyes to accurately fix on a still object in the visual field as the person moves or the head turns.

saccadic fixation: A rapid change of fixation from one point in a visual field to another.

saccule: Organ in the inner ear that transmits information about linear movement in relation to gravity.

sacroiliac: Pertaining to the sacrum and iliac crest.

sacrum: A triangular bone situated between L5 and the coccyx, composed of five vertebrae and creating the posterior portion of the true pelvis.

sadism: Sexual stimulation resulting from demeaning behavior to others.

safe house: Place for protection of battered women and their children.

safe period: Days of the menstrual cycle which fall on either side of the period of ovulation and are considered "safe" for sexual relations while avoiding pregnancy.

safe sex: Use of barrier protection whenever relations include exchange of body fluid, semen, blood, or vaginal secretions.

sagittal plane: Runs from front to back, dividing the body into left and right segments.

sagittal suture: Connective tissue between the parietal bones and extending from the anterior to the posterior fontanel.

salpingo-oophorectomy: Excision of an ovary and fallopian tube.

sandwich generation: Adults who have caregiving responsibilities for their dependent children and their aging parents.

sarcoidosis: A disorder that may affect any part of the body but most frequently involves the lymph nodes, liver, spleen, lungs, eyes, and small bones of the hands and feet; characterized by the presence in all affected organs or tissues of epithelioid cell tubercles, without caseation, and with little or no round-cell reaction, becoming converted, in the older lesions, into a rather hyaline featureless fibrous tissue.

sarcoma: Malignant tissue that originates in connective tissue and spreads through the bloodstream, often attacking bones.

scab: Dried exudate covering superficial wounds.

scapegoat: A symbolic person or thing blamed for other problems.

scapula: Flattened, triangular bone found on the posterior aspect of the body.

schemata: Basic units of all knowledge.

schemes: Structural elements of cognition; plans, designs, or programs to be followed.

schizophrenia: Pervasive psychosis that affects a variety of psychological processes involving cognition, affect, and behavior and is characterized by hallucinations, delusions, bizarre behavior, and illogical thinking.

Schultze's mechanism: Delivery of the placenta with the shiny (fetal) surface presenting first.

sciatica: Nerve inflammation characterized by sharp pains along the sciatic nerve and its branches; area extends from the hip down the back of the thigh and surrounding parts.

scissors gait: Gait in which the legs cross the midline upon advancement.

scleroderma: Disease characterized by chronic hardening and shrinking of the connective tissue of any organ in the body.

scoliosis: Abnormal lateral curvature of the spine. Usually consists of two curves, the original abnormal curve and a compensatory curve in the opposite direction.

screening: The process of examining a population, usually a high risk population, for a given state or disease.

scrotum: Sac containing the testes and parts of the spermatic cords.

seasonal affective disorder (SAD): Mood disorder associated with shorter days and longer nights of autumn and winter. Symptoms include lethargy, depression, social withdrawal, and work difficulties.

seborrhea: Disease of the sebaceous glands marked by the increase in amount and quality of their secretions.

second stage of labor: Includes the time from 10 cm of dilation until the birth of the baby.

secondary aging: Changes in physical functioning, as a result of aging, that are not universal or inevitable but are commonly shared by humans as a result of environmental conditions or circumstances.

secondary care: Intervention provided once a disease state has been identified (e.g., treating hypertension).

secondary conditions: Also called secondary disabilities. Pathology, impairment, or functional limitations derived from the primary condition.

secondary prevention: Efforts directed at populations who are considered at risk by early detection of potential health problems, followed by the interventions to halt, reverse, or at least slow the progression of that condition.

secretion: The process of elaborating a specific product as a result of the activity of a gland. This activity may range from separating a specific substance of the blood to the elaboration of a new chemical substance.

secretory phase of menstrual cycle: Postovulatory or premenstrual phase of the menstrual cycle (14 days in length).

secundines: Afterbirth including fetal membranes and placenta.

seizure disorders: Presence of abrupt irrepressible episodes of electrical hyperactivity in the brain.

selected abstraction: Thinking based on conclusions being made on only one portion of information.

self-actualization: Process of striving to achieve one's ultimate potential in life with accompanying feelings of accomplishment and personal growth.

self-care: The set of activities that make up daily living, such as bed mobility, transfers, ambulation, dressing, grooming, bathing, eating, and toileting.

self-concept: Developing the value of the physical, emotional, and sexual self; view one has of oneself (e.g., ideas, feelings, attitudes, identity, worth, capabilities, and limitations).

self-control: The ability to control one's behaviors. Modifying one's own behavior in response to environmental needs, demands, constraints, personal aspirations, and feedback from others.

self-deprecator: Type of person who seeks praise by devaluing him- or herself; successful "attention getter" initially, but fails over the longer term when other group members become aware of circumstances.

self-determination: Process of making one's own choices.

self-efficacy: An individual's belief that he or she is capable of successfully performing a certain set of behaviors.

self-esteem: An individual's overall feeling of worth.

self-expectancy: The part of one's identify that is that person's view of what he/she wants to be or do.

self-expression: An individual's ability to make his or her thoughts and feelings known. Using a variety of styles and skills to express thoughts, feelings, and needs.

self-fulfilling prophecy: A principle that refers to a belief in or the expectation of a particular outcome as a factor that contributes to its fulfillment.

self-help: Various methods by which individuals attempt to remedy their difficulties without making use of formal care providers (e.g., Alcoholics Anonymous).

self-identity skill: The ability to perceive one's self as holistic and autonomous and to have permanence and continuity over time.

self-image: Internalized view a person holds of him- or herself that usually varies with changing social situations over one's life span.

self-monitoring: Process whereby the client notes specific behaviors or thoughts as they occur.

self-report: Type of assessment approach in which the individual reports on his or her level of function or performance.

semantic memory: Memory for general knowledge.

semantics: The study of language with special attention to the meanings of words and other symbols.

semen: The fluid containing sperm.

semen analysis: In infertility work up, the examination of fluid to determine liquefaction, normal morphology, pH, sperm density, and volume.

semi-autonomous: Individual is partially dependent upon another for the satisfaction of needs.

semicircular canal: Organ in the inner ear that transmits information about head position.

senescence: Aging; growing older. The process or condition of growing old.

senile dementia: An organic mental disorder resulting from generalized atrophy of the brain with no evidence of cerebrovascular disease.

senile plaque: *See* neuritic plaque.

sensation: Receiving conscious sensory impressions through direct stimulation of the body, such as hearing, seeing, touching, etc.

sense of control: Perception of being able to direct and regulate.

sense of security: Feeling of comfort in being able to trust and know that there is predictability in the environment.

sensitivity: Capacity to feel, transmit, and react to a stimulus; rating of how well changes will be measured on subsequent tests to show improvement.

sensitivity to stimuli: Responding in a hyperactive manner due to low thresholds.

sensitization: An acquired reaction; the process of a receptor becoming more susceptible to a given stimulus.

sensory: Having to do with sensations or the senses; including peripheral sensory processing (e.g., sensitivity to touch) and cortical sensory processing (e.g., two-point and sharp/dull discrimination).

sensory behavior: Related to the five senses, indicating a readiness for social interaction.

sensory deprivation: An involuntary loss of physical awareness caused by detachment from external sensory stimuli which can result in psychological disturbances. An enforced absence of the usual repertoire of sensory stimuli producing severe mental changes, including hallucinations, anxiety, depression, and insanity.

sensory impairment: Decrease in functioning of one of the five basic senses.

sensory neuron: Nerve cell that sends signals to the spinal cord or brain.

sensory or body disregard: Condition characterized by lack of awareness of one side of the body.

sensory processing: The brain's ability to receive information and respond appropriately by interpreting sensory stimuli.

sepsis: Poisoning that is caused by the products of a putrefactive process. Infection of the bloodstream.

septic abortion: *See* abortion, septic.

septicemia: Systemic disease associated with the presence and persistence of pathogenic microorganisms or toxins in the blood.

sequela: Morbid condition resulting from another condition or event.

sequencing: Putting things in order. The ability to accomplish a task in a logistical manner by placing information, concepts, and actions in order.

sequestrum: Fragment of necrosed bone that has become separated from the surrounding tissue.

seroconversion: Detection of antibodies in blood in response to disease or vaccination.

serology: The study of blood serum.

serous: Producing a serous secretion or containing serum.

set: A belief or expectation one has about a person, place, or thing.

severe retardation: Within an IQ range of 20 to 34.

sex chromosome: The X (female) and Y (male) chromosomes associated with gender identification; the normal female has two X chromosomes and the normal male has one X and one Y chromosome.

sex identification: Assigning of a masculine or feminine connotation to a given activity.

sexual history: Information collected regarding health conditions, lifestyle behaviors, knowledge, and attitudes related to sex and sexuality.

sexual response cycle: The phases of physical changes and response to sexual stimulation and tension release.

sexuality: The behaviors that relate psychological, cultural, emotional, and physical responses to the need to reproduce.

sexually transmitted disease (STD): A contagious disease usually acquired by sexual intercourse or genital contact.

shaken baby syndrome: A condition of whiplash-type injuries, ranging from bruises on the arms and trunk to retinal hemorrhages or convulsions, as observed in infants and children who have been violently shaken; a form of child abuse that often results in intracranial bleeding from tearing of cerebral blood vessels.

shake test: A "foam" test for lung maturity in the fetus.

shaman: Native American healer; medicine man.

shaping: Learning based on reinforcement in increasing proximity to desired behavior.

shear: Pressure exerted against the surface and layers of the skin as tissues slide in opposite but parallel planes. Trauma caused by tissue layers sliding against each other; results in disruption or angulation of blood vessels.

Sheehan syndrome: Postpartum necrosis of the pituitary gland as a result of DIC (disseminated intravascular coagulation) or hypovolemic shock.

sheltered housing: Living arrangements that provide structure and supervision for individuals who do not require institutionalization but are not fully capable of independent living (e.g., group homes).

shingles: Viral disease of the peripheral nerves with the eruption of skin vesicles along the path of the nerve.

shock therapy: Induced by delivering an electric current through the brain; a procedure used for treating depression.

short-term memory: Limited capacity memory store that holds information for a brief period of time; the so-called "working memory."

shoulder dystocia: Occurs during delivery when the presenting part in the pelvic inlet is the fetal shoulder, thereby arresting normal progression of labor.

shoulder separation: Separation of the acromioclavicular joint due to trauma, injury, or disease.

shoulder subluxation: Incomplete downward, usually partial, dislocation of the humerus out of the glenohumeral joint caused by weakness, stretch, or abnormal tone in the scapulohumeral and/or scapular muscles.

show: Refers to the blood and mucous plug that is extruded from the vagina in early labor.

shunt: Passage between two natural channels, especially blood vessels.

sibling rivalry: Brothers and sisters exhibiting negative behaviors toward a new baby or each other.

sickle-cell hemoglobinopathy: Abnormal crescent-shaped red blood corpuscles found in the blood.

side effect: Other than the desired action (e.g., effect produced by a medication).

sigmoidoscopy: Examination of lower colon using a lighted instrument.

sign: Clinically noted as the objective findings associated with an illness or dysfunction. Objective evidence of physical abnormality.

signage: Displayed verbal, symbolic, tactile, or pictorial information.

silent killer: High blood pressure because it is often asymptomatic.

Sim's position: Patient lies on the left side with the right knee and thigh drawn upward toward the chest.

simple fracture: Bone is broken internally but does not pierce the skin so that it can be seen.

simple reflex: Reflex with a motor nerve component that involves only one muscle.

single-parent family: Family in which there is only one parent (either male or female) with the children. A result of death, divorce, separation, desertion, or birth or adoption of a child to a single parent.

single room maternity care (SRMC): All care given to mother and infant during the hospital birthing stay (labor, delivery, recovery, and postpartum), occurs in the same room and often provided by the same caregiver (also known as LDRP).

singleton: A single fetus.

sitz bath: Sitting in a bath of warm water to obtain moist heat to the perineum.

skeletal demineralization: The loss of bone mass due to loss of minerals from the bone as seen in conditions such as osteoporosis.

skeletal system: Supporting framework for the body that comprises the axial and appendicular divisions.

skilled nursing facility (SNF): Institution or part of an institution that meets criteria for accreditation established by the sections of the Social Security Act that determine the basis for Medicaid and Medicare reimbursement. Provides care that must be rendered by or under the supervision of professional personnel such as a registered nurse. Requirements include care must be required daily and must be a continuation of the care begun in the hospital.

skin: The largest body organ. *See* dermal.

skin fold measurement: Method for estimating percentage of body fat by measuring subcutaneous fat with skin fold calipers.

slander: Oral sharing of information detrimental to a person's reputation.

sleep apnea: Disorder characterized by period of an absence of attempts to breathe; the person is momentarily unable to move respiratory muscles or maintain air flow through his or her nose and mouth.

sleep paralysis: Temporary inability to talk or move when falling asleep or waking up.

sleep-wake cycle: Differing states of newborn consciousness.

slough: Loose, stringy, necrotic tissue.

small for gestational age (SGA): Inadequate weight gain for gestational age in newborns.

smegma: White secretion of the labia minora and under the foreskin of the penis.

Smoking index: pack/day, number of years; estimates are 5–11 minutes of life lost for every cigarette smoked.

SOAP (e, er) (subjective, objective, and assessment plan, and evaluation or evaluation and reassessment): The parts of a written account of a health problem.

social: Having to do with human beings living together as a group in a situation in which their dealings with one another affect their common welfare.

social age: Definition of age emphasizing the functional level of social interaction skills rather than calendar time.

social distance: Cultural space acceptable in interaction among people in social settings. US standard is 4 to 12 feet.

social identity theory: Social psychologist Henry Taifel's theory that when individuals are assigned to a group, they invariably think of that group as an in-group for them. Occurs because individuals want to have a positive image.

social indicators: An approach to needs assessment that examines data from public records: census, county health department, police records, and housing offices.

socialization: Accessing opportunities and interacting with other people in appropriate contextual and cultural ways to meet emotional and physical needs. Development of the individual as a social being and a participant in society that results from a continuing, changing interaction between a person and those who attempt to influence him or her.

social learning theory: View of psychologists who emphasize behavior, environment, and cognition as the key factors for development.

social modeling theory: Maintains that learning is accomplished through observing others. A person may learn a behavior or its consequences by watching another person experience that behavior.

social systems: Organized interactions among individuals, as within marriages, families, communities, and organizations, both formal and informal.

sociological aging: Age-specific roles a person adopts within his or her context of society and individual environment. Includes changes of a person's roles and functions and reflected behavior of these changes within society throughout life.

socket: A hollow in a joint into which another part or organ fits such as a bone socket or an eye socket.

soft neurological signs: Mild or slight neurological abnormalities that are difficult to detect.

soft tissue: All neuromusculoskeletal tissues except bone and articular cartilage.

soft tissue integrity: Health of the connective tissue of the body.

soma: Cell body of a nerve that contains the nucleus.

somatic nervous system: Portion of the nervous system composed of a motor division that excites skeletal muscles and a sensory division that receives and processes sensory input from the sense organs.

somatization: Coping by developing physical symptoms.

somatoform disorders: Group of mental disorders characterized by loss or alteration in physical functioning, for which there is no physiological explanation; evidence that psychological factors have caused the physical symptoms; lack of voluntary control over physical symptoms; and indifference by the patient to the physical loss.

somatosensory evoked potential (SEP): Peripheral nerve stimulation produces potentials that can be recorded from the scalp, over the spine, or the periphery.

somatotopic: Organization of cells in the somatosensory system that enables one to identify the exact skin surface touched.

somnolence: Sleepiness or drowsiness characterized by excitability or disorientation.

sonogram: *See* ultrasound.

soufflé: A murmur or soft blowing sound heard by auscultation; **funic soufflé:** Sound produced by blood rushing through the umbilical vessels and is synchronous with FHTs; **placental soufflé:** Murmur caused by the placental blood current and is synchronous with the maternal pulse; **uterine soufflé:** Sound made by the blood in the arteries of the pregnant uterus and synchronous with the maternal pulse.

spasm: An involuntary muscle contraction.

spastic gait: Stiff movement, toes drag, legs are together, and hip and knee joints are slightly flexed.

spasticity: A result of an upper motor neuron lesion in either the spinal cord or brain which causes velocity, dependent increased muscle tone, exaggerated tendon jerks, and clonus.

spatial awareness: The ability to orient oneself in space, visualize what an object looks like from all angles, know from where sounds are coming, and know where body parts are in space.

spatial relations: Determining the position of objects relative to each other; the ability to perceive the self in relation to other objects.

speculum: An instrument used to hold open or dilate an orifice such as the vagina or nares during inspection.

speech: The meaningful production and sequencing of sounds by the speech sensorimotor system (i.e., lips, tongue, etc.) for the transmission of spoken language.

sperm: Male sex cell.

spermatogenesis: Process by which mature spermatozoa are formed.

spermicide: Chemical substance that kills sperm.

sphygmomanometer: Instrument used to measure arterial blood pressure indirectly.

spina bifida cystica: A lack of union of the laminae and the vertebrae causing a congenital defect that can result in urinary incontinence, limb anesthesia, gait disturbances, and structural changes in the pelvis.

spina bifida occulta: Congenital anomaly of the spine in which a portion of the vertebrae fails to close but without herniation or the spinal cord or meninges through the defect. Often only a dimple seen at the site.

spinal: An injection of anesthesia into the spinal fluid to produce numbness.

spinal fusion: Joining together spinal vertebrae to prevent damage to the bones or spinal cord from disease processes.

spinal nerve: The nerve extending from the spinal cord.

spinocerebellar tracts: Dorsal tract consisting of the afferent ipsilateral ascending tract to the cerebellum, serving most lower extremities for touch, pressure, and proprioception. The ventral tract consisting of the afferent contralateral ascending tract to the cerebellum serving lower extremities for proprioception.

spinothalamic tract: Afferent contralateral and ipsilateral ascending tract to the thalamus for sensation of pain, temperature, and light touch; also known as the anterolateral system (ALS).

spiritual: Nonphysical and nonmaterial aspect of existence that contributes insight into the nature and meaning of a person's life.

spirometry: The measurement of air inspired and expired.

splanchnic engorgement: Excessive pooling of blood within the visceral vasculature occurring after removal of pressure from the abdomen in such instances as birth of a baby, removal of excess urine, or a large tumor.

splint: Supportive device used to immobilize, fix, or prevent deformities or assist in motion.

splitting: Defense mechanism of splitting the world into two types of people: good or bad. Common in borderline personality disorder.

spondylitis: Inflammation of the vertebrae.

spondylolisthesis: Forward displacement of one vertebra over another, usually of the fifth lumbar vertebra over the body of the sacrum or the fourth lumbar over the fifth.

spontaneous abortion: *See* abortion, spontaneous.

spontaneous remission: Unusual occurrence (e.g., when cancer cells revert to normal without aid or apparent cause).

spontaneous rupture of membranes (SROM): Natural rupture of membranes.

sprain: Injury to a joint that causes pain and disability, with the severity depending on the degree of injury to ligaments or tendons.

sputum: Substance expelled by coughing or clearing the throat. Matter ejected from the lungs, bronchi, and trachea through the mouth.

squamocolumnar junction: Site for collection of cells for Pap smear; juncture in endocervical canal where columnar epithelium and squamous epithelium meet.

squamous intraepithelial lesion (SIL): Neoplastic changes of the cervix.

stabilizer: Equipment or device used to maintain a particular position.

staging: Classification of tumors by their spread through the body.

standard assessment: Tests and evaluation approaches with specific norms, standards, and protocol.

standard deviation: Mathematically determined value used to derive standard scores and compare raw scores to a unit normal distribution.

standard error: Amount by which a score might vary in different measurements.

standard precautions: Centers for Disease Control and Prevention guidelines to reduce risk of spread of organisms through body fluids. *See* Reminder Section.

standard scores: Raw scores mathematically converted to a scale that facilitates comparison.

stasis: Stagnation of blood caused by venous congestion.

state-related behaviors: Varying behavioral responses dependent on state of the patient/client.

static equilibrium: The ability of an individual to adjust to displacements of his or her center of gravity while maintaining a constant base of support.

static flexibility: Range of motion in degrees that a joint will allow.

statics: The study of objects at rest.

static splint: Rigid orthosis used for the prevention of movement of a joint or for the fixation of a displaced part.

station: Relationship of the presenting part of the fetus to an imaginary line drawn through the pelvic ischial spines.

statutory rape: Illegal intercourse between a man (older than 16 years) and a female under age of consent.

stature: Height of body in upright position.

steatorrhea: Fatty stools, seen in pancreatic diseases; increased secretion of the sebaceous glands.

stenosis: A narrowing of any canal (e.g., spinal stenosis denoting a state of decreased diameter of the spinal canal and the intervertebral foramen).

stent: Any material used to hold in place or to provide a support for a graft or anastomosis while healing takes place; to maintain open blood vessels.

step test: Graded exercise test in which a person is required to rhythmically step up and down steps of gradually increasing heights.

sterility: Free from living organisms; inability to produce children.

stereognosis: Identifying objects through proprioception, cognition, and the sense of touch; the ability to identify common objects by touch with vision occluded.

stereopsis: Quality of visual fusion.

stereotypic behavior: Repeated, persistent postures or movements, including vocalizations.

stereotyping: Applying generalized and oversimplified labels of characteristics, actions, or attitudes to a specific socioeconomic, cultural, religious, or ethnic group. Often used to belittle or discount a particular group.

stertorous: Respiratory effort that is strenuous and struggling; sounds like snoring.

stethoscope: Instrument used to listen to heart and lung sounds.

stigma: An undesirable difference that becomes a basis for separating an individual bearing such traits from the rest of society.

stillbirth: Refers to the birth of a baby who has died in utero.

stimulation: Arousal of attention, interest, or tension.

stimulus–arousal properties: Alerting potential of various sensory stimuli, generally thought to be related to their intensity, pace, and novelty.

storage fat: Adipose tissue found primarily subcutaneously and surrounding the major organs.

strabismus: Oculomotor misalignment of one eye.

strain: Usually a muscular injury caused by the excessive physical effort that leads to a forcible stretch. Refers to the percent change in original length of a deformed tissue.

streptokinase: An enzyme produced by streptococci that catalyzes the conversion of plasminogen to plasmin.

stress: An individual's general reaction to external demands or stressors. Stress results in psychological as well as physiological reactions; **biomechanical:** The force developed in a deformed tissue divided by the tissue's cross-sectional area.

stress incontinence: A type of urinary incontinence that occurs when the intravesicular pressure exceeds bladder resistance and sphincter activity is weak or absent.

stress management techniques: Methods of relieving or controlling chronic stress by interrupting reflexive neurologic stress reactions.

stressors: External events that place demands on an individual above the ordinary.

striae gravidarum: Stretch marks appearing on the distended skin caused by the rupture of elastic fibers due to excessive distention; often found in pregnant women.

stridor: A harsh, high-pitched respiratory sound, such as the inspiratory sound often heard in laryngeal or bronchial obstruction. Sometimes heard through a tracheostomy tube.

strip: A term used in wound care that denotes the removal of epidermis by mechanical means. Synonym: denude.

stripping and ligation: Removal and tying off of a vein.

stroke: Syndrome characterized by a sudden onset in which blood vessels in the brain have become narrowed or blocked. Synonym: cerebrovascular accident.

stroke volume (SV): The amount of blood ejected from the left ventricle on one beat. Maximum stroke volume is highest volume of blood expelled from the heart during a single beat. Usually reached when exercise is only about 40% to 50% of maximum exercise capacity.

structural theory: Dividing of the mind into three structures: the id, the ego, and the superego.

sty, stye: Localized circumscribed inflammatory swelling of one of the sebaceous glands of the eyelid. Synonym: hordeolum.

subacute care: Short-term, comprehensive inpatient level of care provided in places other than the traditional hospital setting.

subcortical: Region beneath the cerebral cortex.

subculture: Ethnic, regional, economic, or social group exhibiting characteristic patterns of behavior sufficient to distinguish it from others within an embracing culture or society. Does not usually include rejection of the larger culture. Most people are members of several subcultures.

subinvolution: Failure of an organ or part to return to its normal size after enlarging or stretching from a normal functional process such as pregnancy.

subjective measure: Assessment designed to identify the client's own view of problems and performance.

sublimation: Rechanneling unacceptable desires into activities that are more acceptable and constructive.

sublingual: Under the tongue.

subluxation: Partial or incomplete dislocation (e.g., shoulder, tempero-mandibular joint).

suboccipitobregmatic diameter: The smallest diameter of the fetal head.

substance abuse: Misuse of a substance to the point it disrupts normal living.

sudomotor: Stimulating the sweat glands.

suffix: Word element of one or more syllables added to the end of a combining form in order to change its meaning.

summative: Evaluation at the conclusion of a program.

sundowning: Condition in which persons tend to become more confused or disoriented at the end of the day.

sunrise syndrome: Condition of unstable cognitive ability on arising in the morning.

superego: In psychoanalytic theory, one of three personality components. Houses one's values, ethics, standards, and conscience; an analytic concept that equates roughly to the conscience.

superficial: Area of the body that is located closest to the surface.

superior: Toward the head or upper portion of a part or structure. Synonym: cephalad.

supination (sup): The act of assuming the supine position. Rotation of the forearm laterally so the palm is facing up toward the ceiling. Applied to the foot, implies movement resulting in raising of the medial margin of the foot, hence of the longitudinal arch, so that the plantar surface of the foot is facing inward.

supine: Lying on the spine with the face up.

supine hypotension: A fall in blood pressure due to pressure on the inferior vena cava; occurs in pregnant women when they lie in the supine position.

support system: People, programs, organizations that provide resources a person needs. Typically in health care, those who provide emotional support or services needed but not available through another source.

supportive devices: External supports to protect weak or ineffective joints or muscles.

suppression: The ability of the central nervous system to screen out certain stimuli so that others may be attended to more carefully.

surfactant: A surface agent that lowers surface tension, given to relieve respiratory distress.

surrogate: A person or thing that replaces another (e.g., substitute parental figure).

symbiotic relationship: Intense connectedness with another person. Normal relationship between infant and mother; otherwise, considered unhealthy.

symbols: Abstract representations of perceived reality.

symmetrical: Equal in size and shape; very similar in relative placement or arrangement about an axis.

sympathetic nervous system: Autonomic nervous system that mobilizes the body's resources during stressful situations.

sympatholytic: An agent that opposes the effects of impulses conveyed by adrenergic postganglionic fibers of the sympathetic nervous system.

sympathomimetic: Mimicking the effects of impulses conveyed by adrenergic postganglionic fibers of the sympathetic nervous system. An agent (e.g., medication) may be used to do this.

sympathy: Actually sharing another's thoughts and behaviors.

symphysis pubis: Fibrocartilaginous connection of the pubic bones in the midline.

symptom (Sx): Subjective indication of a disease or a change in condition as perceived by the individual. Clinically noted as the subjective findings associated with an illness or dysfunction.

symptom management: Controlling the manifestations of the underlying condition.

synapse: Minuscule space that exists between the end of the axon of one nerve cell and the cell body or dendrites of another.

synaptogenesis: The process of forming "synaptic connections" between nerve cells, or between nerve cells and muscle fibers; the basis of neuronal communication.

syncope: Fainting or brief lapse in consciousness caused by transient cerebral hypoxia.

synchrony: Coordinated response or interaction between the one person's cues and another's response.

syndactyly: Webbing of the fingers (or toes) involving only the skin or in complex cases the fusing of adjacent bones. Syndactyly is usually seen in children and can be surgically corrected.

syndrome: Combination of symptoms resulting from a single course or commonly occurring together that they constitute a distinct clinical picture; numerous conditions comprised of such symptoms.

synergism: Action of two or more substances, organs, or organisms to achieve an effect of which each is not individually capable.

synergist: Any muscle that functions to inhibit extraneous action from a muscle that would interfere with the action of a prime mover.

synergy: Action of two or more agents, muscles, or organs working co-operatively and in coordination with each other; acting in harmony with another element/entity.

synovectomy: Excision of the synovial membrane (e.g., as in the knee joint).

syphilis: Sexually transmitted spirochetic (*T. pallidum*) disease resulting in chancre on skin or mucous membranes.

syringomyelia: Chronic progressive degenerative disorder of the spinal cord characterized by the development of an irregular cavity within the spinal cord.

systematic desensitization: Behavioral procedure that uses relaxation paired with an anxiety-provoking stimulus in an attempt to reduce the anxiety response.

systemic: Involving the whole system, such as in systemic rheumatoid arthritis.

systemic analgesia: Analgesics that cross the blood–brain barrier providing central effects; can be administered either IV or IM.

systemic lupus erythematosus (SLE): A chronic inflammatory collagen disease that affects many body systems including renal, nervous, and integumentary.

systemic vascular resistance (SVR): The tension required for the ejection of blood from the left ventricle into the circulatory system.

systems interactions: The ways various systems affect or interact with each other to provide a more integrative and functional system.

systems model: A conceptual representation that incorporates a set of major functional divisions or systems that interlock and interrelate to create the functional whole. Each division may be considered a whole with multiple subsystems interlocking to form its entire division; each major component or division influences and is influenced by all others.

systems model/approach: A cyclical framework for understanding postural control that includes environmental stimuli; sensory reception, perception, and organization; and motor planning, execution, and modification.

systems theory: A theory describing how divisions or systems create a functional whole.

systole: Contraction of the heart, especially of the ventricles, during which blood is forced into the aorta and pulmonary artery. Systolic blood pressure occurs during systole.

T cell: A heterogeneous population of lymphocytes comprising helper/inducer T cells and cytotoxic/suppressor T cells.

T score: Converted standard score in which the mean equals 50 and the standard deviation equals 10.

T-test: Parametric statistical test comparing differences of two data sets.

taboo: Forbidden by society, improper or unacceptable.

tachycardia: Rapid heartbeat.

tachypnea: Excessively rapid respiration marked by quick, shallow breathing.

tacit: Implied understanding that is not verbalized.

tactile: Interpreting light touch, pressure, temperature, pain, and vibration through skin contact/receptors.

tactile fremitus: A thrill or vibration that is perceptible on palpation. A thrill, as in the chest wall, that may be felt by a hand applied to the thorax while the patient is speaking.

taking-hold phase: Period several days after birth when maternal role adoption occurs and a mother becomes more independent, learns infant care skills, and becomes competent in the maternal role.

taking-in: Immediate postpartum period when the mother is very dependent on family and caregivers and is focused inwardly on her own needs. The mother reviewing the birth experience is of paramount importance at this time.

talipes: Deformities of the foot, especially those congenital in origin. Synonym: clubfoot. *See also* equinovarus.

tamponade: Acute compression of the heart due to effusion of fluid into the pericardium or collection of blood in the pericardium from rupture of the heart or a coronary vessel.

tangentiality: Inability to get to point of a story.

tardive dyskinesia: Movements exhibited as antipsychotic side effects. May include tongue, neck, fingers, trunk, and legs.

target pulse rate: The rate calculated as optimal for a person to achieve during exercise.

target site: Desired site for a medication's action within the body.

taxonomy: Laws and principles for classification of living things and organisms; also used for learning objectives.

telangiectatic nevi ("stork bites"): Clusters of small, red, localized areas of capillary dilation that can be found in the necks, lower occiput, upper eyelids, and nasal bridge of neonates.

telecommunication device for the deaf (TDD) or teletypewriter (TTY): Device connected to a telephone by a special adapter that allows telephone communication between a hearing person and a person with impaired hearing.

telehealth: Provision of consultant services by off-site health care professionals to those on the scene using closed-circuit television.

telereceptive: The exteroceptors of hearing, sight, and smell that are sensitive to distant stimuli.

temperament: Inborn personality characteristics influencing behavior.

temporal environment: Manner in which social and cultural expectations influence behavior by organizing the time during which activities occur and the amount of time devoted to them.

tendon: Bands of strong, fibrous tissue that attach muscles to bones.

tenodesis: Surgical fixation of a tendon.

tenotomy: Surgical section of a tendon used, in some cases, to treat severe spasticity and contractures.

teratogen: Any agent that causes malformation in a developing embryo (e.g., radiation, chemicals, drugs, alcohol, and pollutants).

teratogenic agents: A drug, virus, or irradiation which can cause malformations and disorders in the fetus when the mother is exposed to them.

teratoma: A congenital tumor which can contain three of the primary embryonic germ layers as well as hair, teeth, and endodermal elements.

term infant: Infant born between 38 and 42 weeks of gestation.

term pregnancy: Pregnancy which proceeds to at least 38 weeks gestation.

terminally ill: Having less than 6 months to live.

territoriality: Tendency of individuals to own space.

tertiary care: Rehabilitation of disabilities resulting from disease/pathology to optimize and maximize an individual's functional status (e.g., for hypertension leading to stroke, tertiary care would prevent progression of disability).

tertiary prevention: Rehabilitation after treatment to return to as near normal as possible.

test protocol: Specific procedures that must be followed when assessing a patient; formal testing procedures.

test-retest reliability: Extent to which repeated administrations of a test to the same people produce the same results.

testis: One of the glands that produces the sperm and the male hormone, testosterone, and found in the scrotum.

tests and measures: Specific standardized methods and techniques used to gather data about the patient/client after the history and systems review have been performed.

tetany: A syndrome manifested by sharp flexion of joints, especially the wrist and ankle joints, muscle twitching, cramps, and convulsions, sometimes with attacks of difficult breathing; **uterine tetany:** Prolonged uterine contractions, usually greater than 2 minutes.

tetraplegia: Impairment or loss of motor and/or sensory function in the cervical segments of the spinal cord due to damage of neural elements within the spinal cord.

text-to-speech synthesis: Translation of written communication into speech sounds and messages.

thalamic pain: Central nervous system pain caused by injury to the thalamus and characterized by contralateral and sometime migratory pain brought on by peripheral stimulation.

thalamotomy: Surgical destruction of part of the thalamus to reduce tremors of Parkinson's disease.

thalassemia: Anemia found in Mediterranean and Southeast Asian populations in which there is insufficient globin to fill the red blood cells.

theoretical rationale: Reason, based on theory or empirical evidence, for using a particular intervention for a specific person.

theory: Set of interrelated concepts used to describe, explain, or predict phenomena.

therapeutic abortion: *See* abortion, therapeutic.

therapeutic rest: The use of analgesics to provide a rest period after the onset of labor contractions including greatly reduced pain particularly when there is hypertonic uterine dysfunction.

thermal shift: The change in basal body temperature; both the decrease and then the rise that occurs with ovulation.

thermistor probe: The sensor used to monitor skin temperature of infants when they are under radiant warmers.

thermogenesis: Heat production in the human body.

thermoregulation: Control of temperature.

thermotherapy: The use of heat or cold for therapeutic purposes.

third stage of labor: From birth of the baby through the delivery of the placenta.

thoracic: Pertaining to the chest.

thoracocentesis: Surgical puncture of the chest wall with drainage of fluid.

thought disorder: Disturbance in thinking, including distorted content (e.g., ideas, beliefs, sensory interpretation) and distorted written and spoken language (e.g., word salad, loose associations, echolalia).

threat minimization: Psychological coping strategy in which emotions are managed through "playing down" the importance or significance of a stressor.

threatened abortion: *See* abortion, threatened.

threshold: Level at which a stimulus is recognized by sensory receptors.

thrombin: The enzyme derived from prothrombin that converts fibrinogen to fibrin.

thrombocytopenia: A condition in which the blood platelets are destroyed, causing severe bleeding if injury occurs.

thrombocytopenia purpura: A bleeding disorder in which there is prolonged bleeding time, decreased platelets, increased cell fragility, and purpura resulting in hemorrhage into the skin, mucous membranes, organs, and other tissues.

thromboembolism: When a blood vessel is blocked by a clot that originated someplace else and broke free.

thrombolytic: Dissolving or splitting up a thrombus.

thrombophlebitis: Inflammation of a vein associated with thrombus formation.

thromboplastin: Enzyme that assists in the process of blood clotting.

thrombosis: Coagulation of the blood in the heart or a blood vessel forming a clot.

thrombus: A blood clot obstructing a blood vessel that stays at its site of origin.

thrush: A fungal infection found in the mouth or throat of the neonate. White patches are formed on a red, moist, inflamed mucous membrane and caused by the organism, *Candida albicans.*

thyrotropin releasing hormone: A hormone of the anterior pituitary gland having an affinity for and specifically stimulating the thyroid gland.

tic: Spasmodic muscular contraction usually involving the face, head, or neck.

time out: Removing an individual from the environment where an unacceptable behavior is being demonstrated.

tinnitus: Subjective ringing or tinkling sound in the ear.

tissue plasminogen activator (tPA): Medication to destroy vascular thrombi.

titer: The required quantity of a substance needed to produce a reaction to a given amount of another substance. Synonymous with level.

titration: Volumetric determinations by means of standard solutions of known strength.

tocolytic therapy: Drugs used to relax the uterus, as in suppression of labor or relaxation so the fetus can be turned (version).

tocotransducer: An electrical device that measures contractions and fetal heart tones abdominally.

tolerance: Physiological and psychological accommodation or adaptation to a chemical agent over time.

tone: State of muscle contraction at rest.

tongue-thrust swallow: An immature form of swallowing in which the tongue is projected forward instead of retracted during swallowing.

tonic-clonic: Muscle stiffening and falling into unconsciousness followed by rhythmic jerking, breathing problems, drooling, loss of bladder control, and finally confusion, and sleepiness.

tonic labyrinthine reflex: A normal postural reflex in animals, abnormally accentuated in decerebrate humans, characterized by extension of all four limbs when the head is positioned in space at an angle above the horizontal in quadrupeds or in the neutral, erect position in humans. Synonym: decerebrate rigidity.

tonic neck reflex: A normal response in newborns to extend the arm and the leg on the side of the body to which the head is quickly turned while the infant is supine and to flex the limbs of the opposite side. Integrated at 3 to 4 months of age. Absence or persistence of the reflex may indicate central nervous system damage. Synonym: asymmetric tonic neck reflex.

tonotopic: Organization of cells within the auditory system that enables one to identify the exact sound heard.

top-down processing: When processing starts with higher-order stored knowledge and depends upon contextual information or is conceptually driven.

topographic: Organization of cells in the visual system that enables one to identify the exact location and features of the stimulus.

TORCH infections: A group of organisms that cause infection and damage to the embryo or fetus including toxoplasmosis, syphilis, rubella, cytomegalovirus, and herpes simplex.

torque: Rotating tendency of force; equals the product of force and the perpendicular distance from the axis of a lever to the point of application of the same force.

tort: Wrongful conduct that has caused harm.

torticollis: Irresistible turning of the head that becomes more persistent, so that eventually the head is held continually to one side. Spasm of muscles often painful. Condition may be caused by a birth injury to the sternocleidomastoid muscle. Synonym: wryneck.

total hip arthroplasty: Type of hip surgery involving the removal of the head and neck of the femur and replacement with a prosthetic appliance.

total lymphoid irradiation (TLI): Radiation therapy targeted to the body's lymph nodes; the goal is to suppress immune system functioning (reduce the number of lymphocytes in the blood).

toxemia: Hypertensive states of pregnancy from mild to severe (also eclampsia).

toxicology: Branch of pharmacology that examines harmful chemicals and their effects on the body.

toxicology screen: Laboratory analysis of body fluids such as blood or urine to determine presence of alcohol or drugs. Urine most commonly used because of noninvasiveness.

toxic shock syndrome: A syndrome similar to septic shock and caused by an infection usually involving *Staphylococcus aureus* and associated with the use of tampons during heavy menstruation.

tracheoesophageal fistula: Congenital anomaly that creates a passageway between the trachea and esophagus.

tracheotomy: Incision of the trachea through the skin and muscles of the neck for establishment of an airway, exploration, removal of a foreign body, obtainment of a biopsy specimen, or removal of a local lesion.

trachoma: Chronic infectious eye disease of the conjunctiva and cornea.

traction: The therapeutic use of manual or mechanical tension created by a pulling force to produce a combination of distraction and gliding to relieve pain and increase tissue flexibility.

trajectory: Path to be taken as in trajectory of illness to predict anticipated outcomes.

transmission-based precautions: Centers for Disease Control and Prevention guidelines to prevent transmission of pathogens. Types are airborne, droplet, and contact.

transition period—newborn: Period from birth to the first 4–6 hours; infant passes through period of reactivity, sleep, and second period of reactivity. Breast-fed infants put to breast.

transition phase: From 8 to 10 cm cervical dilatation during labor.

transition to parenthood: Period of time from preconception parenthood decision through the first months after birth of the baby; parents work on their roles and adjust to parenthood.

tranquilizer: Medication that produces a calming effect, relieving tension and anxiety. Referred to also as anxiolytic.

transactional: Ongoing interaction of individual with environment.

transcutaneous electrical nerve stimulation (TENS): The use of electrical energy to stimulate cutaneous and peripheral nerves via electrodes on the skin's surface. A procedure in which electrodes are placed on the surface of the skin over specific nerves and electrical stimulation is done in a manner that is thought to improve central nervous system function, reduce spasticity, and control pain.

transfer: The process of relocating a body from one object or surface to another (e.g., getting into or out of bed, moving from a wheelchair to a chair).

transfer of learning: Practice and learning of one task can influence the learning of another task.

transient ischemic attack (TIA): Episode of temporary cerebral dysfunction caused by impaired blood flow to the brain. Have many symptoms, such as dizziness, weakness, numbness, or paralysis of a limb or half of the body. May last only a few minutes or up to 24 hours but does not have any persistent neurologic deficits.

transillumination spectrography (TIS): Visualization substitute for mammography.

transsexualism: Disorder of gender identity where the anatomical structures of one gender are present but identity is with the opposite gender.

transudate: A fluid substance that has passed through a membrane or been extruded from a tissue, sometimes as a result of inflammation. Transudate, in contrast to exudate, is characterized by high fluidity and a low content of protein, cells, or of solid materials derived from cells.

transvestic fetishism/transvestite: Recurrent desire to dress in clothing of the opposite gender.

traumatic brain injury (TBI): Injury caused by impact to the head. An insult to the brain caused by an external physical force that may produce a diminished or altered state of consciousness that results in impairment of cognitive abilities or physical functioning.

treatment: The sum of all interventions provided to a patient/client during an episode of care. Application of or involvement in activities and stimulation to effect improvement in abilities for self-directed activities or self-care.

tremor: Involuntary shaking or trembling.

Trendelenburg's position: A position in which the patient's head is placed lower than the legs and feet. There is usually a 30–40° difference between the legs and feet and the head.

trephination: Process of making a circular hole in the skull.

trial of labor (TOL): An assessment of whether a laboring woman is likely to deliver vaginally.

trichomonas vaginalis: Vaginal infection caused by *Trichomonas vaginalis*, a parasitic protozoon, and characterized by burning and itching of the vulvae and a frothy white discharge.

trichotillomania: Recurrent pulling out of one's hair.

tricylic antidepressants: Classification of drugs to block reuptake of neurotransmitters.

trigeminal neuralgia: A neurologic condition of the trigeminal facial nerve characterized by a brief but frequent flashing, stablike pain radiating usually throughout mandibular and maxillary regions. Caused by degeneration of the nerve or pressure on it; also known as tic douloureux.

trigeminy: The condition of occurring in threes, especially the occurrence of three pulse beats in rapid succession.

trigger point: Highly sensitive point within the muscle or myofascial tissue.

triglyceride: Any of a group of esters, derived from glycerol and 3 fatty acid radicals; the chief component of fats and oils.

trigonal: Relating to a triangular shape.

trimester: Three periods of 3 months each into which a pregnancy is divided.

trisomy: Whenever a chromosome appears in triplicate rather than the normal double pattern.

trophic: Changes that occur as a result of inadequate circulation, such as loss of hair, thinning of skin, and ridging of nail.

trophoblast: Outer layer of cells of the developing blastodermic vesicle; they establish the nutrient relationship with the uterine endometrium.

trophoblastic disease: The trophoblastic cells covering the chorionic villa proliferate and may become malignant.

trophotropic: Combination of parasympathetic nervous system activity, somatic muscle relaxation, and cortical beta rhythm synchronization. Resting or sleep state.

truncal ataxia: Uncoordinated movement of the trunk.

truth: Faithful to facts and reality.

tubal ligation: A sterilization procedure for women in which the fallopian tubes are tied off and a section is removed to interrupt tubal continuity. This can be done surgically or with laparoscopy.

tubercles of Montgomery: Small papillae on the female nipple that secrete a fatty substance that lubricates the nipple.

tuberosity: Medium-sized protrusion on a bone.

tunnel vision: The visual field is limited to one side; the peripheral fields are lost, usually due to damage to the optic chiasm.

twins: Two infants from the same pregnancy and uterus at the same time; **conjoined twins:** Twins who are physically united (Siamese twins); **disparate twins:** Twins who are of significantly different weight; **dizygotic twins:** Twins who develop from two separate ova and fertilized by two different sperm; **monozygotic twins:** Twins developed from one ovum; identical twins.

two-tail (nondirectional) test: A statistical test of the null hypothesis in which both tails of the distribution are utilized.

tympany: A tympanic, or bell-like, percussion note. A modified tympanic note heard on percussion of the chest in some cases of pneumothorax.

type A behavior: A cluster of personality traits that include high achievement motivation, drive, and a fast-paced lifestyle.

type B behavior: A cluster of personality traits that include low achievement motivation, laziness, and a laid-back lifestyle.

ulcer: An open sore on the skin or mucous membrane characterized by the disintegration of tissue and, often, the discharge of serous drainage.

ultrasound: A diagnostic or therapeutic technique using high-frequency sound waves to produce a picture of the internal organ, or in obstetrics, the fetus; **pulsed:** The application of therapeutic ultrasound using predetermined interrupted frequencies and producing heat.

ultrasound transducer: External electronic signal receptor to monitor fetal heart tones.

ultraviolet: A form of radiant energy using light rays with wavelengths beyond the violet end of the visible spectrum.

umbilical cord (funis): A gelatinous substance containing one artery and two veins that connects the placenta to the fetus carrying nutrients and gases. At birth, the cord is tied and cut; the stump dries and falls off in 4–10 days.

umbilicus: The navel, a depressed point midabdomen that marks the site of attachment of the umbilical cord during intrauterine life.

unconditional positive regard: Unconditional love and acceptance.

undermine: Tissue destruction underlying intact skin along wound margins.

universal: Pertaining to any group, need, or environment.

universal precautions: An approach to infection control designed to prevent transmission of blood-borne and body fluid diseases such as AIDS and hepatitis B; includes specific recommendations for the use of gloves, protective eye wear, and masks.

unlicensed assistive personnel (UAP): Persons providing direct care who have some training that is inconsistent across settings and regions.

unobtrusive observation: Observation for assessment that minimizes reactivity.

unripe: Describes a cervix that is not soft and not ready for labor.

unusual occurrence report: The internal document for an organization to validate any instance that was not anticipated in terms of patient care. Includes such events as medication misadministration, falls, failure of services to respond, or observed inappropriate behavior of staff.

upper motor neuron (UMN): Neurons of the cerebral cortex that conduct stimuli from the motor cortex of the brain to motor nuclei of cerebral nerves of the ventral gray columns of the spinal cord.

uremia: Toxic condition associated with renal insufficiency in which renal byproducts normally excreted by the kidney are present in the blood.

urethra: Small tubular structure that drains urine from the bladder.

urethrocele: Prolapse of the urethra with bulging into the vaginal opening.

urgency: Need to excrete urine immediately.

urinary frequency: The urgent desire to void at frequent intervals.

urinary incontinence (UI): Uncontrolled expulsion of urine, especially when abdominal pressure is increased in coughing, sneezing, and laughing.

urinary meatus: The opening of the urethra.

urinary tract infection (UTI): Bacterial infection of kidney and/or bladder.

urogenital diaphragm: The perineal membrane; the deep muscle layer of the deep fascial layer that supports the pelvic organs.

urokinase: A substance found in the urine of mammals, including humans, that activates the fibrinolytic system, acting enzymatically by splitting plasminogen.

uterine atony: Relaxation of the uterus that can lead to postpartum hemorrhage.

uterine bruit: Murmur heard while auscultating the uterus.

uterine dysfunction: The inability of the uterus to contract and relax in a coordinated fashion.

uterine ischemia: Decreased blood supply to the uterus leading to the death of some cells.

uterine inversion: *See* inverted uterus.

uterus: The pear-shaped organ in which the fetus grows; also called the womb; **Couvelaire uterus:** Interstitial myometrial hemorrhage after placenta abruption; the uterus becomes boardlike and bluish in color.

utilitarianism: Ethical theory principle that prioritizes actions to produce greatest good for the greatest number of people.

vaccination: Injected with vaccine to stimulate creation of antibodies to establish resistance to that specific disease.

vacuum-assisted birth: The use of negative pressure in a vacuum cup attached to the fetal head to assist in birth of the baby.

vacuum curettage: Aspiration of the uterus as a method of early abortion.

vagina: A mucous membrane tube that forms the passageway between the uterus and the vaginal opening/introitis.

vaginal birth after cesarean (VBAC): Vaginal birth after having had a cesarean birth.

vaginismus: Involuntary constriction of outer third of vagina that results in inability for penile penetration to occur.

values clarification: Self-discovery of one's values and their priorities.

varicella: Acute infection resulting in scattered pattern rash predominantly over face and chest.

validity: Degree to which a test measures what it is intended to measure.

Valsalva's maneuver: A process in which the intra-abdominal pressure is increased by holding the breath and pushing down during exertion or excretion.

values: Identifying ideas or beliefs that are important to self and others; operational beliefs that one accepts as one's own and that determine behavior.

valvuloplasty: Replacement of a cardiac valve with a prosthetic valve.

valvulotomy: Incision of a valve, such as valve of the heart.

variability: Normal variance in fetal cardiac rhythm.

variance: Measure that demonstrates how scores in a distribution deviates from the mean.

varicella: Can be seen in infectious diseases such as chickenpox.

varicocele: Enlargement of the veins in the spermatic cord.

varicose veins: Refers to the enlargement of veins when the valves in the veins become swollen and have retrograde flow within them.

vasectomy: Ligation and or removal of a segment of the vas deferens to produce sterility in males.

vasomotor center: A regulatory center in the lower pons and medulla oblongata that regulates the diameter of blood vessels, especially the arterioles.

vasopneumatic compression device: A device to decrease edema by using compressive forces that are applied to the body part.

vasopressor: Stimulating contraction of the muscular tissue of the capillaries and arteries. An agent that stimulates the contraction of the muscular tissue of the capillaries and arteries.

VDRL test: Venereal Disease Research Laboratories. A test for syphilis, more commonly replaced by rapid plasma reagin.

vector: Arrow that indicates direction and magnitude of a force.

ventilation: The circulation of air; to aerate (blood); oxygenate. Mechanical ventilation is the use of equipment to circulate oxygen to the respiratory system.

ventilatory equivalent (VE/VO$_2$): The ratio of minute ventilation to oxygen consumption. The normal ratio is 25:1, meaning that for 25 L of air breathed, 1 L of oxygen has been consumed.

ventilatory pump: Thoracic skeleton and skeletal muscles and their innervations responsible for ventilation. Includes the diaphragm; the intercostal, scalene, and sternocleidomastoid muscles; accessory muscles of ventilation; and the abdominal, triangular, and quadratus lumborum muscles.

ventilatory pump dysfunction: Abnormalities of the thoracic skeleton, respiratory muscles, airways, or lungs that interrupt or interfere with the work of breathing or ventilation.

ventral: In terms of anatomical position, located toward the front or the belly.

veracity: Obligation of the client and the therapist to tell the truth at all times.

verbal communication: Process of interpreting another's words and expressing one's own thoughts and emotions through words.

verbal rating scale: A pain intensity measurement in which patients/clients rate pain on a continuum that is subdivided into gradually increasing pain intensities.

verbal therapies: Any therapy in which talk and discussion are the primary modes of intervention.

vergence: Movement of the two eyes in the opposite direction.

vermis: Forms the unpaired medial region of the cerebellum.

vernix caseosa: Gray-white, cheesy substance covering the fetus as a protective coating.

version: Turning the fetus in utero to change the position and thus the presenting part to facilitate the birth process; **podalic version:** Change the position so the feet are the presenting part.

vertex: Crown of the head; **vertex presentation:** The fetal head is the presenting part.

vertigo: One's sensation of revolving in space or of having objects move around him or her.

very low birth weight infant (VLBW): An infant that weighs less than 1500 gm at birth.

vestibular: Pertaining to a vestibule, a cavity, or space at the entrance of a canal, such as the inner ear. Describing the sense of balance located in the inner ear. Interpreting stimuli regarding head position and movement based on the shift of fluid and inner ear receptors.

vestibular-bilateral disorder: A sensory integrative dysfunction characterized by shortened duration nystagmus, poor integration of the two sides of the body and brain, and difficulty in learning to read or compute. Disorder caused by underreactive vestibular responses.

vestibular function: Pertaining to the sense of balance.

vestibulocochlear nerve: Combined portions of the eighth cranial nerve.

vestibulo-ocular reflex: A normal reflex in which eye position compensates for movement of the head, induced by excitation of vestibular apparatus.

viable: Capable of living. The fetus reaches a maturational point where it can live outside of the uterus, usually approximately 22 weeks gestation.

vicarious reinforcement: Idea that one person's observation of another person's experiencing a positive consequence as a result of a particular behavior increases the probability that the observer will exhibit that behavior.

videofluoroscopy: Radiological study that allows visualization of the pharyngeal and esophageal phases of swallowing.

vigilance: Monitoring events in the environment or person for a sustained time period.

visceral pain: Abdominal discomfort from some abnormality with internal organs.

viscosity: Describes the extent to which a tissue's resistance to deformation is dependent on the rate of the deforming force.

visual: Connected with or used in seeing. Interpreting stimuli through the eyes, including peripheral vision and acuity.

visual acuity: Measure of visual discrimination of fine details of high contrast.

visual agnosia: The inability to name objects as viewed.

visual analog scale: A tool used in a pain examination that allows the patient/client to indicate his or her degree of pain or other feeling by pointing to a visual representation of pain intensity.

visual evoked response (VER): Presentation of a particular visual stimulus evokes consistent electrocortical activity that can be recorded from electrodes placed on the scalp.

visualization: An effective means of deepening relaxation and desensitizing a real-life situation that is generally met with stress and tension.

visual motor coordination: The ability to coordinate vision with the movements of the body or parts of the body.

visual orientation: Awareness and location of objects in the environment and their relationship to each other and to one's self.

visual perception: The brain's ability to understand sensory input to determine size, shape, distance, and form of objects.

vision screening: Can include distance and near visual acuities, oculomotilities, eye alignment or posture, depth perception, and visual fields.

vital capacity (VC): Measurement of the amount of air that can be expelled at the normal rate of exhalation after a maximum inspiration, representing the greatest possible breathing capacity.

vital signs: Measurements of pulse rate, respiration rate, and body temperature.

VO_2 max: Maximum oxygen consumption, usually expressed as a volume of oxygen consumed per minute. Used as a measure of patient exercise capacity.

volar: Palm of the hand or the sole of the foot.

Volkmann's contracture: Permanent contracture of a muscle due to replacement of destroyed muscle cells with fibrous tissue that lacks the ability to stretch.

volvulus: Twisting of the bowel upon itself.

voyeurism: Sexual urges involving observing unsuspecting people in acts of undressing or sexual activity.

vulva: External female genitalia.

vulvodynia: Painful intercourse (in females only).

vulvar self-examination (VSE): Examination of the vulva by the client.

vulvectomy: Surgical removal of all or some parts of the vulva.

wallerian degeneration: The physical and biochemical changes that occur in a nerve because of the loss of axonal continuity following trauma.

wandering: Repetitive walking without purpose, frequently seen in dementia.

wandering cells: Connective cells usually involved with short-term activities, such as protection and repair.

waxy rigidity: Symptom of catatonia in which an individual will assume any position in which he or she is placed and remain there until moved again.

wear-and-tear theory: Theory that describes the biological effects of aging as the body deteriorates.

weaning: Changing from breast feeding or bottle feeding to taking liquids from a cup.

weapons of mass destruction: Any nuclear, chemical, or biological agent that is designed as a weapon against living organisms.

weight shift: Bearing the body's weight from one leg to another; shifting the center of gravity.

wellness: Dynamic state of health in which an individual progresses toward a higher level of functioning, achieving an optimum balance between internal and external environments.

Wernicke's encephalopathy: Brain disorder associated with thiamine deficiency.

Wharton's jelly: Connective tissue with a jellylike quality within the umbilical cord that supports the umbilical vessels.

wheeze: A whistling sound made in breathing resulting from constriction and/or partial obstruction of the airways. Heard on auscultation; however, in severe cases of asthma and chronic obstructive pulmonary disease, can often be audible without use of a stethoscope.

whey proteins: The protein content of mother's milk.

whiplash injury: Injury caused by sudden hyperextension and flexion of the neck, traumatizing cervical ligaments; common in rear-end car accidents or falls.

white coat phenomenon: Condition whereby pulse and blood pressure may be elevated as well as other behaviors due to anxiety about health care services.

white matter: Area of the central nervous system that contains the axons of the cells.

witch's milk: Secretion of whitish substance from the breast tissue in the neonate, stimulated by maternal hormones.

withdrawal: Unpleasant symptoms occurring as a result of lessening or stopping a medication; withdrawing the penis from the vagina prior to ejaculation as a form of birth control (coitus interruptus).

within normal limits (WNL): The normally expected findings in physical examination.

word salad: Group of words constructed in random manner with no logical connection.

womb: *See* uterus.

workup: The process of performing a complete evaluation of an individual, including history, physical examination, laboratory test, and X-ray or other diagnostic procedures, to acquire an accurate database on which a diagnosis and treatment plan may be established.

wound: An area of disrupted or discontinuous skin or tissue.

wound base: Uppermost viable tissue layer of a wound; may be covered with slough or eschar.

wound care: Procedures used to achieve a clean wound bed, promote a moist environment, facilitate autolytic debridement, or absorb excessive exudation from a wound complex.

wound management: Comprehensive intervention to reduce pressure points and manage the interdisciplinary efforts to facilitate wound care and healing.

wound margin: Rim or border of a wound.

wound repair: Healing process. Partial thickness involves epithelialization; full thickness involves contraction granulation and epithelialization.

X chromosome: Human sex chromosomes; there are two in females and one in males.

xenophobia: Fear and/or hatred of any person or thing that is strange or
    foreign.
xeroderma: Condition of rough and dry skin.
X-linked recessive: Trait transmitted by a gene located on the X chro-
    mosome. These traits are passed on by a carrier mother to an af-
    fected son.

Y chromosome: The human male sex chromosome, required for the de-
    velopment of the male gonads.
yin and yang: Basis of Asian health practices of opposing forces of en-
    ergy: negative/positive, hot/cold, dark/light. Focus is on restoring
    balance.
yoga: System of beliefs designed to unite human spirit with universe.
yolk sac: The highly vascularized umbilical vesicle surrounding the yolk
    of the embryo.
young old: Persons between 60 and 75 years of age.

z score (standard score): Numerical value from the transformation of a
    raw score into units of standard deviation.
ZIFT: Zygote intrafallopian transfer.
zona pellucida: Thick membranous envelope of the ovum.
zone of proximal development: Difference between what a child can
    do alone and what he or she can do with the assistance of a more
    skilled helper.
zygote: Single cell formed at conception by the union of the 23 chro-
    mosomes of the sperm and the 23 chromosomes of the ovum.

Abbreviations and Acronyms

This is a list of abbreviations and acronyms most commonly used.
**Caution: Many health care organizations are discontinuing the
practice of abbreviations out of a concern for patient safety.** When
an asterisk (*) appears after an abbreviation, it denotes that the *2004
National Patient Safety Goals* indicates that such an item requires a longer
form to avoid confusion. Expect other abbreviations to be included in
this category as more research about documentation is conducted. This
section is provided as a guide for practice in those situations where abbreviations are still used.

a	*ante* (before)
aa	of each
AA	automobile accident; Alcoholics Anonymous; or arachidonic acid
AAA	abdominal aortic aneurysm
Ab	antibody
ABC	airway, breathing, circulation
abd	abdomen
ABG	arterial blood gases
abn	abnormal
abp	arterial blood pressure
ABO	the main blood group system
ac	*ante cibum* (before meals)
ACE	angiotensin-converting enzyme
ACL	anterior cruciate ligament
ACLS	advanced cardiac life support
ACT	activated clotting time
ACTH	adrenocorticotropic hormone
AD*	autosomal dominant; or atopic dermatitis; or *auris dextra** (right ear)
ADD	attention deficit disorder
ADDH	attention deficit disorder, hyperactivity
ADH	antidiuretic hormone
ADHD	attention deficit-hyperactivity disorder
ADL	activities of daily living
ad lib	*ad libitum* (as desired)
adm	admission, administration
ADP	adenosine diphosphate
ADR	adverse drug reaction
ADS	attention deficit syndrome; or antidiuretic substance
AEP	auditory evoked potential
AF	atrial fibrillation; or aortic femoral
AFB	acid-fast bacillus
AFDC	aid to families with dependent children
AFP	alpha-fetoprotein
AFV	amniotic fluid volume
Ag	antigen; argentums (silver)
A-G ratio	albumin–globulin ration

AGA	appropriate for gestational age
AGC	absolute granulocyte count
AGN	acute glomerulonephritis
AHC	acute hemorrhagic conjunctivitis
AHD	autoimmune hemolytic disease
AHF	antihemophilic factor; or antihemolytic factor
AHG	antihemophilic globulin; antihuman globulin
AI	aortic insufficiency; adequate intake
AID	artificial insemination by donor
AIDS	acquired immunodeficiency syndrome
AIH	artificial insemination by husband
AIOD	aorta iliac occlusive disease
AK	above the knee
AKA	above the knee amputation
ALG	antilymphocytic globulin
ALL	acute lymphoid leukemia
ALS	advanced life support; or amyotrophic lateral sclerosis (Lou Gehrig's disease)
ALT	alanine aminotransferase
AM	*ante meridiem* (morning)
AMA	against medical advice
amb	ambulatory
AMI	acute myocardial infarction
AML	acute monocytic leukemia
amp	ampule; or amputation
AMP	adenosine monophosphate
amt	amount
ANA	antinuclear antibody (test)
ANAD	anorexia nervosa and associated disorders
ANLL	acute nonlymphocytic anemia
ANRED	anorexia nervosa and related eating disorders
ANS	autonomic nervous system; anterior nasal spine
A & O	alert and oriented
AODA	alcohol and other drug abuse
AOM	acute otitis media
AP	antepartum; or anteroposterior; or atrioperitoneal
A & P	auscultation & percussion; or anterior posterior
A2P2	aortic and pulmonic

APIB	assessment of premature infant behavior
approx	approximately
appy	appendectomy
APN/APRN	advanced practice nurse; advanced practice registered nurse
ARBD	alcohol-related birth defects
AR	autosomal recessive
ARC	AIDS-related complex
ARF	acute renal failure; or acute respiratory failure
AROM	artificial rupture of membranes
ARD	acute respiratory distress
ARDS	adult (or acute) respiratory distress syndrome
ART	assistive reproduction technology
ARV	AIDS-associated retrovirus
AS*	aortic stenosis; or aortic sound; or aqueous solution; or aqueous suspension; or astigmatism; or ankylosing spondylitis; or *auris sinistra** (left ear)
ASA	acetylsalicylic acid
ASAP	as soon as possible
ASD	atrial septal defect
ASDH	acute subdural hematoma
ASH	asymmetric septal hypertrophy
ASHD	arteriosclerotic heart disease
ASK	antistreptokinase
ASO	antistreptolysin O
ATG	antithymocyte globulin
ATN	acute tubular necrosis
ATP	adenosine triphosphate; or autoimmune thrombocytopenia (purpura)
ATV	all-terrain vehicle
AU*	*auris uterque* (each ear)
AUB	abnormal uterine bleeding
Av	average; avoirdupois
AV (A-V)	atrioventricular
AVM	arteriovenous malformation
AVF	acute ventilatory failure
AVN	avascular necrosis
AVR	aortic valve replacement
AWD	abdominal wall defect

BA	bronchial asthma; or bone age; or barium
BAC	blood alcohol concentration
BAEP	brainstem auditory evoked potential
BAER	brainstem auditory evoked response
BAT	brown adipose tissue
BB	breakthrough bleeding
BBB	blood–brain barrier
BBT	basal body temperature
BC	blood culture
BCG	Bacille Calmette-Guérin (tuberculin vaccine)
BCS	battered child syndrome
BD	bronchial drainage; or birthday; or birth defect
BE	base excess; or barium enema
BEAM	brain electrical activity map
BEI	butanol-extractable iodine
BFP	biologic false positive
BG	blood glucose
B-hCG	beta human chorionic gonadotropin
BHI	biosynthetic human insulin
bid	*bis in die* (twice a day)
BINS	Bayley Infant Neurodevelopmental Screen
BiPap	bi-level positive airway pressure
BK	below the knee
BKA	below the knee amputation
BL	bleeding; or baseline; or blood loss
BM	bowel movement; or bone marrow
BMD	bone mineral density; or bone marrow depression
BMR	basal metabolic rate
BNBAS	Brazelton Neonatal Behavioral Assessment Scale
BOA	behavioral observation audiometry; or born out of asepsis
BP	blood pressure; or bathroom privileges; or birthplace
BPD	bronchopulmonary dysplasia
BMI	body mass index
BPH	benign prostatic hypertrophy
bpm	beats per minute
BPP	biophysical profile
BR	bedrest

BRAT	bananas, rice cereal, applesauce, toast (diet for diarrhea)
BRATY	bananas, rice, applesauce, tea, and yogurt (diet for diarrhea)
BRBPR	bright red blood per rectum
BRP	bed rest; or bathroom privileges
BS	blood sugar; or bowel sounds; or breath sounds
BSA	body surface area; or bovine serum albumin
BSE	breast self-examination
BSER	brainstem evoked response
BSI	biologic substance(s) isolation; body substance isolation
BSID	Bayley Scales of Infant Development
BT	bleeding time
BUBBLE-HE	breasts, uterus, bladder, bowel, lochia, episiotomy, Homan's Sign, emotional status
BUN	blood urea nitrogen
BW	birth weight
BWS	battered woman syndrome
Bx	biopsy
c	*cum* (with)
C	centigrade; or Celsius; or calorie
Ca (CA)	cancer; or calcium; or chronological age
C & A	Clinitest & Acetest
CABG	coronary artery bypass graph
CAD	coronary artery disease
CAH	congenital adrenal hyperplasia; or chronic active hepatitis
CAL	chronic airflow limitation
CAM	complementary and alternative medicine
cAMP	cyclic adenosine monophosphate
cap	capsule
CAPD	continuous ambulatory peritoneal dialysis
CAT	computed axial tomography
CAV	congenital absence of a vagina; or croup-associated virus
CAVH	continuous arteriovenous hemofiltration
CB	chronic bronchitis

CBA	congenital biliary atresia
CBC	complete blood count
CBD	closed bladder drainage
CBF	cerebral blood flow
CBI	continuous bladder irrigation
CBPU	care by parent unit
CBR	complete bedrest
CBS	chronic brain syndrome
CBV	cerebral blood volume; or central blood flow (velocity)
cc*	cubic centimeter
CC	chief complaint; or Caucasian child; or common cold; or critical condition; or color and circulation; or creatinine clearance
CCMS	clean catch midstream specimen
Ccr	creatinine clearance
CCU	coronary care unit
CD	communicable disease
CDH	congenital diaphragmatic hernia; or congenital dislocated hip
CDP	continuous distending pressure
C-E	croup-epiglottitis syndrome
CEA	carotid endarterectomy
CF	cystic fibrosis; or cardiac failure; or complement fixation
CFU	colony-forming units
C-H	crown-heel
CHB	complete heart block
CHC	child health conference; or community health center
CHD	congenital heart disease; or childhood disease; or coronary heart disease
CHF	congestive heart failure
CHL	crown-heel length
CHO	carbohydrate
CI	cardiac index; or cardiac insufficiency; or cerebral infarction
CID	cytomegalic inclusion disease; or combined immune deficiency
CIE	countercurrent immunoelectrophoresis

CINAHL	Cumulative Index to Nursing and Allied Health Literature
CIS	carcinoma in situ
CK	creatinine kinase
cl	clear liquid diet
CL	client
CL (P)	cleft lip with or without cleft palate
CLP	cleft lip and cleft palate
CLBBB	complete left bundle branch block
CLD	chronic lung disease; or chronic liver disease
cm	centimeter
CMA	cow's milk allergy
CMC	carpal-metacarpal
CMI	cell-mediated immunity
CML	chronic myelocytic leukemia
CMPI	cow's milk protein intolerance
CMR	cerebral metabolic rate
CMV	cytomegalovirus
CNM	certified nurse midwife
CNS	central nervous system; or clinical nurse specialist
CNSD	chronic nonspecific diarrhea
CO	cardiac output
c/o	complains of
CO_2	carbon dioxide
COA	children of alcoholics
COC	combined oral contraceptive
cocci	coccidioidomycosis
COHb	carboxyhemoglobin
COLD	chronic obstructive lung disease
COPD	chronic obstructive pulmonary disease
CP	cerebral palsy
CPAP	continuous positive airway pressure
CPAV	continuous positive airway ventilation
CPD	cephalopelvic disproportion; or childhood polycystic disease
CPK	creatine phosphokinase
CPM	continuous passive motion
CPP	cerebral perfusion pressure

CPPV	continuous positive pressure ventilation
CPR	cardiopulmonary resuscitation
CPS	cycles per second
CPT	chest physiotherapy
CR	crown-rump
CRBBB	complete right bundle branch block
CRD	child restraint devices
CRF	corticotrophin releasing factor
CRP	c-reactive protein
crit	hematocrit
CRS	congenital rubella syndrome
CS	clinical specialist; or cesarean section
C & S	culture and sensitivity
CS	central supply or culture and sensitivity
CSA	colony-stimulating activity
CSD	cat scratch disease
C-sec	cesarean section
CSF	cerebrospinal fluid; or cerebral spinal fluid
CSII	continuous subcutaneous insulin infusion
CST	convulsive shock therapy
CSW	certified social worker
COSM	chronic serous otitis media
CST	contraction stress test
CT	computed tomography; or complementary therapy; or circulation time; clotting time; or coated tablet; or compressed tablet; or corneal transplant; or Coombs test
CTT	computerized transaxial tomography
CUG	cystourethrogram
CV	closing volume; or cell volume; or central venous
CVA	cerebrovascular accident; or costal vertebral angle
CVD	cardiovascular disease
CVO_2	mixed venous oxygen content
CVP	central venous pressure
CVR	cerebral vascular resistance
CVS	chorionic villus sampling; or clean voided specimen
CW	crutch walking
C/W	consistent with

CXR	chest X-ray
cysto	cystoscopy
d	day
DA	developmental age
DASE	Denver Articulation Screening Examination
DAT	diet as tolerated
DAW	dispense as written
db	decibel; or diabetes
DC*	discontinue; or discharge*; or dichorionic
D & C	dilation and curettage
DCT	Direct Coombs Test
DD	dry dressing; or differential diagnosis; or discharge diagnosis; or discharge by death; or diaper dermatitis
D & E	dilation and evacuation
DDH	developmental dysplasia of the hip
DDST	Denver Developmental Screening Test
DDST-R	Denver Developmental Screening Test, revised
DES	diethylstilbesterol
DFA	diet for age
DFE	dietary folate equivalent
DG	diagnosis; or diastolic gallop
DH	diaphragmatic hernia
D/I	direct/indirect ratio (bilirubin)
DIC	disseminated intravascular coagulation
Diff	differential (lab work)
DIP	desquamated interstitial pneumonitis
DJD	degenerative joint disease
DKA	diabetic ketoacidosis
dl	deciliter
DM	diabetes mellitus; or diastolic murmur
DME	Durable medical equipment
DMPA	depot medroxyprogesterone acetate; or Depo-Provera
DMSO	dimethyl sulfoxide
DNA	deoxyribonucleic acid
DNR	do not resuscitate
DOA	date of admission; or dead on arrival

DOB	date of birth
DOD	date of discharge; or date of death
DOE	dyspnea on exertion
DP	dorsalis pedis (artery)
DPT	diphtheria-pertussis-tetanus (vaccine)
DQ	developmental quotient
dr	*drachma* (dram)
DRG	diagnosis-related groups
DRI	dietary reference intake
drsg	dressing
DRV	daily reference value
DS	Down's syndrome
DSA	digital subtraction angiography
DSD	dry sterile dressing
DSDB	direct self-destructive behavior
DSM#	Diagnostic and Statistical Manual of Mental Disorders (# = version of manual)
DT	delirium tremens
DTR	deep tendon reflexes
DU	diagnosis undetermined; or duodenal ulcer
DUB	dysfunctional uterine bleeding
DV	daily value; or dilute volume
D & V	diarrhea and vomiting
DW	distilled water
D5W	dextrose 5% in water
Dx	diagnosis
DZ	dizygotic
EA	esophageal atresia; or each
EAM	external acoustic meatus
EBL	estimated blood loss
EBM	expressed breast milk
EBV	Epstein-Barr virus
ECC	emergency cardiac care; or extracorporeal circulation
ECF	extracellular fluid; or extended care facility
ECG (EKG)	electro(k)cardiogram
ECI	early childhood intervention
ECM	erythema chronicum migrans

ECMO	extracorporeal membrane oxygenation
ECT	electroconvulsive therapy
ED	emergency department
EDB	expected date of birth
EDC	expected date of confinement
EDD	expected date of delivery
ED/ER	emergency department/room
EDNP	energy-dense, nutrient-poor
EEE	eastern equine encephalitis
EEG	electroencephalogram
EENT	eye, ear, nose, throat
EF	extended field (irradiation)
EFA	essential fatty acid
EFE	endocardial fibroelastosis
EFM	electronic fetal monitoring
EGS	electric galvanic stimulator
EHBA	extrahepatic biliary atresia
EIP	early intervention program
E-IVP	enhanced (potency)-IVP
EKG	*see* ECG
EL	elixir
ELBW	extremely low birth weight
ELISA	enzyme-linked immunosorbent assay
elix	elixir
EMG	electromyography
EMI	electromagnetic interference
EMM	expressed mother's milk
EMS	emergency medical services
EMT	emergency medical technician
ENA	extractable nuclear antigens
(E)ENT	(eyes) ears, nose, throat
EOA	examination, opinion, and advice
EOM	extraocular movement; extraocular muscle
EP	extraperitoneal; or evoked potential; or erythrocyte protoporphyrin; or ectopic pregnancy
EPA	erect posteroanterior
ER	estrogen receptors; or external rotation; expiratory reserve; equivalent roentgen (unit)

ERA	electric response audiometry
ERG	electroretinography
ERPF	effective renal plasma flow
ERT	estrogen replacement therapy
ERV	expiratory reserve volume
ESI	Early Screening Inventory
ESP	extrasensory perception
ESR	erythrocyte sedimentation rate
ESRD	end-stage renal disease
EST	electroshock therapy
ET	embryo transfer; or endotracheal; or esotropia; or eustachian tube
ETA	estimated time of arrival
ETCO$_2$	end-tidal carbon dioxide concentration
ETOH	ethyl alcohol
ETT	endotracheal tube
ET TUBE	endotracheal tube
EV	enterovirus
F	Fahrenheit
FAE	fetal alcohol effects
FAS	fetal acoustic stimulation; fetal alcohol syndrome
FB	foreign body; or finger breadth
FBA	foreign body aspiration
FBP	femoral blood pressure
FBS	fasting blood sugar
FCMC	family-centered maternity care
FD	fatal dose; or forceps delivery
FEP	free erythrocyte porphyrins
FET	forced expiratory technique
FEV	forced expiratory volume
FEV1	forced expiratory volume, 1 second
FEV5	forced expiratory volume, 5 seconds
FEVC	forced expiratory volume capacity
FFA	free fatty acid
FFN	fetal fibronectin
FFP	fresh frozen plasma
FH, FHx	familial hypercholesterolemia; or family history

FHR	fetal heart rate
FHS	fetal hydantoin syndrome
FHT	fetal heart tone
FIO_2, Fio2	forced inspiratory oxygen; or fraction of inspired oxygen
FISH	fluorescent in situ hybridization
fld	fluid
FLM	fetal lung maturity
FMC	fetal movement counting
FMD	fibromuscular dysplasia
FMH	family medical history
FMS	fat-mobilizing substance
FNP	family nurse practitioner
FOBT	fetal occult blood test
FOC	frontal-occipital circumference
FP	femoral-popliteal
FPAL	full-term deliveries/preterm deliveries/abortion/living children
FRC	functional residual capacity
FS	full strength
FSE	fetal scalp electrode
FSH	follicle stimulating hormone
FSP	fibrin split products
FSS	family short stature
FTA-ABS	fluorescent treponemal antibody absorption (test)
ftc	footcandle
FTSG	full-thickness skin graft
FTT	failure to thrive
F/U	follow-up
FUE	fever of unknown etiology
FUO	fever of unknown origin
FVC	forced vital capacity
FWB	full weight bearing
Fx	fracture
FHx	family history
FYI	for your information
g	gram
G & P	gravida (#); para (#)

GA	gestational age; or general anesthesia
GABHS	group A B-hemolytic streptococci
GAS	group A streptococci
GB	gallbladder
GBS	group B *Streptococcus*
GC	gonococcal culture
GCS	Glasgow Coma Scale
GCT	genetic counseling team
G & D	growth and development
GDM	gestational diabetes mellitus
GER	gastroesophageal reflux
GERD	gastroesophageal reflux disease
GFR	glomerular filtration rate
GGT, GGTP	gamma-glutamyl transpeptidase
GH	growth hormone
GHB,GHb	glycosylated hemoglobin
GHD	growth hormone deficiency
GHRF	growth hormone releasing factor
GH-RH	growth hormone releasing hormone
GI	gastrointestinal
GIFT	gamete intrafallopian transfer
gm	gram
GNP	gross national product
GnRH	gonadotropin releasing hormone
GOT	glutamic-oxaloacetic transaminase
G6PD	glucose-6-phosphate dehydrogenase
Grav1	gravida 1; or first pregnancy
GSE	gluten-sensitive enteropathy
GSW	gunshot wound
gtt	*guttal* (drops)
GTT	glucose tolerance test
GU	genitourinary
GVH	graft-vs-host
GVHD	graft-vs-host disease
GVHR	graft-vs-host rejection
GYN	gynecology
h	*hora* (hours)
H & H	hematocrit and hemoglobin

HA	headache
H-A	Hartmannella-Acanthamoeba
HAV	hepatitis A virus
HB/HGB	hemoglobin
HBGM	home blood glucose monitoring
HbeAg	hepatitis B e antigen
HBIG	hepatitis B immune globulin
HbO_2	oxyhemoglobin
HBO	hyperbaric oxygen
HbOC	Haemophilus b conjugate vaccine (diphtheria CRM19–protein conjugate)
HBP	high blood pressure
HbsAg	hepatitis B surface antigen
HBV	hepatitis B virus; or honeybee venom
HC	hyperosmolar coma
HC/AC	head-abdomen circumference
hCG	human chorionic gonadotropin
HCI	home care instructions
HCO_3	bicarbonate
Hct	hematocrit
HCTZ	hydrochlorothiazide
HD	heart disease
HCDV	human diploid cell virus
HDL	high-density lipoprotein
HDN	hemolytic disease of the newborn
HEENT	head/eyes/ears/nose/throat
HELLP	hemolysis, elevated liver enzymes, low platelets
HexA	hexosaminidase
HFJV	high-frequency jet ventilator
HFO	high-frequency oscillation
HFOV	high-frequency oscillation ventilation
HFPPV	high-frequency positive pressure ventilation
HFV	high-frequency ventilation
Hgb	hemoglobin
HGH (hGH)	human growth hormone
HGP	Human Genome Project
HGPRT	hypoxanthine-guanine phosphoribosyl-transferase
HHHO	hypothyroidism, hypoxia, hypogonadism, obesity

HHNC	hyperosmolar, hyperglycemic, nonketogenic, coma
H/I	hypoxia-ischemic
Hib (HIB)	*Hemophilus influenzae* type B
HIE	hypoxic-ischemic encephalopathy
HISG	human immune serum globulin
HIV	human immunodeficiency virus
HL	hearing level
HLA	human leukocytic antigen; or histocompatibility locus antigen
HMD	hyaline membrane disease
HMG	hydroxymethylglutaryl
HMO	health maintenance organization
H_2O	water
HO	house officer
HOB	head of bed
HOPI	history of previous (prior) illness
HPA	hypothalamic-pituitary-adrenal (axis)
hPL	human placental lactogen
HPLC	high-powered liquid chromatography
HPN	hypertension
HPV	human papillomavirus; or human parvovirus
HR	heart rate; or hospital record
HRA	health risk appraisal
HRF	health related facility
HRIG	human rabies immune globulin
HRT	hormone replacement therapy
hs*	*hora somni* (hour of sleep; bedtime)
HS	heart sounds
HSA	human serum albumin; or health systems agency
HSBG	heel stick blood gases
HSE	herpes simplex encephalitis
HSN	herpes simplex neonatorum
HSP	Henoch-Schonlein purpura
HSV	herpes simplex virus
HT	healing touch
HTLV-1*	human T-cell leukemia virus type 1

HTLV-III	human T-lymphotropic virus type III
HTN	hypertension
HTPN	home total parenteral nutrition
HTSI	human thyroid stimulator immunoglobulin
HUS	hemolytic uremic syndrome
Hx	history
hypo	hypodermic
IA	imperforate anus; or internal auditory; or intraarterial; or intraarticular; or infantile apnea
IAA	insulin autoantibodies
IABP	intra-aortic balloon pump
IAFI	infantile amaurotic familial idiocy
IAR	interagency referral
IBC	iron-binding capacity
IBD	inflammatory bowel disease
IBO	in behalf of
IBS	irritable bowel syndrome
IBW	ideal body weight
IC	intracutaneous
ICA	islet cell antibodies
ICC	intermittent clean catheterization
ICD#	International Classification of Diseases (# = version of manual)
ICF	intracellular fluid
ICH	intracranial hemorrhage
ICN	intensive care nursery
ICP	intermittent catheterization program; or intracranial pressure
ICS	intercostal space
ICSH	interstitial cell-stimulating hormone
ICSI	intracytoplasmic sperm injection
ICP	intercranial pressure
ICU	intensive care unit
ID	identification; or intradermal; initial dose; or infective dose; or ineffective dose; or inside diameter; or infant death
I & D	incision and drainage
IDD	insulin-dependent diabetic

IDDM	insulin-dependent diabetes mellitus
IDM	infant of a diabetic mother
IDP	infant development program
I/E ratio	inspiratory-expiratory ratio
IEP	individualized education program; or immunoelectrophoresis
IF	involved field (irradiation); immunofluoresence
IFA	indirect fluorescent antibody
IFSP	individualized family service plan
Ig (IG)	immune globulin
IgA	immunoglobulin A
IgG	immunoglobulin G
IgS	immunoglobulin system
IGIV	immune globulin intravenous
IGT	impaired glucose tolerance
IH	infectious hepatitis
IHA	indirect hemagglutination
IHSS	idiopathic hypertrophic subaortic stenosis
IIA	interrupted infantile apnea
IICP	increased intracranial pressure
ILP	interstitial lymphocytic pneumonia
IM	intramuscular; or infectious mononucleosis
IMR	infant mortality rate
IMV	intermittent mandatory ventilation
in	inch
IND	investigational new drug
INH	isoniazid
INV	influenza vaccine
I & O	intake and output
IOL	intraocular lens
IOP	intraocular pressure
IPPB	intermittent positive pressure breathing
IPPD	intermedial purified protein derivative (tuberculin test)
IPV	inactivated poliovirus (vaccine)
IQ	intelligence quotient
IRB	institutional review board
Irr	irregular
IRV	inspiratory reserve volume

IS	in situ; or intercostal space
ISADH	inappropriate secretion of ADH
ISC	intermittent self-catheterization; or intermittent servo control
ISDB	indirect self-destructive behavior
ISF	interstitial fluid
ISG	immune serum globulin
ITP	idiopathic thrombocytopenic purpura
ITT	insulin tolerance test
IUD	intrauterine device
IUFD	intrauterine fetal demise
IUGR	intrauterine growth retardation
IUPC	intrauterine pressure catheter
IV	intravenous
IVC	inferior vena cava
IVCD	intraventricular conductive defect
IVDU	intravenous drug use
IVF	in vitro fertilization
IVGG	intravenous gamma-globulin
IVH	intraventricular hemorrhage
IVP	intravenous pyelogram; or intravenous push (medication)
IVPB	intravenous piggyback
IVT	intravenous transfusion
IWL	insensible water loss
JA	juvenile arthritis
JAS	juvenile ankylosing spondylitis
JCP	juvenile chronic polyarthritis
JND	just noticeable difference
JOD	juvenile-onset diabetes
JODM	juvenile-onset diabetes mellitus
JRA	juvenile rheumatoid arthritis
JV	jugular vein
JVD	jugular vein distention
K	absolute zero; Kelvin
KD	Kawasaki disease

KC	kangaroo care
kg	kilogram
17-KGS	17-ketogenic steroids
KIDS	Kansas Infant Development Screen
KOH	potassium hydroxide
17-KS	17-ketosteroids
KUB	kidneys/ureters/bladder
KVO	keep vein open
L	left
LA	left atrium; or lactic acid; or left arm
LAB	laboratory
LAE	left atrial enlargement
LAD	left anterior descending
LAM	lactational amenorrhea method
LAP	left arterial pressure
lat	lateral
LATS	long-acting thyroid stimulator
LAV	lymphadenopathy-associated virus
lb	pound
LBCD	left border of cardiac dullness (sternal border)
LBM	lean body mass
LBW	low birth weight; or lean body weight
LCA	left coronary artery
LCM	left costal margin
LD	lethal dose; or light difference (perception); or left deltoid
L & D	labor & delivery
LDH	lactate dehydrogenase
LDL	low-density lipoprotein
LDR	labor, delivery, recovery
LDRP	labor, delivery, recovery, postpartum
LE	lupus erythematosus; or left eye; or LE prep; or lower extremity
LES	lower esophageal sphincter; or Life Expectancy Survey
LFD	large for dates
LFT	liver function test

LG	left gluteal
LGA	large for gestational age
LGI	lower gastrointestinal tract
LH	luteinizing hormone
LH-RH	luteinizing hormone releasing hormone
LIP	lymphoid interstitial pneumonitis
liq	liquid
LJM	limited joint movement
LKS	liver, kidneys, spleen
LLBCD	left-lower border of cardiac dullness
LLE	left-lower extremity
LLL	left-lower lobe
LLQ	left-lower quadrant
LLT	left-lateral thigh
LMA	left-mentum-anterior
LMC	left midclavicular line
LMD	local medical doctor
LML	left medial lateral (as in incision or episiotomy site)
LMN	lower motor neuron
LMP	left-mentum-posterior; or last menstrual period
LMQ	left-middle quadrant
LMT	left-mentum-transverse
LNMP	last normal menstrual period
LOA	left-occiput-anterior
LOC	level of consciousness; or loss of consciousness; or locus of control; or loss of movement; or limitation of motion
LOM	left otitis media; or loss of movement; or limitation of motion
LOP	left-occiput-posterior
LOS	length of stay
LOT	left-occiput-transverse
LP	lumbar puncture
LPH	lipotrophic hormone
LPN	licensed practical nurse
LQ	lower quadrant
LRE	least restrictive environment
LRI	lower respiratory infection

LSA	left-sacrum-anterior
LSB	left sternal border; or left scapular border
LSP	left-sacrum-posterior
LST	left-sacrum-transverse
LTB	laryngotracheobronchitis
LTH	luteotropic hormone
LTV	long-term variability
LUE	left-upper extremity
LUL	left-upper lobe
LUOQ	left-upper outer quadrant
LUQ	left-upper quadrant
LV	left ventricle
LVG	left ventrogluteal
LVH	left ventricular hypertrophy
LVN	licensed vocational nurse
LVO	left ventricular output
m	meter
M	molar; or mean; or muscle; or male
M2	meters squared (square meters)
MA	mental age; or menstrual age
MABP	mean arterial blood pressure
MAC	maximum allowable concentration
MAI	Maternal Attachment Inventory
MAP	mean arterial pressure
MAR	medication administration record
MAS	meconium aspiration syndrome
MAWP	mean arterial wedge pressure
MBC	minimum bactericidal concentration
MBP	mean blood pressure
MC	mucocutaneous lymph node syndrome; or maternal child; or monochorionic
MCDI	Minnesota Child Development Inventory
mcg	microgram
MCH	mean corpuscular (cell) hemoglobin; or maternal and child health
MCHC	mean corpuscular (cell) hemoglobin concentration
MCL	midclavicular line

MCSA	McCarthy Scales of Children's Abilities
MCT	medium-chain triglyceride; or mean circulatory time
MCV	mean corpuscular volume; or mean clinical value
MD	muscular dystrophy; or medical doctor; or manic depression; or myocardial disease
MDA	minimal daily allowance
MDI	metered dose inhaler
ME	medical examiner; or middle ear
MED	minimal effective dose
Meds	medications
mEQ	milli-equivalents
MFD	minimal fatal dose
mg	milligram
Mg*	magnesium
MGN	membranous glomerulonephritis
MH	melanocytic hormone
MHC	major histocompatibility complex
MI	myocardial infarction; or mitral insufficiency; or myocardial ischemia; or mental illness
MIF	migration-inhibiting factor
ml	milliliter; midline
MLC	mixed lymphocyte culture
MLD	minimum lethal dose; or median lethal dose
MLE	midline episiotomy
MLNS	minimal lesion nephritic syndrome
MM	mucous membrane; or multiple melanoma
MMEF	maximal midexpiratory flow
mmHG	millimeters of mercury
MMPI	Minnesota Multiphasic Personality Inventory
MMR	morbidity and mortality report
MNF	multiple neurofibromatosis
MNP	mononuclear phagocyte
MO	medical officer
mod	moderate
MOD	March of Dimes
MODM	mature-onset diabetes mellitus

MODS	multiple organ dysfunction syndrome
MOF	multiple organ failure
MOSF	multiple organ system failure
MPAP	mean pulmonary artery pressure
MPD	maximum permissible dose
MPI	McGill Pain Index; or Minnesota Preschool Inventory
MPS	mucopolysaccharidosis; or mononuclear phagocytic system
MPV	microprocessor ventilator
MR	mental retardation; or may repeat; or measles, rubella; or mitral regurgitation; or magnetic resonance
MRD	minimum reacting dose
MRFIT	Multiple Risk Factor Intervention Trial
MRI	magnet resonance imaging
MRSA	methicillin-resistant *Staph aureans*
MS	mitral stenosis; or multiple sclerosis; or mitral sounds; or musculoskeletal
MS-1	hepatitis A
MS-2	hepatitis B
MSAF	meconium-stained amniotic fluid
MSAFP	maternal serum alpha-fetoprotein
MSDA	material safety data sheet
MSG	monosodium glutamate
MSL	midsternal line
MSP	Munchausen syndrome by proxy
MST	McCarthy Screening Tests
MTT	mean transit time
MV	mitral valve
MVA	motor vehicle accident
MVP	moisture vapor permeable (dressing)
MVV	maximum voluntary ventilation
MVU	montivideo unit
MZ	monozygotic
N	normal
n	number

NA	nutritional assessment; or not applicable
NAD	no abnormalities noted; or no appreciable disease
NAI	nonaccidental injury
NANBH	non-A, non-B hepatitis
NANDAI	North American Nursing Diagnosis Association-International
NAS	no added salt
NB	newborn
NBAS	Neonatal Behavioral Assessment Scale
NBN	newborn nursery
NC	no casualty; or not cultured
NCAST	Nursing Child Assessment Satellite Training
NCPAP	nasal continuous positive airway pressure
NCS	nerve conduction studies
NCVS	nerve condition velocity studies
ND	not done; or normal delivery
NE	niacin equivalent; or no effect; or not evaluated
NEC	necrotizing enterocolitis
neg	negative
N/F	negative respiratory force
NFT	nonorganic failure to thrive
NG	nasogastric
NGU	nongonococcal urethritis
NH	nursing home
NI	no information; or not identified
NICU	neonatal intensive care unit
NIDCAP	Newborn Individualized Developmental Care Assessment Program
NIDDM	non-insulin-dependent diabetes mellitus
NIHF	nonimmune hydrops fetalis
nil(o)	none
NIPS	Neonatal Infant Pain Scale
NIPPV	noninvasive intermittent positive pressure ventilation
NKA	no known allergies
nl	normal (value)
NLTR	non-life-threatening reaction
NM	neonatal mortality
NMR	nuclear magnetic resonance; or neonatal mortality rates

NMDS	nursing minimum data set
NMR	numeric rating scale
NND	new and nonofficial drugs
NNS	nonnutritive sucking
NO	nitric oxide
NOFT	nonorganic failure to thrive
NOP	not otherwise provided for
NOS	not otherwise specified
NP	nasopharynx; or new patient; or not palpable; or nerve palsy; or nurse practitioner
NPO	*nil per os*; nothing by mouth
NPN	nonprotein nitrogen
NR	normal range; or nonreactive; or no report; or no respirations; or not remarkable; or no resuscitation; or not refillable; or normal reaction
NREM	nonrapid eye movement
NS	normal saline; or not significant
NSAID	nonsteroidal anti-inflammatory drugs
NSFTD	normal spontaneous full-term delivery
NSR	normal sinus rhythm
NST	nonstress test
NSU	nonspecific urethritis
NT	nasotracheal
NTB	necrotizing tracheobronchitis
NTG	nitroglycerin
NTD	neural tube defect
NTP	normal temperature and pressure
NUG	necrotizing ulcerative gingivitis
NVD	nausea and vomiting of pregnancy; neck vein distension
NVSS	normal variant short stature
NWB	non-weight-bearing
NYD	not yet diagnosed
O_2	oxygen
OASDL	ordinary activities and skills of daily living
OASIS	outcome assessment information sets
OBS	organic brain syndrome

OB	obstetrics
OC	oral contraceptive; or oculocephalic (doll's eye reflex); or on call; or office call
OCA	oral contraceptive agent
OCD	over-the-counter drug; obsessive-compulsive disorder
OCP	oral contraceptive pill
OD*	*oculus dexter** (right eye); or once daily; or overdose; or outside diameter; optical density
OFC	occipitofrontal circumference
OG	orogastric
OHS	orally administered hydration solution (s)
OI	osteogenesis imperfecta
OME	otitis media with effusion
OOB	out of bed
OP	osmotic pressure
O & P	ova and parasites
OPC	outpatient client
OPD	outpatient department
OR	operating room
ORIF	open reduction internal fixation
os	mouth
OS*	*oculus sinister* (left eye)
OSA	obstructive sleep apnea
OSB	open spina bifida
OT	occupational therapy; or orotracheal; or old tuberculin; or old term
OTC	over-the-counter
OU*	*oculi unitas* (both eyes)
OV	oculovestibular (cold water caloric test)
oz	ounce
P	phosphorus; or probability; or protein
PA	physician's assistant; or pathology; or primary anemia; or pulmonary artery
P & A	posterior & anterior
P/PR	pulse/pulse rate
PAC	premature atrial contraction

PaCO$_2$	partial pressure of arterial carbon dioxide
PACU	postanesthesia care unit
PAI	Prenatal Attachment Inventory
PAIDS	pediatric AIDS
PALS	pediatric advanced life support
PANESS	physical and neurologic examination for soft signs
PaO$_2$	partial pressure of arterial oxygen
PAP	primary atypical pneumonia; or Papanicolaou smear; or passive-aggressive personality; or pulmonary artery pressure
PAPVR	partial anomalous pulmonary venous return
PAR	post anesthesia room
PAT	pain assessment tool
PAWP	pulmonary artery wedge pressure
PBB	polybromated biphenyl
pc	*post cibum* (after meals)
PCA	patient controlled analgesia
PCO$_2$	partial pressure of carbon dioxide
PCOS	polycystic ovary syndrome
PCP	polymerase chain reaction; or patient care plan; or *Pneumocystis carinii* pneumonia
PCP	primary care provider/primary care physician
PCR	polymerase chain reaction
PCT	prothrombin consumption test
PCV	packed cell volume
PCWP	pulmonary capillary wedge pressure
PD	papillary distance; or postural drainage; or poorly differentiated
PDA	patent ductus arteriosis
PDC	private diagnostic clinic
PDI	Preschool Development Inventory
PDNB	penile dorsal nerve block
PDQ	Prescreening Developmental Questionnaire
PDR	*Physicians' Desk Reference*
PE	Physical examination; or pressure equalizing; or probable error; or pulmonary embolism; or port of entry; or physical education; or pelvic examination
per	by or through

PEEP	positive end expiratory pressure
PEEX	Pediatric Early Elementary Examination
PEFR	peak expiratory flow rate
PEG	percutaneous endoscopic gastrostomy; or pneumoencephalogram
PEN	parenteral/enteral nutrition
PEPI	postmenopausal estrogen/progestin interventions
PERL	pupils equal and react to light
per os	by mouth
PERRLA	pupils equal, round, react to light and accommodation
PET	positron emission tomography
PETT	positron emission transaxial tomography
PETCO$_2$	partial pressure of end tidal carbon dioxide
PF	pulmonary flow
PFC	persistent fetal circulation
PFNB	percutaneous fine needle biopsy
PFT	pulmonary function test
PG	phosphatidylglycerol; or prostaglandin
PGE2	prostaglandin E2
PGIS	Perinatal Grief Intensity Scale
pH	free hydrogen ion concentration; power of hydrogen
PH	past history; or previous history; or public health
PHA	phytohemagglutinin
PHN	public health nurse
PHV	peak height velocity
PI	pulmonary insufficiency; or present illness; or pulmonary infarction
PICC	percutaneously inserted central catheter
PICU	pediatric intensive care unit
PID	pelvic inflammatory disease
PIE	pulmonary interstitial emphysema
PIH	pregnancy-induced hypertension
PIP	peak inspiratory pressure; or proximal interphalangeal
PIPP	Premature Infant Pain Profile
PKD	polycystic kidney disease
PKU	phenylketonuria

PLH	pulmonary lymphoid hyperplasia
PM	post mortem; *post meridiem* (afternoon)
PMC	pseudomembranous colitis
PMH	past medical history
PMI	point of maximum impulse; or posterior myocardial infarction
PMN	polymorphonuclear neutrophil
PMR	polymyalgia rheumatica; or psychomotor retardation; or perinatal mortality rate; or physical medicine and rehabilitation
PMS	premenstrual syndrome
PN	pneumonia
PND	postural nocturnal dyspnea; or postnasal drip
PNI	psychoneuroimmunology
PNM	postnatal mortality
PNP	pediatric nurse practitioner
PNPR	positive-negative pressure respiration
PNI	psychoneuroimmunology
p.o.	*per os* (by mouth)
PO	post operative; or phone order
PO_2	partial pressure of oxygen
POA	primary optic atrophy
poly	many
POMR	problem-oriented medical record
POR	problem-oriented record
POS	point of service
postop	post operative
PP	partial pressure; or patient profile; or peripheral pulses; or postpartum; postprandial; or presenting problem
PPC	progressive patient care
PPD	purified protein derivative
PPHN	persistent pulmonary hypertension of the newborn
PPLO	pleuropneumonia-like organism
PPO	preferred provider organization
PPPA	Poison Prevention Packaging Act
PPROM	preterm premature rupture of membranes

PPS	peripheral pulmonic stenosis
PPT	partial prothrombin time
PPV	positive pressure ventilation
PR	perfusion rate; or peripheral resistance; or progress report; or pulse rate; or public relations
PRA	plasma rennin activity
PRBC	packed red blood cells
preop	preoperative
prep	preparation
PRESS	Preschool Readiness Experimental Screening Scale
PROM	premature rupture of membranes; passive range of motion
PRN	*pro re nata* (as necessary); or circumstance may require
PRP	persistent recurrent pneumonia
PS	pulmonic stenosis; or pyloric stenosis; or physical status
PSA	prostate specific antigen
PSDA	Patient Self Determination Act
P/SH	personal social history
PSMA	progressive spinal muscular atrophy
PSP	phenolsulfonphthalein test
PSR	psychological stimulus response
PT	prothrombin time; or physical therapist; or patient
PTA	prior to admission; plasma thromboplastin antecedent; or percutaneous transluminal angioplasty
PTC	plasma thromboplastin component; or phenylthiocarbamide
PTCA	percutaneous transluminal coronary angioplasty
PTH	parathyroid hormone; pseudohyperparathyroidism
PTL	preterm labor
PTSD	post-traumatic stress disorder
PTT	partial thromboplastin time
PTU	propylthiouracil
PUBS	percutaneous umbilical blood sampling
PUD	peptic ulcer disease
PUO	pyrexia of undetermined (unknown) origin

PUPPP	pruritic urticarial papules and plaques of pregnancy
PV	parainfluenza virus; or peripheral vascular; or peripheral vein
PVC	premature ventricular contraction; or polyvinyl chloride
$PVCO_2$	partial pressure of venous carbon dioxide
PVD	percussion, vibration, and drainage; or peripheral vascular disease
PVH	periventricular hemorrhage
PVP	pulmonary venous pressure
PVR	pulmonary vascular resistance; or peripheral vascular resistance
PVS	percussion, vibration, and suction
PWB	partial weight bearing
PWP	pulmonary wedge pressure
PWS	port-wine stain; or Prader-Willi syndrome
PX	pneumothorax; or prognosis
q	*quaque* (every)
qd*	*quaque die* (every day)
qh	*quaque hora* (every hour)
q2h	every 2 hours
qhs	*quaque hora somni*; every night at bedtime
qid	*quarter in die* (four times a day)
qn	every night
qns	quantity not sufficient
qod*	every other day
QPIT	quantitative pilocarpine iontophoresis test
qs	quantity sufficient
R	right
R/RR	respirations/respiratory rate
RA	rheumatoid arthritis; or return appointment; or renal artery; or right arm; or right atrium; or repeat action; or rectal atresia; or room air
RAE	right atrial enlargement
RAP	recurrent abdominal pain

RAST	radioallergosorbent test
RATG	rabbit antithymocytic globulin
RBC	red blood cells
RBD	right border dullness
RBE	relative biologic effectiveness
RBF	renal blood flow
RBRVS	resource-based relative value scale
RBS	random blood sugar
RC	rice cereal; or red cell
RCC	red cell concentrate
RCM	right costal margin
RD	registered dietitian
RDA	recommended daily allowance
RDI	reference daily intake
RDS	respiratory distress syndrome
RDSI	Revised Developmental Screening Inventory
RE	regional enteritis; or rear end (accident); or right eye; or rectal examination
REE	resting energy expenditure
REEDA	redness, edema, ecchymosis, discharge, approximation
REM	rapid eye movement
req	requisition
RF	rheumatoid factor; or rheumatoid factor
RG	right gluteal
Rh	rhesus factor
RHD	rheumatic heart disease; or relative hepatic dullness
RhoGam	Rho(D) immune globulin
RIA	radioimmunoassay; radioactive immunoassay
RICE	rest, ice, compression, elevation
RICM	right intercostal margin
RLE	right-lower extremity
RLF	retrolental fibroplasia
RLQ	right-lower quadrant
RLT	right-lateral thigh
RMA	right-mentum-anterior; or rhythmic motor activities
RML	right mediolateral (as in episiotomy); or right-middle lobe

RMP	right-mentum-posterior
RMR	resting metabolic rate
RMSF	Rocky Mountain spotted fever
RMT	right-mentum-transverse
RN	registered nurse
RNA	ribonucleic acid
R/O	rule out; or routine order
ROA	right-occiput-anterior
ROM	range of motion; or right otitis media; or rupture of membranes
ROP	right-occiput-posterior; or retinopathy of prematurity
ROS	review of systems
ROT	right-occiput-transverse
RP	resting pressure
R-PDQ	Revised Prescreening Developmental Questionnaire
RPF	renal plasma flow
RR	respiratory rate; or recovery room; or radiation response; or rust ring
RS	review of symptoms; or Reye syndrome; Reiter syndrome
RSA	right-sacrum-anterior
RSB	right sternal border
RSP	right-sacrum-posterior
RSR	regular sinus rhythm
RST	right-sacrum-transverse
RSV	respiratory syncytial virus
RT	respiratory therapy (therapist); or room temperature
RTA	renal tubular acidosis
RTI	respiratory tract infection
RTUS	real-time ultrasound
RUE	right-upper extremity
RUL	right-upper lobe
RUOQ	right-upper outer quadrant
RUQ	right-upper quadrant
RV	residual volume; or right ventricle
Rv	rotavirus
RVG	right ventrogluteal

RVH	right ventricular hypertrophy
RVV	rubella vaccine virus
Rx	prescription; *recipe* (take); or treatment
s	*sine* (without)
s&s	signs and symptoms
SAC	short arm cast
SAD	sugar and acetone determination
SAH	subarachnoid hemorrhage
SAM	surface active material
SaO2	saturation of arterial oxygen
sb	strabismus
SB	sternal border; or stillborn
SBE	subacute bacterial endocarditis
SBO	small bowel obstruction
SBR	strict bed rest
SC*	subcutaneous*; or servocontrol
SCB	strictly confined to bed
SC disease	sickle-cell-hemoglobin C disease
SCD	sickle-cell disease; sudden cardiac death
SCFE	slipped capital femoral epiphysis
SCID	severe combined immune deficiency disease
SCM	sternocleidomastoid muscle
SCU	special care unit
SCV	smooth, capsulated, virulent
SD	standard deviation; or septal defect; or spontaneous delivery; or sudden death; or shoulder disarticulation; or shoulder dystocia
SDA	specific dynamic action
SES	socioeconomic status
SF	spinal fluid; or scarlet fever
SFAO	superficial femoral artery occlusion
SFD	small for dates
SG	specific gravity; or Swan-Ganz catheter; or skin graph
SGA	small for gestational age
SGOT	serum glutamic-oxaloacetic transaminase
SGPT	serum glutamic-pyruvic transaminase

SH	social history; or self-help; or serum hepatitis; or shoulder; or sex hormone
SIADH	syndrome of inappropriate ADH
SIDS	sudden infant death syndrome
SIG	serum immune globulin
sIgA	secretory immunoglobulin A
SILV	synchronous independent lung ventilation
SIMV	synchronous intermittent mandatory ventilation
SIRS	system inflammatory response syndrome
SKL	serum killing levels
SKSD	streptokinase/streptodornase (control test)
SLC	short leg cast
SLD	specific learning disability
SLE	systemic lupus erythematosus; or St. Louis encephalitis
SLUD	salivation, lacrimation, urination, defecation
SLWC	short leg walking cast
SM	simple mastectomy; or systolic murmur
SMA	smooth muscle antibodies; or sequential multiple analyzer
SMBG	self-monitoring blood glucose
SM-C	somatomedin-C
SNF	skilled nursing facility
SNS	sympathetic nervous system
SO	salpingo-oophorectomy
SOAP	subjective, objective, assessment, plan
SOB	shortness of breath
SOM	serous otitis media
S/P	status post
SPA	suprapubic aspiration; or salt poor albumin
spec	specimen
SPF	sun protection factor
SPEP	serum protein electrophoresis
sp gr	specific gravity
SPL	sound pressure levels
SpO_2	saturation of arterial capillary hemoglobin

SPT	sweat patch test
SQ*	subcutaneous
SR	system review; or sinus rhythm; or sedimentation rate; or stretch reflex; or schizophrenic reaction; or stimulus-response
S-R	stimulus-response
SRI	systemic reaction index
SRSA	slow reacting substance of anaphylaxis
ss	*semis* (one half)
S/S	signs and symptoms
SS disease	sickle-cell disease
SSE	soapsuds enema; or soap solution enema
SSEP	somatosensory evoked potential
SSI	segmental spinal instrumentation
SSSS	staphylococcal-scalded skin syndrome
stat	*statim* (immediately)
STC	serum theophylline concentration
STD	sexually transmitted disease; or skin test dose; or standard test dose
STORCH	syphilis, toxoplasmosis, other infections, rubella, cytomegalovirus, herpes
STS	serologic test for syphilis
STSG	split-thickness skin graft
STU	skin test unit
STV	short-term variability
SubQ	subcutaneous
supp	suppository
susp	suspension
SV	spontaneous ventilation or stroke volume
SVC	superior vena cava
SVD	spontaneous vaginal delivery
SVE	sterile vaginal examination
SVR	systemic vascular resistance
SVT	sinus ventricular tachycardia; or supraventricular tachycardia
SUD	sudden unexplained death
Sx	symptoms
SxH	sexual history; symptom history

T3	triiodothyronine
T4	thyroxine
TA/TAT	toxin-antitoxin; or tricuspid atresia; or truncus arteriosus
T & A	tonsillectomy and adenoidectomy
tab	tablet
TAPVR	total anomalous pulmonary venous return
T/TMP	temperature
TB	tuberculosis
TBG	thyroxine-binding globulin
TBI	traumatic brain injury; or total body irradiation
TBLC	term birth, living child
TBM	total body mass
Tbn	tuberculin
TBSA	total body surface
TBT	tracheobronchial tree
TBW	total body water
TC	total cholesterol
TCDB	turn, cough, deep breath
TCM	traditional Chinese medicine
$TcPaCO_2$	transcutaneous carbon dioxide pressure (tension)
$TcPaO_2$	transcutaneous oxygen pressure (tension)
TCU	transitional care unit
Td	adult tetanus and diphtheria
TD	typhoid dysentery
TDM	therapeutic drug monitoring
T3	expiratory time
TE	tracheoesophageal; or tetanus
TEF	tracheoesophageal fistula
TEN	toxic epidermal necrolysis
TENS	transcutaneous electrical nerve stimulation
TEV	talipes equinovarus
TEWL	transevaporative water loss
Tg	thyroglobulin
TG	triglyceride(s)
TGA	transposition of great arteries
TGE	theoretical growth evaluation
TGV	transposition of great vessels

THF	tetrahydrofolate
TI	tricuspid insufficiency
TIA	transient ischemic attack
tid	*ter in die* (three times a day)
TIPP	The Injury Prevention Program
TKO	to keep open
TL	team leader
TLC	tender loving care; or total lung capacity; or total lymphocyte count; or thin layer chromatography
TM	tympanic membrane; or temperature by mouth; or tender midline; or transmetatarsal; or temporomandibular
TMR	trainable mentally retarded
TNI	total nodal irradiation
TNM	tumor, nodal involvement and metastasis
TNR	tonic neck reflex
TO	target organ; or telephone order
TOF	tetralogy of Fallot
TOLAC	trial of labor after cesarean
TORCHS	toxoplasmosis, rubella, cytomegalovirus, herpes simplex, syphilis
Torr	millimeters of mercury
tPA	tissue plasminogen activator
TPR	temperature, pulse, respirations; or total perfusion resistance
Tr.	tincture
TRH	thyrotropin releasing hormone
TSA	tumor-specific antigen
TSB	total serum bilirubin
TSD	Tay-Sachs disease
TSE	testicular self-examination
TSF	triceps skinfold
TSH	thyroid stimulating hormone
TSS	toxic shock syndrome
TT	therapeutic touch; or transit time
TTN	transient tachypnea of the newborn
TU	tuberculin units; or toxic unit; or transmission unit
Tx	treatment
TV	tidal volume; or total volume

UA	urinalysis
UAC	umbilical artery catheters
UAP	unlicensed assistive personnel
UC	uterine contraction
UCHD	usual childhood illnesses (diseases)
UD	urethral discharge
UDT	undescended testicle
uE3	unconjugated estrogen
UGI	upper gastrointestinal
UI	urinary incontinence
UIL	upper intake level
U/L	upper-lower body ratio
UMN	upper motor neuron
UO	urine output
UP	universal precautions
UPC	unplanned pregnancy counseling
URI	upper respiratory infection
UQ	upper quadrant
UrA	uric acid
URI	upper respiratory infection
US	ultrasonography
USA	ultrasonic aerosol (nebulization)
UTI	urinary tract infection
UV	ultraviolet
UAV	ultraviolet A
UAB	ultraviolet B
V	vein; or volume; or vision
VA	visual acuity
VACTERL	vertebral, anal, congenital heart defect, tracheoesophageal atresia or fistula, renal anomalies, and limb deformities
VAD	ventricular assist device
VAR	visual-aural range
VATER	vertebral, anal, tracheoesophageal atresia or fistula, and renal anomalies
VB	viable birth
VBAC	vaginal birth after cesarean
VC	vital capacity

VCA	viral capsid antigen
VCG	vectorcardiograph
VCT	venous clotting time
VCUG	voiding cystourethrogram
VD	venereal disease
VDG	venereal disease, gonorrhea
VDRL	Venereal Disease Research Laboratory
VDRR	vitamin D-resistant rickets
VDS	venereal disease, syphilis
VDT	video display terminal
VE	vesicular exanthema
VEP	visual evoked stimuli
VF	visual fields; or ventricular fibrillation
VG	ventricular gallop
VH	vaginal hysterectomy; or viral hepatitis
VIG	vaccinia immune globulin
VLBW	very low birth weight
VLDL	very low-density lipoprotein
VM	vasomotor; or vestibular membrane
VO	verbal order
VP	ventricular-peritoneal; or venous pressure
VCP	ventricular premature complex
VR	valve replacement; or venous return
VRA	visual reinforced audiometry
VPS	ventricular peritoneal shunt
Vr	tidal volume
VS	vital signs
VSD	ventricular septal defect
VSGA	very small for gestational age
VSS	vital signs stable
VT	ventricular tachycardia
VUR	vesicoureteral reflux
VZ	varicella-zoster
VZIG	varicella-zoster immune globulin
VZV	varicella-zoster virus
w	watt; or weight; or wife; or week
WAIS	Wechsler Adult Intelligence Scale

WB	whole blood; or weight bearing
WBC	white blood cell count
w/c	wheelchair
WC	whooping cough; or ward clerk
WD	well developed; or well differentiated
WEE	western equine encephalitis
WHM	women's health movement
WIC	women, infants, and children
WIPI	word intelligibility by picture identification
WISC-R	Wechsler Intelligence Scale for Children, revised
WM	white male
WN	well nourished
WNL	within normal limits
WPPSI	Wechsler Preschool and Primary Scale of Intelligence
WPW	Wolff-Parkinson-White syndrome
WR	Wasserman reactions
WRAT	Wide Range Achievement Test
WT	weight; white
XLMR	X-linked mental retardation
XLR	X-linked recessive
XTB	X-ray treated blood
YF	yellow fever
YO	years old
YRBSS	youth risk behavior surveillance system
ZIG	zoster immune globulin
ZIP	zoster immune plasma

PART 2

Basic Processes

Communication

Professional communication is designed to accomplish two goals. The first is to be clear, comforting, and caring in our communication with patients. The second is to be precise in our interdisciplinary and intradisciplinary communications so that patients may benefit. Sharing personal perspectives about life in general may be the goal for some patients. Irrespective of what we share personally, we must be able to communicate clearly about health care matters. There are four parts to this section. The first relates to key messages and guidelines we can use on a regular basis and includes examples of what we can say as professionals. The second is medically oriented Spanish, the second most prevalent spoken language in the United States. The third is sign language, the third most prevalent language in the United States. The fourth is the Braille alphabet.

Key Messages and Guidelines
Communication Guidelines

1. Understand the HIPAA (Health Insurance Portability and Accountability Act) expectations. Although the act is designed to assure portability of insurance and patient confidentiality, how the law is implemented varies dramatically across institutions. ⌐ www.hipaa.org or www.hhs.gov/ocr/hipaa.
2. Determine the level of understanding of the patient or family member. Assume responsibility for the flow of the communication process.
3. Be open. Share your thoughts and feelings carefully— particularly about the patient and situation.
4. Create a balance in the conversation of both serious aspects and lighter humorous aspects. Some "small talk" can be helpful and natural, for instance if traffic or driving time is prolonged or difficult, ask if there were problems. If the weather has been particularly severe, ask about the effect upon them or their neighborhood.
5. Support the patient/client and the family by acknowledging, encouraging, and even praising them, e.g., when the patient or family presents a plan for some aspect of care, visiting, or home care, acknowledge them for whatever

aspect of the idea works and then seek clarification if some aspect of the idea may have potential difficulties.

6. Avoid asking yes or no questions unless this is appropriate for conditions such as limited energy, language capability, or difficulty in speaking.

7. Avoid asking "why" questions. They often make people defensive. Rather, ask "what" questions, such as, "What made you think that the doctor was going to operate tomorrow?"

8. Use technical terms if appropriate or necessary, and follow those with the common terms used by the public, e.g., "The procedure the doctor is planning is a CABG, commonly known as heart surgery."

9. Be honest, but not alarming, e.g., "I am caring for many patients" (rather than saying, "We are really short staffed.")

10. Talk to patients and family as equals. Refrain from talking down to them.

Guidelines for Active Listening

- Convey interest in what the other person is saying through nonverbal affirmations and verbal responses, as in nodding your head, smiling, or verbal feedback such as "I hear what you're saying," or "I understand."

- Encourage the person to expand his/her thinking; ask such questions as, "What more can you tell me about. . . ?"

- Seek clarity by reflecting or paraphrasing what the person has said, e.g., "Then the problem, as you see it is. . ."

- Refrain from making judgments or "labeling" the person. Rather, understand the perspective of the other person as he/she tells you his/her story, as in "This is a person who wants me to understand her" as opposed to "This is an old woman who is losing her faculties and is clearly a hypochondriac."

- Respond to the person's feelings rather than to the words, e.g., "You feel strongly about the lack of interaction you had with the anesthesiologist."
- Listen to the words the patients use and reflect those words to your patients, e.g., say "long bone" as opposed to thigh bone or femur when patients use that term.
- Summarize specific points in the interaction and check to make sure the patient agrees with the summary, as in "You feel distressed about the diagnosis and you are unclear how you will manage once you return home?"

Special Considerations in Communicating

The Hearing-Impaired Patient

1. Stand directly in front of the patient. Speak slowly and distinctly in a normal volume. Do not yell or raise your voice.
2. Make sure the patient/client can see you; many people are hearing impaired and read lips.
3. Check for a hearing aid and the status of the batteries.
4. Keep paper and pencil close at hand and write notes, particularly if privacy is an issue.
5. Check to see if the person uses sign language.
6. Should all these efforts fail, act out what you want to convey.

Aphasic Patients

- Use active listening skills.
- Take time with the patient.
- Encourage the patient to repeat if necessary and do not rush.
- Use pencil and paper as necessary.
- Consult with the family if this is a long-standing condition, such as a stroke, to determine what has worked for them.
- Consult with a speech therapist for ideas and help.

PART 2

Tracheostomy Patients

1. Be prepared to cover the trach opening for brief periods to support communication.
2. Always prepare the patient for what you are going to do prior to taking action.
3. If covering the trach is not effective, offer paper and a pencil or other nonoral devices.
4. Try a dry erase board with pens or a small chalkboard for the patient to write on.
5. Devise and use a code. Eye blinks (one blink for no and two blinks for yes) and hand signals can be used.

Intubated Patients

Similar strategies as those for the trach patient can be used except, of course, for covering the tube opening.

Unconscious Patients

- Remember that the first sense to return from an unconscious state is hearing. Thus, it is critical to talk to the unconscious patient throughout the delivery of care.
- A radio with news and music may be helpful.
- Encourage family members to talk to the patient as if he or she could understand everything.

Cultural Considerations

1. Be receptive to patient information about how the family and significant others interrelate.
2. Be an active listener and an observant communicator. (Note for example use of gestures associated with speech, physical contact with others, and eye contact.)
3. Speak clearly and carefully; use gestures and actual objects to enhance the message when there is a language barrier.
4. Be respectful of the family's presence and their preference for how they would be addressed.

5. Explain why information is needed, especially if it seems to be of a private nature.
6. Use an interpreter whenever possible (if needed), and make certain the patient and family know that this service is available.
7. Learn basic words and remember that people appreciate attempts to speak in their language.
8. Be honest, even if that means saying you are unable to answer a question. Trust is important when communication is complex.
9. Note religious symbols and practices and incorporate them into care as possible.
10. Avoid stereotyping a patient or family based on any cultural considerations such as religion, ethnicity, socioeconomic, gender, or other factor.

Medically Oriented Spanish

1. What is your name?
   Como se llama?
2. My name is_____ and I am your nurse (female).
   Me llama es_____ y soy su enfemera.
3. What day is it?
   Que dia es hoy?
4. What time is it?
   Que hora es?
5. Where are you?
   Donde esta usted?
6. Where do you live?
   Donde vive usted?
7. How old are you?
   Cuantos años tiene?
8. Are you taking any medications?
   Esta usted tornando algun medicamento?
9. Do you have any allergies?
   Padece usted de alguna alergia?

10. Have you ever had any surgeries and/or been admitted to the hospital?
   Ha sido usted operada en alguna occasion o ingresada en el hospitale?
11. Where is your pain?
   Donde esta dolor?
12. Do you have pain?
   Tiene usted dolor?
13. Do you need to go to the bathroom?
   Necesita ir al bano?
14. Can you breathe okay?
   Dificultad al respirar?
15. Are you having contractions? (labor)
   Tiene contracciones?
16. When did they start?
   Cuando empezaron?
17. How far apart are the contractions?
   Las contracciones estan a cuantos minutos aparte?
18. Push; Don't Push
   Empuje!; No empuje!
19. Breathe!
   Respiré!

Sign Language

Sign language can help with communication when a patient is unable to speak. While using sign language may be a slow process, it is important to share information between the patient and the nurse.

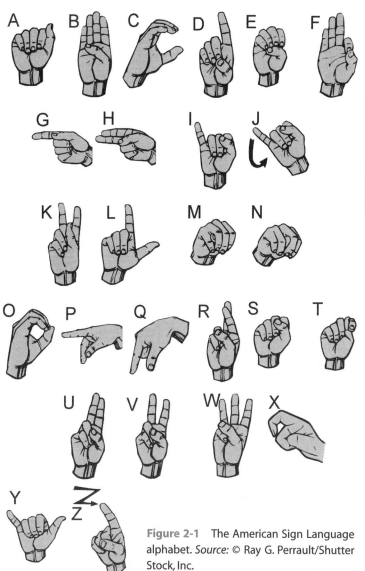

Figure 2-1 The American Sign Language alphabet. *Source:* © Ray G. Perrault/Shutter Stock, Inc.

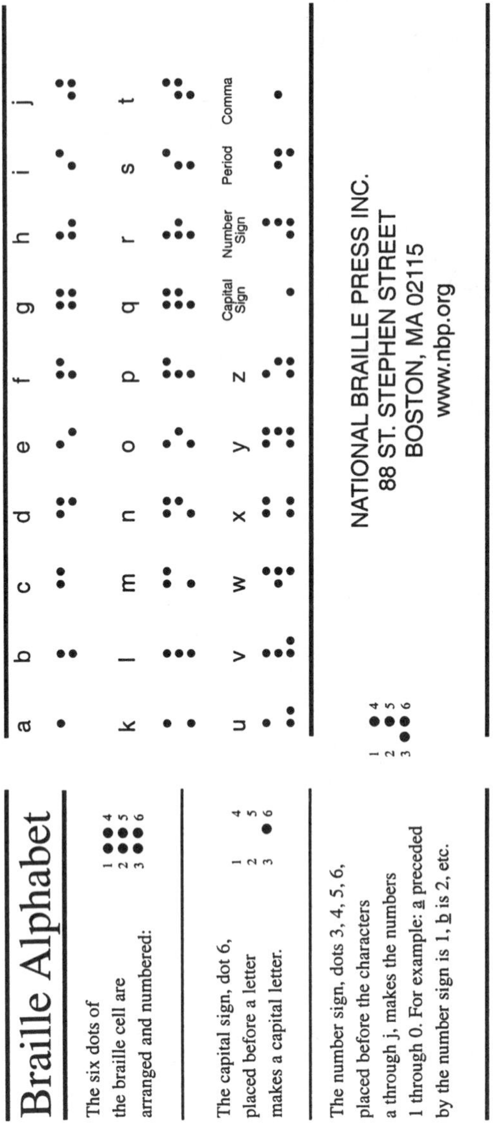

Braille Alphabet

The six dots of
the braille cell are
arranged and numbered:

```
1  • 4
2  • 5
3  • 6
```

The capital sign, dot 6,
placed before a letter
makes a capital letter.

```
1    4
2    5
3  • 6
```

The number sign, dots 3, 4, 5, 6,
placed before the characters
a through j, makes the numbers
1 through 0. For example: a preceded
by the number sign is 1, b is 2, etc.

```
1    4
2    5
3  • • 6
```

a	b	c	d	e	f	g	h	i	j

k	l	m	n	o	p	q	r	s	t

u	v	w	x	y	z	Capital Sign	Number Sign	Period	Comma

NATIONAL BRAILLE PRESS INC.
88 ST. STEPHEN STREET
BOSTON, MA 02115
www.nbp.org

Figure 2-2   The Braille alphabet. *Source:* Courtesy of the National Braille Press.

Braille Alphabet

The Braille alphabet may be useful when an individual is sightless and must read something. Normally it is not the nurse's responsibility to validate or create Braille documents. In the event of an emergency, however, this tool may be useful.

The Nursing Process

The nursing process represents a systematic approach to determining what an individual, family, or group needs from nursing care and how to provide and evaluate the outcomes geared toward health improvement. The nursing process forms the basis for the National Council Licensure Examination for Registered Nurses (NCLEX-RN) and thus provides a foundation for understanding the way in which registered nurses determine, provide, and evaluate care. Because patients (whether individual, family, or group) are dynamic entities, so is the nursing process. It is an approach to be used on an ongoing basis so that nursing actions best fit the current situation and needs.

Numerous views exist about the exact steps of the process. Various authors and various schools of nursing have a preferred view about the number of steps, what is contained in each, and what key words should appear in which step. Irrespective, the following content should appear somewhere in the process. Some health care organizations use specific formats for documenting the process. If these exist, they should be used.

Assessment

This initial element is designed to create a profile. It includes physical and emotional data that are collected and analyzed in terms of normal or acceptable standards, including age, socioeconomic, gender, and ethnic data and risk factors. This step includes a detailed health history and a head-to-toe assessment. Subsequently, nurses typically focus on updating information that relates to the health issues. It is always useful to end with some question related to gaining any other information that might be viewed as useful but that might have been overlooked. A question such as, "Is there anything else you think I should know about what is happening for you right now?" may help provide insight that wouldn't necessarily be gained by a typical assessment.

Diagnosis

This element focuses on the conclusions about the assessment. It consists of actual and potential problems that then guide what actions nurses take. Typically, some lexicon of terms is standard within a school or health care organization. This text references the NANDA-I (North American Nursing Diagnosis Association-International) standards, because these standards are widely used. NANDA-I diagnoses are patterns reflective of patient responses to a health situation. Subcategories frequently reflect the underlying cause whether it is the patient's actual response or the disease condition or the physiological condition associated with a health situation. For more information, see ⏻ www.nanda. org.

Outcomes Definition

Outcomes are the desired result of the nursing action taken to improve or maintain a person's, family's, or group's health. They must be specific, measurable, and realistic. Outcomes may be addressed in "absence of" statements as well as specific actions or states. An outcome might include numbers, such as walked so many steps, or values, such as pain free. Outcomes may be short term or long term and may be referred to as goals. The key, however, is to think about the outcome before beginning care so that actions are goal oriented and improvement can be measured. Critical pathways and care maps or protocols are usually based on anticipated outcomes. Some desired outcomes will be short term; others, especially those involving chronic disease and rehabilitation, may be long term.

Implementation

This element consists of specific actions or categories of action that the nurse will take in relation to the defined diagnoses that move the patient, family, or group toward desired outcomes. It may also be called *interventions* because it is the set of actions nurses or their delegatees perform to provide care to patients. This step frequently includes procedures that nurses perform either on their own or in accordance with the medical treatment plan. This element is frequently the most documented in the patient record because it is connected with reimbursement, interim evaluation of progress, or legal aspects of assuring appropriate actions were taken. Implementation strategies should be based on evidence whenever possible.

Evaluation

This final element is based on a review of the process in an ongoing manner so that changes and progress toward outcomes may be noted. This element requires professional judgment about the progress made and is not merely a measurement of activities or procedures completed. It is the judgment phase that determines if the current approach should be maintained or revised. Documentation should reflect findings and judgments of evaluation.

Assessment Guides

This section contains information useful in performing specific assessment techniques and strategies. Used in combination with the glossary, the diagrams, and the tests sections, the assessment guide can provide the basis for creating an appropriate nursing assessment.

Health History

Sometimes the health history may be established before your first encounter with the patient. Generally, it is useful to read that history and then discuss specific points for clarification. If no history has been established, you will need to seek the information described below. After introducing yourself, you should explain to the patient what you will do and why. It is useful to establish that the patient's primary oral language is the same as yours. If either you or the patient is able to communicate in a different language when a language barrier exists, it is important to secure a translator or interpreter for the two languages.

Biographic Data

This information is usually found on an admitting office form. It should contain name, address, phone, date of birth, marital status, occupation, religious preference, next of kin, whom to notify in the event of an emergency, and insurance sources.

Chief Complaint

The focus of this discussion is to determine if the person is experiencing an illness, concern, or discomfort, as described in his or her own words. Frequently, the questions asked are: Why did you come here today? What seems to be troubling you?

History

The information gathered in this section is among the most important. It provides the background about how to interpret the patient's current health status and how he or she will likely be able to incorporate any life changes and adapt to temporary changes in a recuperative period.

General

Ask the patient about his or her general perception of health. (Remember that health is the term related to a broad spectrum, not the opposite of wellness.) It will be important to seek clarification about wellness if the patient addresses only illness.

Current History

In this section, you want to target the key concerns as reflected in the chief complaint. Information should include when the patient first became concerned about the current issue (be sure to ask how long it existed before he or she actually became concerned); what, if anything, the patient associates this issue with (e.g., eating certain foods, falling, or activity); the nature of the onset (sudden or gradual); type and location of any pain/discomfort; frequency of the issue (has it happened before, how long between episodes, pattern of recurrence); what makes it better or worse; and the typical response if this isn't an acute episode (e.g., sees a provider for care, takes over-the-counter medication, ignores or changes activity/diet).

Family History

This information is generally related to siblings, parents, and their siblings and grandparents. (It may be important here to remind patients to consider what they know about their biological parents. In addition to people who are adopted, this consideration applies to people born as a result of in vitro fertilization.)

Past History

This section tends to be among the most troublesome for health care providers because many people don't keep records nor were they given any from their parents. The focus of this element is on childhood illnesses, immunizations, accidents, surgeries, transfusions, major illnesses, and hospitalizations. Each of these elements may require follow-up questions to elicit better information. The goal is to determine if there is anything a health care provider needs to know that isn't necessarily related to the current condition but that may influence the way in which care is rendered.

Medication History

Asking the patient about current medications including names, dosages, and frequencies (and the patient's understanding of what the medication is intended to do) is most important. This should include herbal remedies and over-the-counter medications. It is also important to ask what medications have produced any allergic responses.

Allergy History

As more allergens produce more discomfort for people, it is important to determine what might compromise patient care and what might cause discomfort. Questions should relate to medications (see above); products; trees, plants, and weeds; and foods.

Lifestyle History

Lifestyle focuses on living patterns people use. Common questions here focus on tobacco (smoking and chewing), alcohol (including wine, spritzers, beer, and cocktails), drugs, sexual activities/orientation, personal relationships, health practices, exercise, and diet.

Psychosocial/Spiritual History

This area should incorporate questions about family and friends as support systems, special health or religious practices, a general view of life, comfort in the home and neighborhood, major stressors and ways of adaptation, and normal coping strategies.

Review of Systems

The term *review of systems* means that a systematic discussion about each element is conducted using an organized approach (systems) to assure that a comprehensive view is obtained. These data are considered subjective primarily because they rely on what the patient or significant other states in response to statements and questions. The flow can vary based on what the client declares as a primary problem, but an initial assessment includes all of the following elements.

General health: This section focuses on how the patient responds to questioning about how he or she feels in general. It should include energy level, appetite, weight gain or loss, general mood, outlook on life, discomfort, and other systemic descriptions.

Hair: Loss of hair, itching

Skin: Skin diseases, changes in pigmentation or size or shape of moles, bruising, dryness, open sores or cuts that are slow to heal, itching, jaundice, rashes

Head: Headaches, dizziness, loss of consciousness

Eyes: Clarity of vision, pain, drainage, tearing, sensitivity to light, itching, use of glasses or contact lens, any surgery. Last eye examination.

Ears: Clarity of hearing, pain, discomfort, discharge, use of hearing aid

Nose: Ease of breathing (and relational to position), allergies, postnasal drip, tenderness, nosebleeds, colds

Mouth and throat: Sore or bleeding gums; lumps or white spots on mouth, lips, or tongue; toothaches, cavities, or dental work (including dentures); changes in voice or swallowing. Last dental appointment.

Neck: Swollen glands, difficult movement, swelling, pain

Breasts: Shape; discharge, scaling or cracks around nipples, lumps, pain. Pattern of breast self examination. Last mammogram.

Respiratory: Difficulty breathing (including shortness of breath, pain, wheezing, persistent cough), lung disease (such as tuberculosis, emphysema, asthma, bronchitis). History of chest X-rays (purpose, time, results).

Cardiovascular: High blood pressure, varicose veins, palpitations, heart murmur, heart disease (including anemia), leg swelling, or ulcer

PART 2

Gastrointestinal: Heartburn, nausea, vomiting, loss of appetite, indigestion, change in bowel habits (including blood in stool, diarrhea, constipation or presence of a colostomy or ileostomy), pain, excessive gas, hemorrhoids, rectal pain

Genitourinary: Frequency, urgency, dribbling, discoloration (unrelated to food intake), pain or burning, difficulty starting urination, incontinence, infections (including sexually transmitted diseases and infections), presence of a ureterostomy

Females: Age of menarche, last menstrual period, duration, flow, regularity, presence of pain during or between periods, painful intercourse, discharge, itching, use of contraceptives

Males: Discharge, swelling, difficulty with sexual relations, presence of lumps or lesions, use of contraceptives

Musculoskeletal: Pain, soreness, swelling, joint pain or stiffness, leg cramps, bone condition

Neurological: Seizures, tremors, numbness, difficulty walking, tingling, burning, numbness, weakness on one side of body, speech pattern, memory (loss of or forgetfulness), disorientation, changes in emotional state

Endocrine: Tolerance to heat and cold, excessive thirst or eating, past diagnosis of goiter or diabetes

Examination

There are four key techniques for examinations.

- *Inspection:* This is the visualization of the person in a systematic way. This step is always done first.
- *Palpation:* This uses specific touching to determine features and characteristics such as texture, position, size, mobility, presence of pulses, or pain. This step is done next except when checking the abdomen. Then, auscultation is done first.

- *Percussion:* This involves a specific way of striking body surfaces to elicit sounds. This step follows palpation. The five types of sounds are:
  - Dullness (thud): Heart, liver, spleen
  - Flatness (dull): Bone and muscle
  - Hyperresonance (boom): Emphysematous lung
  - Resonance (hollow): Air-filled lung
  - Tympani (drum): Air-filled stomach
- *Auscultation:* This is the process of listening to sounds, usually with the assistance of a stethoscope. This step always follows inspection when examining the abdomen. There are four qualities related to auscultated sounds.
  - Duration: Length of sound
  - Intensity: Strength of sound
  - Pitch: Frequency
  - Quality: Subjective view of sound

Before beginning any assessment, the nurse should explain what is about to happen and secure the patient's consent and cooperation.

Physical Examination (Objective Data)

Vital signs: Temperature, pulse, respirations, blood pressure, pain, height, weight

General appearance: Age, ethnicity, gender, posture, gait, affect

Mental status: Consciousness, orientation to person/place/time, memory, emotional stability, speech clarity (include information about situation)

Skin: Color, integrity, turgor, hygiene, lesions, hair distribution and texture, nail texture and angle, moisture level, petechiae, bruises

Head and neck: Scalp, normocephalic deviations, temporal pulses, trachea position and tug, carotid and jugular quality, thyroid, lymph assessment, range of motion

Eyes: Pupils (PERRLA), eyelids, sclerae, conjunctiva, light reflex, visual fields, fundoscopy, acuity, EOMs, nystagmus

Ears: Lesions, hearing, discharge, otoscope examination findings

Nose: Discharge, septum, turbinates, mucosa, sinuses

Throat and mouth: Lips, teeth, gums, tongue (movement and appearance), palates, tonsils, drainage, uvula, gag reflex, sputum

Breasts: Contour, symmetry, discharge, lumps, masses, axilla lymph node, supra- and infraclavicular, nipples and areolae

Chest and lungs: Movement, expansion, use of accessory muscles, tactile fremitus, crepitus, percussion, auscultation (rales, rhonchi, wheeze, rub), excursion

Heart: PMI, thrills, rate, rhythm, gallops, rubs, murmurs, S1 and S2, splits

Vascular: Cyanosis, clubbing, peripheral pulses, skin, nails, edema

Abdomen: Contour, symmetry, skin, auscultation (bruits and hum), liver span and border, tenderness, masses, spleen, kidneys, aortic pulsation, reflex, percussion, CVA tenderness, femoral pulses, inguinal lymph node, swelling/ascites

Genitalia: Female: Pubic hair, external lesions/discharge, glands, urethra, vaginal walls, cervix, ovaries, uterus
Male: Pubic hair, glans, penis, scrotum, testes, epididymis, discharge, hernia

Rectum/prostate: Anus, sphincter, walls, masses, occult blood

Musculoskeletal: Posture, alignment, symmetry, joint (temperature/swelling/color), muscle tone, ROM, strength/atrophy

Neurologic: Eyes (*see* eyes), eyebrow raise/close, smile, taste, gag, head and neck rotation, shoulder shrug, tongue movement, Rinne and Weber, gait, finger to nose, Romberg, DTR, superficial responses

Assessment Tests and Strategies

ADL Assessment   Activities of daily living include cooking, dressing, driving, eating, exercise, grooming, hygiene, shopping, sleeping, toileting, and walking. These are normally assessed while conducting the health history. The Katz Index, a commonly used ADL assessment tool, uses these categories: bathing, dressing, toileting, transferring, continence, and feeding. The general rule is that there is increased need for care when there is increased need for help in one of the categories (e.g., to the dependency level) and when the overall assessment indicates there are multiple areas needing help, even if none is at the totally dependent level.

Alcohol Dependency Assessment   Note: The best source for current information on all recognized tests is the National Institute on Alcohol Abuse and Alcoholism, ⌐ www.niaaa.nih.gov. The CAGE test (from the American Psychiatric Association) consists of four questions such as, "Have you ever felt you should cut down on your drinking?" The MAST (Michigan Alcohol Screening Test) is a self-administered 22-question test from the National Council on Alcoholism and Drug Dependence. Questions include: Can you stop drinking without difficulty after one or two drinks? Have you ever gotten into trouble at work because of drinking?

APGAR   The APGAR test is a scoring for newborns done at one, five, and ten minutes after birth. The normal score is 7–10 points. The elements consist of activity, pulse, grimace, appearance, and respiration. The score is determined by a point system of 0, 1, or 2 for each of the five items. Examples of these items are respiration: crying would score 2; appearance: acrocyanosis would score 1; and activity: flaccid would score 0.

Babinski   Using a firm instrument such as the handle of a diagnostic hammer, scrape the bottom of the foot from heel to great toe. Flexing of the great toe toward the top of the foot and flaring of the toes is normal until about 2 years old. Afterward, this is an abnormal sign indicative of a neurological disorder.

Braden Scale   This tool consists of an assessment of a patient in six categories: sensory perception, moisture, activity, mobility, nutrition, and friction and shear. The scale is used to determine the potential for pressure ulcers. Each category has a range of scores from 1 to 4. The higher scores indicate lesser potentials for developing pressure ulcers. Health care organizations that use this scale typically have printed forms to allow for routine assessment of these factors (*see* Skin assessment).

Brudzinski's Sign   Passively flex the neck by placing one hand behind the neck and the other on the chest. If flexion of the patient's hips and knees occurs, there is a positive Brudzinski sign. This sign is positive in meningeal disease.

Child Abuse   (*See* pediatric section.)

Clark's Classification of Skin Growths   This is a detailed way to classify skin growths, but the simplified version is to check for four elements on any skin growth. The abnormal findings appear in parentheses: asymmetrical (irregular shape); border (irregular edges); color (irregular color); diameter (larger is of greater concern). Describe any skin growth by indicating these elements and precise measurements.

Cognitive Assessment   This area of assessment is frequently accomplished through the health history and general discussions with patients. It comprises thinking, reasoning, and problem solving. There is some variation with age and with IQ. Severe limits of cognitive abilities are seen in delirium and dementia and other conditions affecting the brain.

Cranial Nerves   (*See* Part 5.)

Cultural Assessment   Individuals respond differently to health issues, frequently based on cultural differences. In the broadest sense culture includes factors related to gender, ethnicity, social status, spirituality, education, language, community, family, habits, customs, and beliefs. Open-ended questions such as: What health practices do you use that we should know about? What do you typically do for this (condition/sign/symptom)? Such questions can help meet the patient's expectation of care.

Edema Press one or two fingers on prominent bones of leg for at least 4 seconds. Score pitting edema using a +1 to +4 scale as follows: +1—slight indentation, responds quickly when pressure released; +2—clear indentation that lasts for at least 10 seconds; +3—deep indentation that may last for up to 1 minute and has presence of obviously swollen extremity; +4—very deep indentation that may not disappear for more than 2 minutes and has presence of obviously swollen and usually distorted extremity.

Elder Abuse Presence of any of the following factors may indicate elder abuse: fear of a family member or caregiver; unusually poor hygiene; unexplained injuries, broken bones, or burns; apparent neglect or mistreatment; signs of physical restraint.

Glasgow Coma Score This scale is based on three aspects of functioning: eye opening, verbal response, and motor response. Record as E#, V#, M#. www.cdc.gov/masstrauma/resources/gcscale.htm. (*See* end of this section.)

Gordon's Functional Health Patterns (*See* end of this section.)

Growth and Development Guidelines (*See* Part 5, Development Data.)

Falls (Morse Fall Scale) This scale is built on six factors. The factors that predict falls are these: a history of falling, a presence of more than one diagnosis, use of ambulatory aid (especially of the unstable variety such as furniture), the presence of an IV/heparin lock or Saline PIID, impaired gait, and disorientation to own abilities.

Heart Murmur Grades of heart murmurs: 1 (barely audible), 2 (soft), 3 (loud, no thrill), 4 (loud with thrill), 5 (loud with light chest contact), 6 (loud with no stethoscope contact).

Homan's Sign Pain in calf when foot is dorsiflexed quickly

Immunization Schedule (*See* Part 3, Medications, CDC Recommendations.) Remember to check the Centers for Disease and Prevention Web site for the most current version at www.cdc.gov/nip.

Katz Index (*See* ADL Assessment.)

PART 2

Kernig's Sign   Place patient in a supine position with hips and knees flexed. Extend the knees (one at a time). The inability to extend beyond 135° without pain is a positive Kernig's Sign. This sign is positive in meningeal disease.

Mini Mental Status Examination   This examination comes in different forms, but it is basically designed to determine a person's orientation to person, place, and date; attention; recall; language and special relationships. It is a relatively easy examination to administer. A printable form of this examination, known as the MMSE, can be found at ⌐ www.lawandpsychiatry.come/html/mini_mental status examination.htm

Neuro Assessment   (cranial and spine) (*See* Part 5, Anatomy and Physiology)

Nutrition   (*See* Part 5, Nutrition.)

Pain   Numerous scales exist for pain assessment. The most common is a scale of 1 to 10 with 1 being no pain and 10 being the worst pain imaginable. Another common scale is the faces scale with a range of smiles to intense frowns. Typically an organization has a standardized tool so that comparisons can be made across time. Quality and duration are two other elements to assess consistently. (*See* Part 3, Pain Management.)

Pressure Ulcer Staging   The following staging is the USDHHS standard for describing pressure ulcers:

* Stage I: Erythema of intact skin
* Stage II: Loss of epidermis and dermis
* Stage III: Loss of structure from epidermis through subcutaneous tissue and into fascia, but not through it, may include necrosis
* Stage IV: Full thickness loss involving muscle and bone, usually extensive destruction is present.

Additionally the Braden and Norton scales are two tools that are commonly used to predict pressure ulcers. Factors such as sensation, moisture, activity, mobility, nutrition and friction/shear are assessed.

Range of Motion   If a patient is able to use joints actively, the examiner should direct the patient in the following movements. Otherwise, the examiner should passively move the joints to determine if there is full or limited range of motion. Never force a joint!

- Thumb: Open hand with fingers straight and cross palm until thumb touches base of the fifth digit. Repeat with each digit.
- Fingers: Open hand with fingers straight and roll tops of fingers to palm until touching. Open and repeat.
- Wrist: Flex and extend wrist, then slide fingers laterally in both directions.
- Elbow: Rest arm flat and bend arm so that fingers approach shoulder. Repeat with opposite side.
- Shoulder: With patient supine, raise arm above head, keeping elbow straight and arm close to ear. Return to beginning position and repeat with opposite side.
- Hip: With patient supine and legs about 6 inches apart, point toes up, slide leg to side, return to beginning position. Repeat with opposite side.
- Hip and knee: With patient supine, support joints and bend knee toward chest. Repeat with opposite side.
- Ankle: With patient supine, place fingers under the heel so that the foot rests on arm. Press gently so that toes are moving toward head and then extend foot so that toes point away from the body. Repeat with opposite side.

Rebound Tenderness   Perform an abdominal palpation and release quickly. If discomfort ensues, the patient has experienced rebound tenderness.

Restraints   If physical restraints are used, specific assessments must be made. The following provide typical guidelines, but organizations that use physical restraints have designated guidelines and these should be used. Typically restraints should not be in place for longer than 12 hours. Patients who are

PART 2

restrained should be checked at least every 30 minutes to determine their safety. Every two hours restraints should be released (not concurrently) and the patient should be repositioned. Skin should be assessed for abrasions and discoloration and should be kept dry.

Seizure Assessment   In addition to asking about a history of prior seizures, the examiner should look for rigid arms and legs, arched back, muscle twitches, dilated pupils, irregular breathing, loss of bowel and bladder control, and excessive salivation ("foaming").

Skin Assessment   The Braden Risk Assessment Scale is a tool designed to assess skin integrity and pressure ulcers. The categories include sensory perception (feeling discomfort), moisture, activity, mobility, nutrition, and friction and shear. A downloadable copy is available at www.webmedtechnology.com/BradenScale-skin.pdf.

Stroke Assessment   Several tools exist to assess the presence of a stroke. Prehospitalization tools focus on facial droop, arm drift, and speech. Additional factors include level of consciousness, orientation, and leg drift. The accumulation of these factors suggests a stroke event and requires immediate attention unless therapeutic intervention has already occurred.

Trauma Survey: Primary and Secondary   This is designed as a routine to be followed in an emergency situation. If at any time during the secondary survey the patient destabilizes, return to the primary survey. Primary: Airway maintenance with cervical spine immobilization; breathing; circulation, including hemorrhage control; neurological assessment; vital signs; trauma scoring (respiration rate and excursion, blood pressure, pulse, and coma status). Secondary: History; complete assessment; apply splints; insert urinary catheter, and describe output and blood presence.

Vital Signs (Blood pressure, pulse, respirations, temperature, and pain):

> Blood pressure: Avoid any limb that is injured or has an IV or shunt in place. Place an appropriate-sized cuff around

a limb above the pulse point. Avoid taking blood pressures when the patient drank alcohol or was smoking or exercising. Inflate the cuff above the highest recorded systolic pressure and release the pressure so the cuff deflates at a steady rate. Readings above 120/80 are now considered to be of concern; 120/90 indicates need for treatment.

Pulse: Take a pulse when the client is at rest (unless the purpose is to determine the pulse rate on exertion). Place index and middle fingers lightly over site (except for apical, which requires a stethoscope). Note rate, rhythm, volume, intensity, and corresponding pulse equality. Normal range: 80–100 (adults). Take irregular pulses for a full minute. There are nine typical sites for determining circulation and pulse. (*See* Part 5, Anatomy and Physiology.)

- Temporal
- Carotid
- Apical*
- Brachial*
- Radial*
- Femoral
- Popliteal
- Posterior tibial
- Pedal

*Most common for pulse

Respirations: Because this is the most easily self-controlled vital sign, attempt to assess this when the patient is unaware of the assessment. Note rate, depth, rhythm, and quality.

Temperature: Unless specified otherwise, most adult temperatures are taken orally. Leave the thermometer in place for a sufficient time. Generally, the patient should not be left alone during this procedure.

Pain: (*See* pain assessment.)

Glasgow Coma Score

E+ (Eye opening)
    4 = spontaneous
    3 = voice activated
    2 = pain activated
    1 = none
V+ (Verbal communication)
    5 = normal communication
    4 = disoriented
    3 = incoherent
    2 = sounds only
    1 = none
M+ (Motor responses)
    6 = normal
    5 = localized to stimulus
    4 = withdraws from stimulus
    3 = decorticate
    2 = decerebrate
    <u>1 = none</u>
Total = E + V + M

Gordon's Functional Health Patterns

This guide is useful in conducting a full health assessment. It is designed to determine patterns of responses rather than specific responses to a specific condition or event. Marjory Gordon devised the pattern areas to assure comprehensive assessment. Sample questions appear in parentheses after each pattern area.

    I. Health Perception and Management (What do you do to improve or maintain your health? How would you describe your current health?)

   II. Nutrition/Metabolism (What are your typical food choices?)

 III. Elimination (How frequently do you go to the bathroom? What does your urine look like?)

IV. Activity/Exercise (What do you do for exercise in a typical week? What are your leisure activities?)

V. Sleep/Rest (Do you sleep during the night? For how many hours?)

VI. Cognition/Perception (Do you have pain? If yes, describe it. Do you have any sensory changes? If yes, are they corrective? e.g., glasses)

VII. Self-Perception/Concept (How would you describe yourself?)

VIII. Role Relationships (Which relationships are most important to you?)

IX. Sexuality/Reproduction (Are you satisfied with your sexuality? Do you have any areas of dysfunction?)

X. Coping/Stress/Tolerance (How do you usually respond to problems? Do you usually feel better or worse after your response?)

XI. Values/Beliefs (What cultural (*see* Cultural Assessment) influences exist for you? What support systems do you have?)

Source: Gordon, M. (2002). *Manual of nursing diagnosis* (10th ed.). St. Louis, MO: Mosby.

PART 2

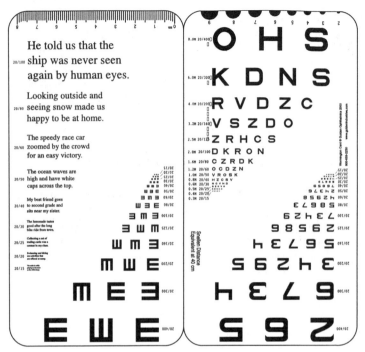

Figure 2-3 The Wormington Eye Test Card. *Source:* Reprinted with permission of Dr. Charles Wormington.

Documentation Guidelines

Documentation in the patient record is guided by standards developed over the years from many sources including the State Nurse Practice Act, professional organizations (such as the ANA and specialty organizations such as the Association of Women's Health, Obstetrical and Neonatal Nursing also known as AWHONN), and the Joint Commission on Accreditation of Healthcare Organizations. Charting is based on the nursing process: assessment, nursing diagnosis, planning, intervention, and evaluation.

Effective Documentation

Documentation must be:

1. **Timely**—Document the care as soon after it is given as possible. Whenever the patient is assessed, it must be documented.
2. **Accurate**—Document only the facts, that is, only what you see, hear, smell, feel, do, or teach. Document only the care you have personally provided or seen provided by a nursing assistant with whom you are working.
3. **Truthful**—Document only what you have observed, and avoid making assumptions.
4. **Appropriate**—Write in the chart only those entries you are comfortable with anyone, including the patient's family, reading. Resist making judgmental statements such as "Uncooperative, defensive, manipulative or difficult." Describe behavior in an impartial way.

Source: Habel, M. (2003). Document it right: Would your charting stand up to scrutiny? *Nurse Week, 14*(1), 20–21.

General Documentation Guidelines (Electronic and Paper Format)

1. Be certain you have the correct patient chart and that each page is correctly stamped. If an online record is used, be sure the documents you are viewing match the patient's name and identification number.
2. Document the patient encounter as soon as it is completed so as to remember the entire event as clearly as possible. Follow the organizational policy for frequency of charting (i.e., after rounds at the beginning of the shift and periodically thereafter, according to the institutional policy).
3. Use specific guidelines as designated by your organization such as:
   a. Write legibly; type correctly.
   b. Use permanent ink pen, usually black (which photocopies well). [paper only]

PART 2

   c. Include date and time with each entry.

   d. Leave no space between entries.

   e. Sign every entry with full name and credentials. Validate your electronic signature (or its equivalent) in electronic records.

   f. Leave *no* space between entries (draw a line through any blank spaces). [paper only]

   g. Use complete and concise documentation including approved phrases and abbreviations.

   h. Use quotation marks for direct patient comments such as "I have intense pain."

4. If an error is made, cross out the error with one single line, write the word *void* (or *error*), and your initials above the error. Date, time, and sign the correction. Follow the institutional policy for correcting electronic entries that have already been saved.

5. Never change another person's entry.

6. Document in chronological order.

7. Document all phone calls concerning the patient. Use the "write down, read back" method, which means you write what you hear and read it back aloud to the individual, especially with telephone orders. Document electronic transmissions of orders according to institutional policy.

8. Record all patient and family teaching.

9. *Remember:* Legally, if you didn't chart it, you didn't do it.

10. *Do not* chart: "An incident report was completed."

Source: White, L. (2003). *Documentation and the nursing process* (p. 94). Clifton Park, NY: Thomson, Delmar Learning.

Documentation in Crisis or Emergency Situations

1. Describe the patient's condition prior to the emergency situation.

2. Describe the precipitating event or the condition of the patient immediately prior to the emergency.

3. Be sure to chart the time of the event.

4. Chart the time of notification of the physician as well as the time of the arrival of medical/physician help.
5. Chart specific interventions and medications and the time for each activity and medication.
6. Chart the patient's response or lack of response to these interventions.
7. Use one designated person who charts all activities and interventions chronologically.

Source: Nurse Service Organization. (2002). When every second counts: How to protect yourself from malpractice. Retrieved December 8, 2002, from http://www.nursingcenter

PART 2

What Constitutes Illegal Documentation?

- Destroying any part of the patient's chart
- Adding to another professional's note
- Adding to an existing note without indicating the addition as a late entry
- Failing to record important details (*see* effective documentation and general documentation guidelines)
- Recording false information—charting anything in the chart prior to its administration (e.g., medications, dressing changes, treatments, etc.) constitutes falsifying the record. You may note the nursing care plan prior to its implementation.
- Charting inaccurate dates or times

Source: Springhouse Corp. (2002). *Chart smart: The A-to-Z guide to better nursing documentation* (pp. 203–301). Springhouse, PA: Author.

Documentation of Medication Error

When a medication error is made:

1. It must be charted on the medication administration record so that other caregivers will not give additional dosages or other medications that might be contraindicated.

2. The error must be documented in the nursing progress notes including:
   a. Name and dosage of the medication
   b. Time given
   c. Patient's response
   d. Physician or other practitioner notified of the error
   e. Time notification occurred
   f. Any nursing or medical interventions to counteract the error
   g. Patient's response to the intervention
3. Most institutions require an incident report or unusual occurrence report for medication errors, and the policy of the organization should be followed.

Source: White, L. (2003). *Documentation and the nursing process.* Albany, NY: Thomson, Delmar Learning.

Guidelines for Patient Charting Essentials

Follow the nursing process when caring for patients and charting: assess, nursing diagnosis, plan, implement, and evaluate, and then revise the plan.

1. Any patient symptoms or physical changes
   a. Any pain, particularly when it is severe or unrelieved. Evaluate with a standard pain scale.
   b. Any condition that tends to reoccur or persist such as skin problems or wound problems
   c. Anything that deviates from normal, such as fever or abnormal laboratory results
   d. A deteriorating situation, such as weight loss or progressive lethargy
   e. Any sign of poor health habits, such as lack of cleanliness or lice
   f. Any known health danger signs, such as severe varicosities or a breast lump

2. Any nursing interventions provided for the patient or family
   a. Activities of daily living, such as bath, a.m. or p.m. care, and associated assessments
   b. Any prescribed therapeutic interventions and their effects or how they were tolerated
   c. Any teaching done with the patient and/or family and the retention of information
3. Any changes in physical functioning
   a. Weakness in extremities
   b. Difficulty in ambulating or difficulty in maintaining balance
   c. Problems in hearing or seeing
4. Any behavioral changes
   a. Indications of strong emotions such as crying, anger, or fear
   b. Marked changes in mood such as manic or depressive behavior
   c. Changes in level of consciousness, e.g., a change from decreased awareness to stupor
   d. Change in relationships with family and friends, such as no longer wishing to see them
5. Any data collected by other health professionals and shared with you including physicians and all other team members, e.g., clergy, PT, social worker, or assistive personnel

Source: VanLeuven, K. (2000). *Clinical companion: Fundamentals of nursing* (6th ed., pp. 225–226). Upper Saddle River, NJ: Prentice Hall Health.

Minimum Data Set Categories

The term *minimum data set* (MDS) refers to areas of documentation required in long-term care settings. The Basic MDS is one that must be complete and current. The Full MDS is to be completed at designated times such as on admission to a long-term care site in which it is a specified requirement.

Basic
Name _____
Gender _____
Birth date _____
Race/Ethnicity _____
Social Security and Medicare numbers _____
Facility provider number _____
Medicaid number _____
Reason for assessment _____
   Time frame: admission, quarterly, annually _____
   Significance: change in status, correction in status _____
   Medicare/Medicaid requirement _____

Full
Identification information _____
Cognitive patterns _____
Communication/Hearing patterns _____
Vision patterns _____
Mood and behavior patterns _____
Psychosocial well-being _____
Physical functioning and structural problems _____
Continence in last 14 days _____
Disease and diagnoses _____
Health conditions _____
Oral/Nutritional status _____
Skin condition _____
Activity pursuit patterns _____
Medications _____
Special treatments and procedures _____
Discharge potential and overall status _____
Assessment information _____
Therapy supplement for Medicare PPS _____
Resident assessment protocol summary _____

Collecting and Organizing Data for Reporting to the Physician Either by Phone or in Person*

1. Use the following modalities when contacting the physician (use the physician's preference if known)
   - Pager number
   - Physician's call service
   - During week days, the physician's office number
   - On weekends and after hours during the week, the physician's home phone
   - Cell phone number
2. Prior to calling the physician check the following list of activities:
   - See and assess the patient yourself prior to calling
   - Discuss the situation with another as needed
   - Review the chart prior to the call
   - Be certain the correct member of the physician group is called (see patient health record)
   - Read the most recent MD progress notes and the notes from the nurse who worked the previous shift.
   - Always have the chart with you when you contact the physician
3. Identify why you are initiating the contact: "Your patient, Mrs. X is experiencing Z change in status. I am concerned. . ."
4. Review the patient's history (briefly) to refresh the physician about which patient this is; include current illness or surgery, medications, treatments, any significant allergies, or comorbidities.
5. State the current clinical situation:
   a. Vital signs
   b. Level of consciousness

---

*Students should seek assistance of preceptor or instructor.

c. Perfusion changes including skin color, O_2 saturation, and urine output
d. Unusual pain
e. Change in behavior such as: irritability or agitation, hallucinations or a sense of impending doom ("I feel like I am going to die")
f. Change in the status of a drain or dressing
g. Laboratory or diagnostic test results that deviate from normal

Source: Carelock, J., & Innerarity, S. (2001). Critical incidents: Effective communication and documentation. *Critical Care Nursing Quarterly, 23*(4), 59–66.

Descriptions of Charting Systems

Health care facilities use a variety of charting systems. You will want to use the one adopted by your facility. The options are compared in the following table.

PART 2

TYPE	HOW	WHERE	WHEN
Narrative charting	Straight chronological accounting of pt. status, nursing interventions performed, & pt. response Organized by: Head to toe Plan of care Body systems	Progress notes, nurses' notes, & flow sheets	Document when: • Changes in pt. condition occurs • Pt. responds to treatment • Lack of improvement • Pt. or family response to info or teaching
Problem-oriented medical record	Focus on specific pt. problem using 5 components • Data base—both subjective and objective data • Problem list including numbered list of current problems	Intake history & physical exam. Progress notes using **SOAP, SOAPIE,** or **SOAPIER.** • **Subjective data:** reason for seeking care • **Objective data:** factual data, e.g.,	Each day/shift or as warranted. When a problem resolves, note date & time.

Continued

TYPE	HOW	WHERE	WHEN
	• Initial plan including expected outcomes & additional data collection, pt. care, & teaching	signs, symptoms, vital signs, test values	
	• Progress notes (*see* SOAP)	• Assessment data: conclusions based on **S & O** and formulated as nursing diagnoses or patient problems	
	• Discharge summary covering each problem and noting resolution or not. Plan identified for unresolved problems and postdischarge care.	• **Plan**: for solving pt. problems from **A**, inc. both short- & long-term actions.	
		• **Interventions**: actions taken to achieve outcomes of **P**	
		• **Evaluation**: analyze effectiveness of **I**	
		• **Revision**: alterations in original plan based	

| Problem-intervention-evaluation (PIE) system | Data organized by pt. problems which are numbered. In progress notes, use **PIE** system.
• **P**roblem: use data from initial assessment and nursing diagnoses; label problem with **P** with #.
• **I**ntervention: actions taken and outcomes
• **E**valuation: pt.'s response to treatment. Label it **E** followed by **P** and #. | Daily assessment flow sheet that includes areas for documenting major areas, e.g., respiration, pain, routine care, & monitoring. Can integrate plan of care with nursing progress notes, which eliminates a separate care plan & provides a nursing record. | Uses flow sheet for treatments, meds, monitoring, pain assessment when they are due. |

Continued

TYPE	HOW	WHERE	WHEN
Focus charting	Organized in patient-centered foci. Organize information in categories: • **D**—data: subjective & objective information • **A**—action: immediate & future nursing actions • **R**—response: Describe pt. response to action.	Use progress notes with columns for date, time, focus, and progress. In focus column, coded problems as nursing diagnosis, sign or symptom, pt. behavior, special needs, change in condition and assessment. All routine data placed on flow sheets & check lists.	Daily/shifts, or as changes occur.
Charting by exception	Document only significant or abnormal findings. Must adhere to guidelines for nursing	• Preprinted nursing diagnosis-based standardized plans of care with individualized plan in blank spaces.	Daily/shifts, or as changes occur.

assessments &
interventions,
standards of practice,
& standardized care
plans.

- Nursing care flow
  sheets used for
  24-hr. period.
- Graphic records for
  vital signs, weight,
  I&Os, & activity
  level.
- Pt. teaching record:
  used to track and
  document teaching
  and outcomes.
- Pt. discharge
  record: pt.
  instructions,
  appointments,
  follow-up care,
  medications & diet
  instructions, signs
  & symptoms to
  report, activity, and
  pt. education.

Continued

TYPE	HOW	WHERE	WHEN
		• Progress notes: document revisions to care plan and anything else that doesn't fit on various flow sheets.	
FACT documentation	System incorporates many CBE principles • Flow sheets • Assessments with baseline parameters • Concise integrated progress notes & flow sheets for patient condition & responses • Timely entries recorded at time of care	• Begins with complete initial assessment • Assessment-action flow sheet: Chart ongoing assessments & interventions—normals printed with planned interventions. • Abnormalities can be charted. • Frequent assessment flow	Chart daily/shift & more often as needed. For progress notes, at least every 24 hours.

Core charting	Focus is on nursing process—most important part of documentation • Database • Plan of care • Flow sheets • Progress notes • Discharge summary	Database & plan of care used as initial assessment & focus on pt.'s body systems and daily activities. • Include summary of pt.'s problems & nursing diagnosis.	sheet: Chart vital signs & frequent assessments. • Progress notes: integrated progress record with narrative notes to chart progress & significant incidents Use Data-action-response method.
			Every shift or more as needed.

Continued

TYPE	HOW	WHERE	WHEN
	Use DAE (data, action, and evaluation or response)	• Flow sheets used for pt. activities, response to nursing interventions, diagnostic procedures, and pt. teaching. • Progress notes: focus on each problem using **DAE.** Discharge summary: includes nursing diagnosis, pt. teaching, and follow-up care.	
Outcome documentation	Present pt. condition related to predetermined outcome in plan of care with focus on	Components: • Database: includes S & O data, identifying pt. problem, &	Every shift and as needed.

learning needs as foundation for continuing evaluation
- Plan of care: establishes priorities, focuses on expected outcomes, nursing interventions, documents the plan
- Use preprinted standardized plans, clinical pathways, & pt. care guidelines.
- Expected outcome statements: Describe desired results, use measurable outcome criteria with target date/time. Learning

desired outcomes rather than problems. Use progress notes, flow sheets, & plans of care (some use separate teaching plan).

Continued

TYPE	HOW	WHERE	WHEN
		outcomes focus on measurable pt. behavior. Outcomes evaluated & problems resolved when outcomes met.	
Computerized charting	Computerized nursing information systems (NISs) can increase efficiency & accuracy for nursing process & help in meeting JCAHO standards. NISs can collect, transmit, and organize information, as well as suggest nsg. diagnoses, provide standardized pt. status, & nsg.	Computerized processes include: • Assessment: Admit data including health status, history, chief complaint, etc., and flag any data deviating from normal. • Nursing diagnosis: Programs list standard diagnoses with signs &	Whenever care is given.

interventions used in care plans & progress notes. Can prompt RN with questions & suggestions.

- Nursing minimum data set (NMDS) program standardizes nursing information in 3 categories: nursing care, pt. demographics, service elements. NMDS allows collection of nursing diagnoses & intervention data and identifies needs of various pt. populations and tracks the outcomes.

symptoms and suggest most appropriate given existing data. Judgment used to confirm appropriateness.

- Planning: Help in writing plan comes from displaying expected outcomes and interventions for each diagnosis.
- Implementation: Record actual interventions. Use computer to input progress notes, medications, vital signs, & treatments.
- Evaluation: Computer records evaluation & pt.'s

Continued

TYPE	HOW	WHERE	WHEN
	Accurate nursing care costs can be identified.

Nursing trends, locally, regionally, & nationally can be compared. | response to nursing care. | |

Source: Springhouse Corp. (2002). *Chart smart: The A-to-Z guide to better nursing documentation* (pp. 432–448). Springhouse, PA: Author.

PART 3

Select Care Issues

PART 3

Patient Teaching

Most institutions have some standard teaching tools and checklists to be used with patient teaching activities. Some of these have been developed by the specific organization; others have been derived from such groups as disease-based associations. In addition to the patient teaching precipitated by a specific event (for instance a clinic visit or a hospitalization), it is often useful to validate the ongoing understanding of health and chronic condition management.

To determine specific needs, the following should be assessed and recorded.

Key Patient Teaching Assessment

One of the expected nursing interventions in all settings and with all disease conditions is teaching. The focus of this effort is based in concerns about patient safety. Although patient teaching is a complex process and recent research focuses mostly on the affective (beliefs and values) domain, there are specific elements that a nurse needs to assess to assist patients. Knowing information about the primary language spoken *and* read (and they may differ) is important in communicating information. Further, it isn't sufficient to know the primary language that is read; it is equally important to know the reading level of the patient. Many printed materials are available and the Internet has opened new avenues of accessing information. Matching those resources with the appropriate reading level is important. Knowing if there are learning encumbrances and what cultural beliefs and practices influence behavior is also important. Some common areas of assistance also need to be assessed.

Language
    Spoken
    Read
Educational level
Reading level
Learning encumbrances (ADD, mental retardation, etc.)
Cultural beliefs and practices (what is valued and used by
    the patient)
Specific areas of assistance:
    Physical
    Emotional
    Knowledge deficits
    Home services
    Ambulation
    Nursing care
    Nutrition
    Transportation

PART 3

Home safety
Cultural practices' conflicts with treatment or care
Financial ability to meet treatment or care costs

Discharge Teaching

Most discharge teaching plans include the following:

Date of discharge
Anticipated
Actual
Discharge location (e.g., home, nursing home, rehabilitation center)
Resources
People
Financial
Equipment and supplies
Transportation
Disease content (e.g., specific care warning signs and symptoms)
Healthy living content (e.g., diet, activity level)
Follow-up care (e.g., medication prescriptions, health care support services, return appointments)

Patient Safety

Patient safety is a broad, encompassing term that includes a variety of elements. The intent of this section is to recall for users what the key hazards are and what nurses need to do to best protect their patients. Known as medical errors, and in extreme situations, sentinel events, issues of safety include errors where a patient receives a wrong medicine or treatment, an incorrect surgical procedure, or an incorrect diagnosis, or when a biohazard exists because of accidental or unintended exposure to dangerous elements, or when an environmental condition exists that is not conducive to patient safety. This latter may include concerns about proper disposal of sharps, obstructed passageways, objects or fluids on the floor that could precipitate falls, faulty equipment, or inattention to emerging hazards such as weather concerns. Every organization has some process for documenting when an error occurs, and that process should be followed. More effective, however, is the prevention of safety. The most important thing to remember about patient safety is that most errors commonly reflect system concerns. In other words, they usually are not the result of one faulty practitioner.

Adverse Drug Events   Multiple strategies for preventing these errors have been considered. The most common suggested prevention is having computerized records that prevent misreading medication orders, that connect the order to the dispensing procedure, and that provide validation of intended action prior to administration.

Surgical Errors   Labeling sites and validating repeatedly the intended procedure and site can decrease the likelihood of this type of error.

Diagnostic Errors   Organizations that provide a particular procedure more frequently than others are less likely to have inaccurate diagnoses.

Standardizing protocols is key to preventing several errors. But more importantly, the attitude of promoting safety is a key factor in preventing errors. If the organization conducts root cause analyses, a structured process of asking why at each step of an event to determine all possible causes and the initiating cause of an error, the outcomes should be known by the staff. Root cause analysis is used to determine what is wrong with the system rather than the response of placing blame on an individual.

Safety can involve basic strategies within the organization, such as the procedure for fire notification, reporting a terrorist threat or security breach, or personnel behavior. It can also include issues of medication administration, falls, risks of infection, adequate delivery of fluids and gases, and informed consent. Perhaps the most fundamental example of safety is whether or not people who touch a patient have washed their hands.

PART 3

The Web site for the Agency for Healthcare Research and Quality (AHRQ) is useful in terms of patient safety issues and can be found at ⌐ www.ahcpr.gov/research/errors.htm.

Key Actions

- Report any faulty equipment; discontinue use for patients; label it as faulty and remove it from patient care areas.
- Report any spills immediately, block off the area, and validate they are cleaned up in a reasonable time. If the spill is a hazardous material, follow the hazardous risk materials policies.
- Be aware of the top medication errors to avoid similar names, incorrect administration routes and dosages, and other commonly documented errors.
- Avoid abbreviations.
- Dispose of any sharps in a secure disposal container that prevents injury to health care providers as well as patients.
- Validate any report, such as laboratory or radiographic, to be certain it was the procedure ordered and that the report belongs to the patient.
- Validate patient identity with at least two means for each therapeutic interaction. (Avoid asking the patient if he or she is Mr(s). . . .)
- Institute practices that are designed to prevent errors, such as labeling surgical sites and repeating intended actions.
- Avoid physical restraints, and if they must be used, check them frequently and follow the organizational policy.
- Use generic names of medications and know common misperceived names. Validate that a prescribed medication fits with the patient's diagnosis and condition.
- Report any suspicious persons or packages to security promptly. In areas with infants or children, be aware of

the organizational policy and procedure for infant or child abduction.
- Know the emergency procedures for fire and severe weather.
- Use the fire acronym:
  - *R*—Rescue clients.
  - *A*—Alert others, pull alarm.
  - *C*—Contain fire.
  - *E*—Extinguish fire.

Pain Management

Pain is a personal experience and therefore nurses are dependent on the information and responses provided by patients in terms of intensity, duration, frequency, quality, precipitating event, and response. Pain should be described in as much detail as possible. The following factors are critical descriptors of pain.

Critical Descriptors

Intensity: The severity of pain, frequently denoted by a 1 to 10 scale (1 being no pain, 10 being the worst pain imaginable). Young children often use the "pieces of hurt" (use of poker chips to quantify pain; useful with children between 3 and 7 years old) or the faces scales (available at 🖱 www.painsourcebook.ca; useful with children between 3 and 12 years old) to represent intensity.

Duration: The length of time since the pain was first noticed (refers to the original episode) and the length of time the current pain has been experienced (refers to the current episode)

Frequency: The interval with which the pain reoccurs

Quality: The use of words (sharp, tingly) or analogies (pin, needles) to describe the type of pain experienced

Precipitating event: Any event associated with the beginning or intensifying of pain. This may include a fall or something eaten or a certain work. It also may be unknown.

PART 3

Response: A descriptor related to what relieves or alleviates pain, how long the relief lasts, and if there are any accompanying signs and symptoms

Numerous interventions are possible, even though the most common is medication. The following list identifies some commonly performed interventions by nurses.

Common Nursing Interventions

Breathing: Slow, focused breathing in through the nose, holding, and blowing out through the mouth.

Massage: Typically using long, slow strokes with sufficient pressure to stimulate circulation.

Medications: Medications, which may be administered through intravenous or intrathecal methods. If medication is administered via a patient-directed device, monitoring the level of the medication available and the description of pain remains important. The key concept is to provide medication frequently enough so that the pain does not require more dramatic action.

Relaxation: A systematic manner of focusing on tensing and relaxing muscle groups in the body. Frequently this is combined with breathing, as described above.

Repositioning: Changing the position of the body to relieve pressure on given spots and to stimulate circulation.

Visualization: A deliberative strategy of mental "viewing" and experiencing places and activities that are associated with positive feelings.

Additionally, other avenues should be considered such as acupressure or acupuncture, biofeedback, and pain clinic interventions, such as electrodes and anesthesia blocks. Noting the use of any of these strategies, as well as others, and the patient's response is important.

Medications

Multiple professionals and technicians are involved in the process of providing a medication to an individual. The physician, nurse practitioner, or other authorized prescriber writes an authorization for a medication. A pharmacy, with professional pharmacists and pharmacy technicians, prepares the medication for administration. In home settings, the medication is given to the individual or his or her representative. In institutional settings, the medication typically is delivered to a care area where nurses or, as in the case of long-term settings, a medication aide, administers the medication. This section focuses on the nursing role in administration of medications. Even if someone else administers the medication, the registered nurse (and thus the nursing student) has the accountability to continue accurate assessments to determine the patient's response to the medication(s).

The Rights of Medication Administration

Prior to preparing a medication for administration, nurses must recall what the patient's diagnoses are, what allergies exist (if any), and what the normal dosages, expected response, negative reactions, and contraindications are for the medication to be administered. The goal of this activity is to assure the most accurate practice in administering medications. Further, the time-honored "Seven Rights" of medication administration should be followed.

The Seven Rights

1. Right drug
2. Right client
3. Right dose
4. Right time
5. Right route
6. Right reason
7. Right documentation

PART 3

Steps in Preparing Medications for Administration

1. Check the medication order sheet with the medication administration record (MAR) to be sure there is agreement. (The order sheet is the key source for validating.)
2. Check the medication with the correct documents (order sheet and MAR).
3. State to yourself what the medication is, what it is intended for, how it acts, what cautions there are (incompatibilities) and why this patient would receive that medication. Don't forget to look it up!

Administering Medications

Medications should remain within your control once administration procedures have begun. Wash hands and, as appropriate, wear gloves.

Gastric Tube/Nasogastric Tube

1. Approach the patient. Check the patient identification, or if it is missing, ask the patient to state his or her full name. Do *not* ask, "Is your name . . . ?" Ask for some other validating information, and be sure to secure patient identification for future use. Two items of identification should be used.
2. Position the patient in a sitting position (at least 30–40° elevation).
3. Assess the patient for feelings of distension, loose stools, eructations, and flatulence.
4. Listen to bowel sounds to determine adequate motility and to stomach sounds to validate the tube is in the stomach and not the lungs.
5. Administer the medication according to expected practice for the medication.
6. Remove the administration unit and dispose of it in a safe disposal device.

7. Document the administration and patient response.
8. Observe for any untoward reaction.

Intradermal

1. To prepare the injection:
   a. Use the standard procedure for validating medication.
   b. Clean the tops of vials with an alcohol wipe.
   c. Open the syringe protection.
   d. If the vial is multidose, retract the syringe and insert an equivalent air volume for the fluid volume to be removed.
   e. Hold the vial upside down with the syringe securely attached and slowly pull back on the plunger while watching the fluid enter the syringe. Note: If the fluid volume is not designated in the medication order, calculate the medication quantity first (*see* subsequent section).
   f. Be sure only fluid is in the syringe—eliminate air bubbles.
   g. Keep the needle sterile.
2. Approach the patient. Follow standard patient validation procedures.
3. Position the patient. Typically, this injection is administered under the skin on the upper arm (allergy testing) or lower arm (ppd).
4. Cleanse the area with an alcohol wipe (or approved agent within the organization).
5. Place the uncapped syringe almost parallel with the skin, bevel up, insert.
6. Slowly and steadily, inject the medication.
7. Remove the syringe quickly and cover the injection area (if appropriate).
8. Dispose of the syringe in a safe disposal device.
9. Document the administration and patient response.
10. Observe for any untoward reaction.

See Figure 3-1.

PART 3

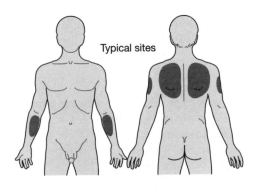

Typical sites

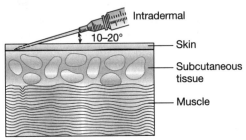

Intradermal

10–20°

Skin

Subcutaneous tissue

Muscle

Note: Expect a bleb under the epidermis.

Figure 3-1   Intradermal Sites and Needle Angles

Intramuscular

1. Follow step 1 and 2 above for medication preparation and patient validation.
2. Position the patient so the intended site muscle is relaxed.
3. Cleanse the area with an alcohol wipe (or approved agent within the organization).
4. Uncap the syringe and place it at a 90° angle to the skin. Place nondominant hand at edges of desired area and spread skin taut. See Figure 3-2 for the Z track method when applicable.

5. Inject the syringe quickly into the center of the area.
6. Aspirate by pulling back on the plunger to determine if blood returns. If blood returns, a new site needs to be selected. Discard needle and syringe and prepare new syringe.
7. Slowly and steadily, inject the medication.
8. Remove the syringe quickly and place the wipe over the area and apply pressure.
9. Dispose of the syringe in a safe disposal device.
10. Document the administration and patient response.
11. Observe for any untoward reaction.

See Figure 3-2.

The preferred sites for children are the vastus lateralis and ventrogluteal. See Figure 3-3.

Subcutaneous

1. Follow the steps above.
2. Alter the angle of administration (see Figure 3-4), typically to a 45–60° angle.

Intravenous/Central Lines (direct or drip administration)

1. Secure medication, and IV tubing if needed, and approach patient.
2. Validate the patient identification as described above.
3. Check existing IV site for sign of infection or infiltration.
4. Check the IV placement and catheter patency by assessing for blood return.
5. Cleanse the ports.
6. Connect the IV medication unit to the appropriate IV port and administer according to expected practices for that medication.
7. Disconnect the medication administration unit when done and dispose in a safe disposal device.
8. Document the administration and patient response.
9. Monitor as indicated by the medication administered.

PART 3

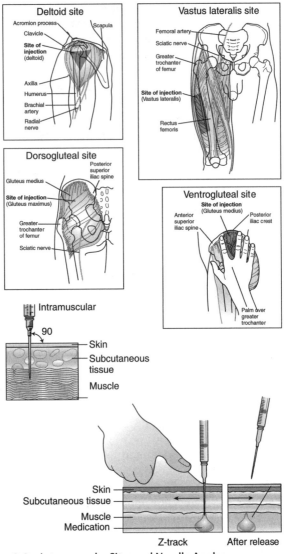

Figure 3-2   Intramuscular Sites and Needle Angles

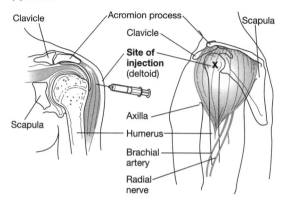

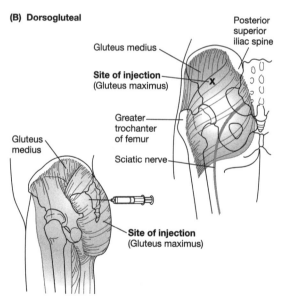

Figure 3-3 Intramuscular Injection Sites in Children. *Source:* Wong, D.L., & Hess, C.S. (2000). *Wong and Whaley's clinical manual of pediatric nursing* (5th ed., pp. 245–246). St. Louis, MO: Mosby. Used with permission.

Vastus lateralis

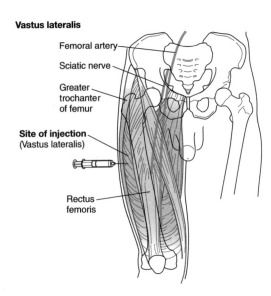

Femoral artery

Sciatic nerve

Greater
trochanter
of femur

Site of injection
(Vastus lateralis)

Rectus
femoris

Ventrogluteal

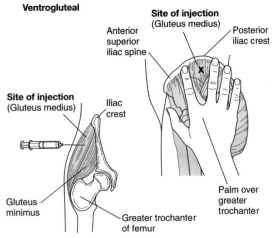

Site of injection
(Gluteus medius)

Anterior
superior
iliac spine

Posterior
iliac crest

Site of injection
(Gluteus medius)

Iliac
crest

Gluteus
minimus

Greater trochanter
of femur

Palm over
greater
trochanter

Figure 3-3   *Continued*

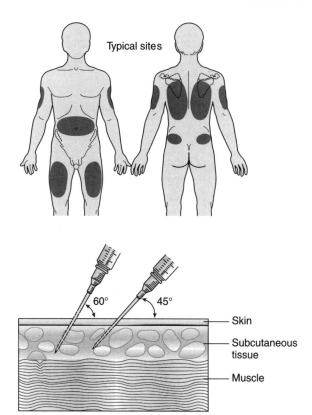

Figure 3-4   Subcutaneous Sites and Needle Angles

Oral Medications

1. Approach the patient and validate identification as described previously. If the medication is to be given after meals or before meals, validate that the patient has or has not eaten.
2. Assist the patient to sit up as best as possible, if this is allowed.

3. Have the patient drink some water.
4. Offer the medication to the patient. Assist as needed.
5. Validate that the medication was swallowed.
6. Return the patient to a desired position.
7. Assess for effects.
8. Document administration and any major effects.

Sublinguals

1. Complete steps 1, 2, and 4 for oral medications administration discussed previously.
2. Remind the patient to place the medication under his or her tongue.
3. Complete steps 7 and 8 of oral medications administration discussed previously.
4. Remind the patient to have nothing by mouth for 15–30 minutes.

Suppositories (Rectal)

1. Complete the patient validation process.
2. Place the patient on the left side unless contraindicated.
3. Remove the suppository from the wrapper, using patient care gloves, and lubricate the end of the suppository with a water-soluble jelly.
4. Insert the suppository followed by the index finger until it is beyond the internal sphincter.
5. Hold buttocks together for 5 to 10 minutes until the urge to expel the suppository passes.

Transdermal

1. Complete steps 1, 2, and 4 for oral medications administration previously mentioned.
2. Cleanse site and remove old patch, if present.
3. Open the sealed envelope at the tear line.

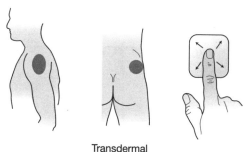
Transdermal

Figure 3-5 Common Transdermal Sites and Administration

4. Remove backing, being careful not to touch the medicated surface.
5. Place the patch at a designated site (site varies with medication).
6. Beginning with the center of the patch and working outward, press the patch to adhere to the skin; apply firm pressure to entire patch for approximately 30 seconds.
7. Document administration.

See Figure 3-5.

Medication Calculation

The basic rule is to create a ratio of known dosage per quantity to required dosage per quantity to be determined.

$$\frac{\text{Known dosage}}{\text{Known quantity}} = \frac{\text{Required dosage}}{\text{Quantity to be determined}}$$

Monitoring Intravenous Fluids

Texts and procedures for children and infants should be consulted on this topic. For adults, the usual rule is 30 cc/Kg/24hr to maintain basic hydration. For every 1° C temperature increase, an additional 15% of fluid quantity should be added.

PART 3

DEPARTMENT OF HEALTH AND HUMAN SERVICES • CENTERS FOR DISEASE CONTROL AND PREVENTION

Recommended Childhood and Adolescent Immunization Schedule UNITED STATES • 2006

Vaccine ▼ Age ▶	Birth	1 month	2 months	4 months	6 months	12 months	15 months	18 months	24 months	4–6 years	11–12 years	13–14 years	15 years	16–18 years
Hepatitis B[1]	HepB	HepB[1]			HepB						HepB Series			
Diphtheria, Tetanus, Pertussis[2]			DTaP	DTaP	DTaP		DTaP	DTaP		DTaP	Tdap		Tdap	
Haemophilus influenzae type b[3]			Hib	Hib	Hib[3]	Hib								
Inactivated Poliovirus			IPV	IPV	IPV					IPV				
Measles, Mumps, Rubella[4]						MMR				MMR	MMR			
Varicella[5]						Varicella					Varicella			
Meningococcal[6]									MPSV4	MPSV4	MCV4		MCV4 / MCV4	
Pneumococcal[7]			PCV	PCV	PCV	PCV	PCV		PCV		PPV			
Influenza[8]					Influenza (Yearly)	Influenza (Yearly)			Influenza (Yearly)		Influenza (Yearly)			
Hepatitis A[9]									HepA Series	HepA Series				

Vaccines within broken line are for selected populations

Legend: Range of recommended ages | Catch-up immunization | 11–12 year old assessment

This schedule indicates the recommended ages for routine administration of currently licensed childhood vaccines, as of December 1, 2005, for children through age 18 years. Any dose not administered at the recommended age should be administered at any subsequent visit when indicated and feasible. ▨ Indicates age groups that warrant special effort to administer those vaccines not previously administered. Additional vaccines may be licensed and recommended during the year. Licensed combination vaccines may be used whenever any components of the combination are indicated and other components of the vaccine are not contraindicated and if approved by the Food and Drug Administration for that dose of the series. Providers should consult the respective ACIP statement for detailed recommendations. Clinically significant adverse events that follow immunization should be reported to the Vaccine Adverse Event Reporting System (VAERS). Guidance about how to obtain and complete a VAERS form is available at www.vaers.hhs.gov or by telephone, **800-822-7967**.

1. **Hepatitis B vaccine (HepB).** *AT BIRTH:* All newborns should receive monovalent HepB soon after birth and before hospital discharge. **Infants born to mothers who are HBsAg-positive** should receive HepB and 0.5 mL of hepatitis B immune globulin (HBIG) within 12 hours of birth. **Infants born to mothers whose HBsAg status is unknown** should receive HepB within 12 hours of birth. The mother should have blood drawn as soon as possible to determine her HBsAg status; if HBsAg-positive, the infant should receive HBIG as soon as possible (no later than age 1 week). **For infants born to HBsAg-negative mothers,** the birth dose can be delayed in rare circumstances but only if a physician's order to withhold the vaccine and a copy of the mother's original HBsAg-negative laboratory report are documented in the infant's medical record. *FOLLOWING THE BIRTHDOSE:* The HepB series should be completed with either monovalent HepB or a combination vaccine containing HepB. The second dose should be administered at age 1–2 months. The final dose should be administered at age ≥24 weeks. It is permissible to administer 4 doses of HepB (e.g., when combination vaccines are given after the birth dose); however, if monovalent HepB is used, a dose at age 4 months is not needed. **Infants born to HBsAg-positive mothers** should be tested for HBsAg and antibody to HBsAg after completion of the HepB series, at age 9–18 months (generally at the next well-child visit after completion of the vaccine series).

2. **Diphtheria and tetanus toxoids and acellular pertussis vaccine (DTaP).** The fourth dose of DTaP may be administered as early as age 12 months, provided 6 months have elapsed since the third dose and the child is unlikely to return at age 15–18 months. The final dose in the series should be given at age ≥4 years.
   Tetanus and diphtheria toxoids and acellular pertussis vaccine (Tdap – adolescent preparation) is recommended at age 11–12 years for those who have completed the recommended childhood DTP/DTaP vaccination series and have not received a Td booster dose. Adolescents 13–18 years who missed the 11–12-year Td/Tdap booster dose should also receive a single dose of Tdap if they have completed the recommended childhood DTP/DTaP vaccination series. Subsequent **tetanus and diphtheria toxoids (Td)** are recommended every 10 years.

3. *Haemophilus influenzae* **type b conjugate vaccine (Hib).** Three Hib conjugate vaccines are licensed for infant use. If PRP-OMP (PedvaxHIB® or ComVax® [Merck]) is administered at ages 2 and 4 months, a dose at age 6 months is not required. DTaP/Hib combination products should not be used for primary immunization in infants at ages 2, 4 or 6 months but can be used as boosters after any Hib vaccine. The final dose in the series should be administered at age ≥12 months.

4. **Measles, mumps, and rubella vaccine (MMR).** The second dose of MMR is recommended routinely at age 4–6 years but may be administered during any visit, provided at least 4 weeks have elapsed since the first dose and both doses are administered beginning at or after age 12 months. Those who have not previously received the second dose should complete the schedule by age 11–12 months.

5. **Varicella vaccine.** Varicella vaccine is recommended at any visit at or after age 12 months for susceptible children (i.e., those who lack a reliable history of chickenpox). Susceptible persons aged ≥13 years should receive 2 doses administered at least 4 weeks apart.

6. **Meningococcal vaccine (MCV4).** Meningococcal conjugate vaccine (MCV4) should be given to all children at the 11–12 year old visit as well as to unvaccinated adolescents at high school entry (15 years of age). Other adolescents who wish to decrease their risk for meningococcal disease may also be vaccinated. All college freshmen living in dormitories should also be vaccinated, preferably with MCV4, although **meningococcal polysaccharide vaccine (MPSV4)** is an acceptable alternative. Vaccination against invasive meningococcal disease is recommended for children and adolescents aged ≥2 years with terminal complement deficiencies or anatomic or functional asplenia and certain other high risk groups (see *MMWR* 2005;54 [RR-7];1-21); use MPSV4 for children aged 2–10 years and MCV4 for older children, although MPSV4 is an acceptable alternative.

7. **Pneumococcal vaccine.** The heptavalent **pneumococcal conjugate vaccine (PCV)** is recommended for all children aged 2–23 months and for certain children aged 24–59 months. The final dose in the series should be given at age ≥12 months. **Pneumococcal polysaccharide vaccine (PPV)** is recommended in addition to PCV for certain high-risk groups. See *MMWR* 2000; 49(RR-9);1-35.

8. **Influenza vaccine.** Influenza vaccine is recommended annually for children aged ≥6 months with certain risk factors (including, but not limited to, asthma, cardiac disease, sickle cell disease, human immunodeficiency virus [HIV], diabetes, and conditions that can compromise respiratory function or handling of respiratory secretions or that can increase the risk for aspiration), healthcare workers, and other persons (including household members) in close contact with persons in groups at high risk (see *MMWR* 2005;54(RR-8);1-55). In addition, healthy children aged 6–23 months and close contacts of healthy children aged 0–5 months are recommended to receive influenza vaccine because children in this age group are at substantially increased risk for influenza-related hospitalizations. For healthy persons aged 5–49 years, the intranasally administered, live, attenuated influenza vaccine (LAIV) is an acceptable alternative to the intramuscular trivalent inactivated influenza vaccine (TIV). See *MMWR* 2005;54(RR-8);1-55. Children receiving TIV should be administered a dosage appropriate for their age (0.25 mL if aged 6–35 months or 0.5 mL if aged ≥3 years). Children aged ≤8 years who are receiving influenza vaccine for the first time should receive 2 doses (separated by at least 4 weeks for TIV and at least 6 weeks for LAIV).

9. **Hepatitis A vaccine (HepA).** HepA is recommended for all children at 1 year of age (i.e., 12–23 months). The 2 doses in the series should be administered at least 6 months apart. States, counties, and communities with existing HepA vaccination programs for children 2–18 years of age are encouraged to maintain these programs. In these areas, new efforts focused on routine vaccination of 1-year-old children will enhance, not replace, ongoing programs directed at a broader population of children. HepA is also recommended for certain high risk groups (see *MMWR* 1999; 48[RR-12];1-37).

The **Childhood and Adolescent Immunization Schedule is approved by:**
Advisory Committee on Immunization Practices www.cdc.gov/nip/acip · American Academy of Pediatrics www.aap.org · American Academy of Family Physicians www.aafp.org

Figure 3-6 Recommended Childhood and Adolescent Immunization Schedule—United States (2006)

Vaccine ▼	Age group ▶	19–49 years	50–64 years	≥ 65 years
Tetanus, diphtheria (Td)*		1-dose booster every 10 yrs		
Measles, mumps, rubella (MMR)[2]*		1 or 2 doses	1 dose	
Varicella[3]*		2 doses (0, 4–8 wks)	2 doses (0, 4–8 wks)	
Influenza[4]*		1 dose annually	1 dose annually	
Pneumococcal (polysaccharide)[5,6]		1–2 doses		1 dose
Hepatitis A[7]*		2 doses (0, 6–12 mos, or 0, 6–18 mos)		
Hepatitis B[8]*		3 doses (0, 1–2, 4–6 mos)		
Meningococcal[9]		1 or more doses		

— — — Vaccines below broken line are for selected populations

NOTE: These recommendations must be read along with the footnotes.
*Covered by the Vaccine Injury Compensation Program.

| For all persons in this category who meet the age requirements and who lack evidence of immunity (e.g., lack documentation of vaccination or have no evidence of prior infection) | Recommended if some other risk factor is present (e.g., based on medical, occupational, lifestyle, or other indications) |

This schedule indicates the recommended age groups and medical indications for routine administration of currently licensed vaccines for persons aged ≥19 years. Licensed combination vaccines may be used whenever any components of the combination are indicated and when the vaccine's other components are not contraindicated. For detailed recommendations, consult the manufacturers' package inserts and the complete statements from the ACIP (www.cdc.gov/nip/publications/acip-list.htm).

Report all clinically significant postvaccination reactions to the Vaccine Adverse Event Reporting System (VAERS). Reporting forms and instructions on filing a VAERS report are available by telephone, 800-822-7967, or from the VAERS website at www.vaers.hhs.gov.

Information on how to file a Vaccine Injury Compensation Program claim is available at www.hrsa.gov/osp/vicp or by telephone, 800-338-2382. To file a claim for vaccine injury, contact the U.S. Court of Federal Claims, 717 Madison Place, N.W., Washington D.C. 20005, telephone 202-357-6400.

Additional information about the vaccines listed above and contraindications for vaccination is also available at www.cdc.gov/nip or from the CDC-INFO Contact Center at 800-CDC-INFO (232-4636) in English and Spanish, 24 hours a day, 7 days a week.

DEPARTMENT OF HEALTH AND HUMAN SERVICES
CENTERS FOR DISEASE CONTROL AND PREVENTION

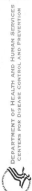

Figure 3-7 Recommended Adult Immunization Schedule, by Vaccine and Age Group—United States (October 2005–September 2006)

Vaccine / Indication ▼	Pregnancy	Congenital immunodeficiency; leukemia;[14] lymphoma; generalized malignancy; cerebrospinal fluid leaks; therapy with alkylating agents, antimetabolites, radiation, or high-dose, long-term corticosteroids	Diabetes; heart disease; chronic pulmonary disease; chronic liver disease, including chronic alcoholism	Asplenia[12] (including elective splenectomy and terminal complement component deficiencies)	Kidney failure, end-stage renal disease, recipients of hemodialysis or clotting factor concentrates	Human immunodeficiency virus (HIV) infection[13]	Healthcare workers
Tetanus, diphtheria (Td)[1]*	1-dose booster every 10 yrs						
Measles, mumps, rubella (MMR)[2]*			1 or 2 doses				
Varicella[3]*			2 doses (0, 4–8 wks)				2 doses
Influenza[4]*	1 dose annually			1 dose annually			
Pneumococcal (polysaccharide)[5,6]	1–2 doses		1–2 doses				1–2 doses
Hepatitis A[7]*	2 doses (0, 6–12 mos, or 0, 6–18 mos)						
Hepatitis B[8]*	3 doses (0, 1–2, 4–6 mos)				3 doses (0, 1–2, 4–6 mos)		
Meningococcal[9]	1 dose			1 dose		1 dose	

NOTE: These recommendations must be read along with the footnotes.
*Covered by the Vaccine Injury Compensation Program.

For all persons in this category who meet the age requirements and who lack evidence of immunity (e.g., lack documentation of vaccination or have no evidence of prior infection)

Recommended if some other risk factor is present (e.g., based on medical, occupational, lifestyle, or other indications)

Contraindicated

Approved by the Advisory Committee on Immunization Practices (ACIP), the American College of Obstetricians and Gynecologists (ACOG), and the American Academy of Family Physicians (AAFP)

PART 3

Figure 3-8 Recommended Adult Immunization Schedule, by Vaccine and Medical and Other Indications—United States (October 2005–September 2006)

1. **Tetanus and Diphtheria (Td) vaccination.** Adults with uncertain histories of a complete primary vaccination series with diphtheria and tetanus toxoid-containing vaccines should receive a primary series using combined Td toxoid. A primary series for adults is 3 doses; administer the first 2 doses at least 4 weeks apart and the third dose 6–12 months after the second. Administer 1 dose if the person received the primary series and if the last vaccination was received ≥10 years previously. Consult ACIP statement for recommendations for administering Td as prophylaxis in wound management (www.cdc.gov/mmwr/preview/mmwrhtml/00041645.htm). The American College of Physicians Task Force on Adult Immunization supports a second option for Td use in adults: a single Td booster at age 50 years for persons who have completed the full pediatric series, including the teenage/young adult booster. A newly licensed tetanus-diphtheria-acellular pertussis vaccine is available for adults. ACIP recommendations for its use will be published.

2. **Measles, Mumps, Rubella (MMR) vaccination.** *Measles component:* adults born before 1957 can be considered immune to measles. Adults born during or after 1957 should receive ≥1 dose of MMR unless they have a medical contraindication, documentation of ≥1 dose, history of measles based on healthcare provider diagnosis, or laboratory evidence of immunity. A second dose of MMR is recommended for adults who 1) were recently exposed to measles or in an outbreak setting, 2) were previously vaccinated with killed measles vaccine, 3) were vaccinated with an unknown type of measles vaccine during 1963–1967, 4) are students in postsecondary educational institutions, 5) work in a healthcare facility, or 6) plan to travel internationally. Withhold MMR or other measles-containing vaccines from HIV-infected persons with severe immunosuppression. *Mumps component:* 1 dose of MMR vaccine should be adequate for protection for those born during or after 1957 who lack a history of mumps based on healthcare provider diagnosis or who lack laboratory evidence of immunity. *Rubella component:* administer 1 dose of MMR vaccine to women whose rubella vaccination history is unreliable or who lack laboratory evidence of immunity. For women of child-bearing age, regardless of birth year, routinely determine rubella immunity and counsel women regarding congenital rubella syndrome. Do not vaccinate women who are pregnant or might become pregnant within 4 weeks of receiving the vaccine. Women who do not have evidence of immunity should receive MMR vaccine upon completion or termination of pregnancy and before discharge from the healthcare facility.

3. **Varicella vaccination.** Varicella vaccination is recommended for all adults without evidence of immunity to varicella. Special consideration should be given to those who 1) have close contact with persons at high risk for severe disease (healthcare workers and family contacts of immunocompromised persons) or 2) are at high risk for exposure or transmission (e.g., teachers of young children; child care employees; residents and staff members of institutional settings, including correctional institutions; college students; military personnel; adolescents and adults living in households with children; nonpregnant women of childbearing age; and international travelers). Evidence of immunity to varicella in adults includes any of the following: 1) documented age-appropriate varicella vaccination (i.e., receipt of 1 dose before age 13 years or receipt of 2 doses [administered at least 4 weeks apart] after age 13 years); 2) born in the United States before 1966; 3) history of varicella disease based on healthcare provider diagnosis or self- or parental report of typical varicella disease for non-U.S.-born persons born before 1966 and all persons born during 1966–1997 (for a patient reporting a history of an atypical, mild case, healthcare providers should seek either an epidemiologic link with a typical varicella case or evidence of laboratory confirmation, if it was performed at the time of acute disease); 4) history of herpes zoster based on healthcare provider diagnosis; or 5) laboratory evidence of immunity. Do not vaccinate women who are pregnant or might become pregnant within 4 weeks of receiving the vaccine. Assess pregnant women for evidence of varicella immunity. Women who do not have evidence of immunity should receive dose 1 of varicella vaccine upon completion or termination of pregnancy and before discharge from the healthcare facility. Dose 2 should be given 4–8 weeks after dose 1.

4. **Influenza vaccination.** *Medical indications:* chronic disorders of the cardiovascular or pulmonary systems, including asthma; chronic metabolic diseases, including diabetes mellitus, renal dysfunction, hemoglobinopathies, or immunosuppression (including immunosuppression caused by medications or by HIV); any condition (e.g., cognitive dysfunction, spinal cord injury, seizure disorder or other neuromuscular disorder) that compromises respiratory function or the handling of respiratory secretions or that can increase the risk of aspiration; and pregnancy during the influenza season. No data exist on the risk for severe or complicated influenza disease among persons with asplenia; however, influenza is a risk factor for secondary bacterial infections that can cause severe disease among persons with asplenia. *Occupational indications:* healthcare workers and employees of long-term care and assisted living facilities. *Other indications:* residents of nursing homes and other long-term care and assisted living facilities; persons likely to transmit influenza to persons at high risk (i.e., in-home household contacts and caregivers of children birth through 23 months of age, or persons of all ages with high-risk conditions); and anyone who wishes to be vaccinated.

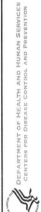

DEPARTMENT OF HEALTH AND HUMAN SERVICES
CENTERS FOR DISEASE CONTROL AND PREVENTION

For healthy nonpregnant persons aged 5–49 years without high-risk conditions who are not contacts of severely immunocompromised persons in special care units, intranasally administered influenza vaccine (FluMist*) may be administered in lieu of inactivated vaccine.

5. **Pneumococcal polysaccharide vaccination.** *Medical indications:* chronic disorders of the pulmonary system (excluding asthma); cardiovascular diseases; diabetes mellitus; chronic liver diseases, including liver disease as a result of alcohol abuse (e.g., cirrhosis); chronic renal failure or nephrotic syndrome; functional or anatomic asplenia (e.g., sickle cell disease or splenectomy [if elective splenectomy is planned, vaccinate at least 2 weeks before surgery]); immunosuppressive conditions (e.g., congenital immunodeficiency, HIV infection [vaccinate as close to diagnosis as possible when CD4 cell counts are highest], leukemia, lymphoma, multiple myeloma, Hodgkin disease, generalized malignancy, organ or bone marrow transplantation); chemotherapy with alkylating agents, antimetabolites, or high-dose, long-term corticosteroids; and cochlear implants. *Other indications:* Alaska Natives and certain American Indian populations; residents of nursing homes and other long-term care facilities.

6. **Revaccination with pneumococcal polysaccharide vaccine.** One-time revaccination after 5 years for persons with chronic renal failure or nephrotic syndrome; functional or anatomic asplenia (e.g., sickle cell disease or splenectomy); immunosuppressive conditions (e.g., congenital immunodeficiency, HIV infection, leukemia, lymphoma, multiple myeloma, Hodgkin disease, generalized malignancy, organ or bone marrow transplantation); or chemotherapy with alkylating agents, antimetabolites, or high-dose, long-term corticosteroids. For persons aged ≥65 years, one-time revaccination if they were vaccinated ≥5 years previously and were aged <65 years at the time of primary vaccination.

7. **Hepatitis A vaccination.** *Medical indications:* persons with clotting factor disorders or chronic liver disease. *Behavioral indications:* men who have sex with men or users of illegal drugs. *Occupational indications:* persons working with hepatitis A virus (HAV)-infected primates or with HAV in a research laboratory setting. *Other indications:* persons traveling to or working in countries that have high or intermediate endemicity of hepatitis A (for list of countries, visit www.cdc.gov/travel/diseases.htm#hepa) as well as any person wishing to obtain immunity. Current vaccines should be given in a 2-dose series at either 0 and 6–12 months, or 0 and 6–18 months. If the combined hepatitis A and hepatitis B vaccine is used, administer 3 doses at 0, 1, and 6 months.

8. **Hepatitis B vaccination.** *Medical indications:* hemodialysis patients (use special formulation [40 μg/mL] or two 20-μg/mL doses) or patients who receive clotting factor concentrates. *Occupational indications:* healthcare workers and public-safety workers who have exposure to blood in the workplace; and persons in training in schools of medicine, dentistry, nursing, laboratory technology, and other allied health professions. *Behavioral indications:* injection-drug users; persons with more than one sex partner in the previous 6 months; persons with a recently acquired sexually transmitted disease (STD); and men who have sex with men. *Other indications:* household contacts and sex partners of persons with chronic hepatitis B virus (HBV) infection; clients and staff of institutions for the developmentally disabled; all clients of STD clinics; inmates of correctional facilities; or international travelers who will be in countries with high or intermediate prevalence of chronic HBV infection for >6 months (for list of countries, visit www.cdc.gov/travel/diseases.htm#hepa).

9. **Meningococcal vaccination.** *Medical indications:* adults with anatomic or functional asplenia, or terminal complement component deficiencies. *Other indications:* first-year college students living in dormitories; microbiologists who are routinely exposed to isolates of *Neisseria meningitidis*; military recruits; and persons who travel to or reside in countries in which meningococcal disease is hyperendemic or epidemic (e.g., the "meningitis belt" of sub-Saharan Africa during the dry season [Dec–June]), particularly if contact with the local populations will be prolonged. Vaccination is required by the government of Saudi Arabia for all travelers to Mecca during the annual Hajj. Meningococcal conjugate vaccine is preferred for adults meeting any of the above indications who are aged ≤55 years, although meningococcal polysaccharide vaccine (MPSV4) is an acceptable alternative. Revaccination after 5 years may be indicated for adults previously vaccinated with MPSV4 who remain at high risk for infection (e.g., persons residing in areas in which disease is epidemic).

10. **Selected conditions for which *Haemophilus influenzae* type b (Hib) vaccine may be used.** *Haemophilus influenzae* type b conjugate vaccines are licensed for children aged 6 weeks–71 months. No efficacy data are available on which to base a recommendation concerning use of Hib vaccine for older children and adults with the chronic conditions associated with an increased risk for Hib disease. However, studies suggest good immunogenicity in patients who have sickle cell disease, leukemia, or HIV infection, or have had splenectomies; administering vaccine to these patients is not contraindicated.

Approved by the Advisory Committee on Immunization Practices (ACIP), the American College of Obstetricians and Gynecologists (ACOG), and the American Academy of Family Physicians (AAFP)

PART 3

Figure 3-8 *Continued*

Many IVs are monitored by an automatic pump. Be sure it is functional. Keep the alarm operative. Respond to any alarm, and readjust the flow and trouble shoot according to standard organizational procedures.

Fluid Tonicity

Isotonic fluids are those consistent with the osmolality of blood (310 mEq/L).

Hypotonic fluids are those with an electrolyte content below 250 mEq/L.

Hypertonic fluids are those with an electrolyte content above 375 mEq/L.

Flow Rate

To calculate flow rates, the rule is:

Rate of flow =

$$\frac{\text{amount of fluid} \times \text{drop factor of tubing}}{\text{administration time stated in total number of minutes}}$$

This formula provides the number of drops per minute to be administered.

Immunizations

Immunizations are a special form of administration that adheres to a prescribed schedule. The CDC standards for both children and adolescents and for adults are on pages 310–315. The adult standards are further categorized by age group and medical conditions. Validate current standards at ⌐ www.cdc.gov.

Bioterrorism

Bioterrorism consists of intentional acts of releasing biologic agents. Accidental release may also occur and is typically responded to in the same manner. Prevention is the most effective strategy, so it is always useful to observe suspicious behavior, packages, and substances. Such observations should be reported to security or law enforcement specialists. It is also important to be alert to any sudden increase in illnesses with reported common symptoms, location, and time. Common signs and symptoms associated with biologic agents are: unexplained fever, sepsis, pneumonia, cough, rash, and flaccid paralysis. The CDC provides up-to-date information about common biologic agents, their clinical manifestations, isolation and decontamination requirements, required clinical tests and recommended therapy ✍ www.cdc.gov. The Agency for Healthcare Research and Quality provides specific details about numerous biologic agents and links to sources that have developed appropriate information ✍ www.ahrq.gov/browse/bioterbr.htm.

A goal with any biologic agent is to contain the source (and thus the patient) and provide monitoring. Only Level II and Level III laboratories are able to handle biologic agents testing. In general, specimen contact requires using laminar flow hoods, protective eyewear, gloves, and protective clothing (or at least closed-front clothing). Clinical contact may require comparable gear and full-isolation strategies. Universal precautions are always used and specific isolation precautions may also be instituted. If an organization does not have a well-defined, clear policy and procedure, the information from the CDC and AHRQ should be used. If a victim is hospitalized, family and friends need to know that visitation should be limited and, in some cases, discouraged (for example if a family member is pregnant). Valuable items should be limited because they may need to be destroyed.

Anthrax

There are three types of anthrax: cutaneous (exposure through open skin surface); inhalation (respiratory—this is usually fatal); gastrointestinal (consumption of contaminated food).

> *Symptoms:* Cutaneous—ulcer with necrosis; Inhalation—sore throat, mild fever, muscle aches; Gastrointestinal—nausea, vomiting, fever, abdominal pain, severe diarrhea

PART 3

Intervention: Preventive vaccination, antimicrobial therapy (or penicillin)

Botulism

There are three types of botulism: food borne (fairly rapid response to preformed toxins); infant (rare, harbored *C. botulinum* in intestinal tract); wound (direct contact with wounds).

Symptoms: Double or blurred vision, slurred speech, difficulty swallowing, descending muscular weakness, including respiratory paralysis
Intervention: Antitoxin

Plague

There are three types of plague: pneumonic (spreads via air or direct contact with respiratory droplets); bubonic (flea bite or direct contact, but does not spread from person to person); septicemic (plague multiplication in blood).

Symptoms: Fever, headache, weakness, shortness of breath, chest pain, cough, and sometimes bloody sputum
Intervention: Antibiotics; wear mask

Smallpox

A viral infection spread through respiratory tract.

Symptoms: Malaise, fever, pharyngitis, rigors, vomiting, headache, backache, delirium, followed by rash and then pustules
Intervention: Vaccine within 3 days of exposure, antibiotics for secondary infections, consider contagious until scabs are gone

Infection Control

The primary issue in infection control is hand hygiene (see ⌲ www.cdc.gov/handhygiene). Washing hands prior to contact with patients protects the patient; washing them afterwards protects the nurse.

Universal/standard precautions can be found in the Reminder Section at the front of this book. The following information is designed to help make quick decisions regarding care; however, organizational manuals will detail the exact expectations about specific conditions.

Common Strategies

Handwashing or Cleaning with Alcohol Washing should be done for at least 15 seconds. Key points to remember are: friction is important; avoid touching anything in the patient care area after washing hands.

Gloves Gloves should be worn whenever contact with body fluids is expected, including contact with equipment exposed to body fluids.

Protective Clothing This set of items, which includes gowns, caps, and boots, should be used whenever potential contact with body fluids is anticipated, especially from splashes or exudates.

Face Protection This set of items includes mask and eye or full-face shield and is worn when contact with mucous membranes is possible. Splashes are special concerns requiring the use of a full-face shield.

Types of Precautions

Standard (Applied to *all* patient situations)

- Wash hands after contact.
- Wear gloves if contacting body fluids.

PART 3

- Wear face protection if contact with body fluids is likely from splashes.
- Contain equipment and linens to prevent exposure to other products or patients.

Airborne (Applied to any patient situation with real or suspected airborne disease)

- Standard plus
- Assign to private room with negative air pressure.
- Wear respiratory protection in room.
- Place mask on patient if transport is required.

Droplet (Applied to any patient situation with real or suspected droplet disease)

- Standard plus
- Assign to private room (or shared with others with same infection).
- Wear respiratory protection if within 3 feet of patient.
- Place mask on patient if transport is required.

Contact (Applied to any patient situation with real or suspected contact disease)

- Standard plus
- Assign to private room (or shared with others with same infection).
- Wear gloves when entering room. Change after direct contact with infective material.
- Wear gown when entering room if contact is anticipated.
- Validate daily cleaning of room, equipment and patient care items; do not remove equipment to other areas.

Seizures

Seizures may constitute an emergency when they alter consciousness and motor and sensory abilities to the extent that the individual is compromised. There are two types of seizures: focal (limited to neurons in one part of the brain); and generalized (multiple neurons involved). Some people experience auras before a seizure begins. These may involve any of the senses. Metallic taste and noxious odors are among the most commonly reported auras. The following is a list of key nursing measures:

- Stay with the person.
- Attempt to maintain a patent airway (place person on a flat, protected surface if possible, turn person on side); *do not* place your hands in the oral cavity; *do not* force clenched jaws apart.
- Prevent injury (protect head, loosen clothing, move nearby objects).
- Note the time of initiation and duration of each seizure and the entire event. Note types of movements (e.g., tremors or clonic/tonic movements) and parts of body (e.g., one area or total body) involved.
- Note if autonomic signs (e.g., lip smacking, grimacing) were present.
- Note position of eyes.
- Note skin color and presence of diaphoresis.
- Note if incontinence occurred.
- Check the Babinski sign. (Was it positive?)
- Note vital signs.
- Secure suctioning equipment, if possible.

After the seizure is over, remember to focus on the airway (keep it clear, check oxygen saturation levels) and the potential for injuries. Staying with the person at this point is important to help with reorientation.

Violence

Violence is one of society's greatest concerns. The World Health Organization (1996) defines violence as: "The intentional use of physical force or power, threatened or actual, against oneself, another person, or against a group or community that either results

322 Part 3: Select Care Issues

in or has a high likelihood of resulting in injury, death, psychological harm, maldevelopment, or deprivation."

Violence can also be thought of as self-directed, other directed, or collective (as in gang behavior). Violence occurs across the age span, socioeconomic groups, and ethnicities, and in both genders and various settings. Violence may be verbal, emotional, physical, or sexual. It is a result of people's limited abilities to cope with frustration and needs in appropriate ways. Whenever a child, and sometimes when an elder, is involved, additional procedures are instituted because they are viewed as vulnerable populations. Violence can range from intimidation to homicide. As a result of early experience with abuse, some people become abusers themselves, and they may also have resultant health issues directly related to abusive experiences. In addition to a detailed health history, reviewing laboratory and radiographic reports is important.

Physical abuse is more easily detected than emotional; but usually a reason is offered for why a physical sign is present. Common physical signs might include:

- Broken bones, especially if repeated breakage is evident
- Abdominal or head injuries
- Burns, especially in shapes suggestive of cigarettes or use of ropes or immersion in hot water
- Cuts or tears, especially of the mouth, genitals, or anus
- Bruises, especially in shapes such as belt buckles

Nonspecific behavioral or emotional problems may relate to abuse, so that should always be a consideration when obtaining health histories.

Children

Children who are abused are often victims of a family member or someone who is well known to the child, especially if the nature of the abuse is sexual. A parent may be concerned but nonspecific, or a parent may fail to acknowledge the potential for abuse.

Unusual fears should always be an alert for possible violence (*see* Child Abuse in pediatric section).

Adults

Asking about prior abuse may help relate important information with current conditions. Because the stories are often painful to hear, all of the best techniques of communication will be valuable. Domestic violence may include control of activities and finances, isolation from other family members and friends, threats toward the individual or children or other family members. The greatest risk period for personal safety is when the victim is beginning to take action to leave or has left. If a patient divulges such recent or impending action, be sure the patient knows how to access the appropriate community supports such as law enforcement agencies and support groups. Sources for help are often posted in public bathrooms, including those located in physicians' offices. Questions to the provider which appear to focus on fear towards the spouse or partner may signal an abusive situation.

Elders

Elderly patients may experience violence because they may be seen as vulnerable. Theft of property may be one of the forms of violence, as well as neglect.

Key Actions

Trust is critical to providing the opportunity for a victim of violence to share concerns. Be sure to be alert to signs that are frequently posted in clinic settings that are designed to elicit information about abuse. To be effective in interactions with patients who may be victims of violence, it is important to:

- Validate that notices about abuse and access to safe sources are available in private places such as an examination room and public restrooms.

- Acknowledge concern for the person's safety, including making certain resources are clear.
- Convey supportive statements that indicate understanding that violence is not a "deserved" situation.
- Share why certain information must be shared with others.
- Provide careful documentation, including patient statements about the situation. In cases of sexual assault, careful documentation is needed especially in relation to the site and time of the assault and the nature of the contact. Specific kits are used in emergency departments that involve controls of reports and specimens to document evidence for subsequent legal action. Specific procedures for reporting are used when the victim is a child or an elderly person. Frequently, the victim can identify the person who was the assaulter, because that person is known to the victim.

Specific Questions to Ask

If there is any reason to suspect violence concerns, the following questions may help a patient assess the safety of the situation.

- Is it safe to return home?
- Are there weapons in the home?
- Does the abuser use drugs or alcohol?
- Has the violence increased either in intensity or frequency or both?
- Has there been any threat of increased violence including potential acts of homicide?
- Has the patient acted on or thought of suicide as an escape from a situation?

Source: WHO. (1996). *Violence: A public health priority.* Geneva: WHO Global Consultation on Violence and Health.

End-of-Life Care

The work of Kübler-Ross, *On Death and Dying* (1969), raised the level of consciousness in the United States regarding the process of dying.

Stages of Death and Dying

- Denial—Denial of the situation and/or the diagnosis, e.g., the tests were wrong or confused with another
- Anger—Hostile with caregivers, excessively demanding, withdrawn or cold or unemotional, resentment or rage, and uncooperative or manipulative
- Bargaining—Bargaining with God or physician, promises to change behavior and lifestyle, feelings of guilt
- Depression—Crying, weeping, a desire to be alone, and actually discussing the upcoming loss
- Acceptance—A calmness or peace, decreased interest in surroundings, or may no longer be interested in visitors

In the last decade, there has been a marked increase in interest in the dying patient due to research that revealed 80% of Americans (as late as 1995) were dying in institutional settings, often in high-cost intensive care units. Even more alarming, they often had intense un-relieved pain and very little communication with physicians who did not take notice of such documents as living wills and orders for no resuscitation. The Commission on Aging discovered that most terminally ill people have five wishes:

1. Identify the person they want to make decisions for them when they cannot.
2. Be able to designate the kind of medical treatment they want and don't want.
3. Request the level of comfort they desire.
4. Designate how they want to be treated.
5. Decide what they want their loved ones to know.

PART 3

It is helpful to differentiate between palliative and curative care. When striving to cure, the approach is analytical, based on a diagnosis, scientific, medical approach, and aimed at the disease. On the other hand, palliative care is focused on controlling the symptoms, aimed at comfort, humanistic, viewing patients as individuals and death as normal.

Thus, the goals in palliative care include:

1. Provide desired physical comfort.
2. Support the dying person to control the decisions regarding medical care and daily routines.
3. Find support and relief for the family so they do not have to be the caregivers for their loved one all the time.
4. Educate the family so they feel confident in the care they do give.
5. Secure emotional support for the family both before and after the death.

The process of dying can require an extended period of time. However there are alerts to the impending event.

Signs and Symptoms of Imminent Death

- Weakness increasing to completely bedbound
- Assistance required with nearly all care
- Physical appearance is gaunt and pale (most prevalent in cancer patients)
- Reduced awareness (including insight and perception) and extreme drowsiness
- Severely limited attention span and difficulty in concentrating and focusing
- Decreased ability to cooperate with caregivers
- Disoriented
- Little interest in food or fluid with significantly diminished intake

- Increased difficulty in swallowing, particularly oral medications
- Loss of consciousness

Nursing Care of Dying Patient

Physical Needs

- Adequate pain medication
- Skin care with an emphasis on massage, lotion, and lip care
- Positioning for greater comfort
- Frequent changing and straightening of linens
- Suctioning if there are excessive oral secretions to promote easier breathing
- Artificial tears as needed

Spiritual Needs

- Clergy visits as requested by patient or family
- Access to Sacrament of the Sick or Holy Communion (or comparable support)
- Religious books and music available
- Cultural or religious practices supported
- Time for family and friends to talk or pray

Preparation of the Family and Friends

- Prepare family and friends for physical changes.
- Facilitate time with patient as both patient and family and friends want.
- Support the family in cultural or religious rituals.
- Keep the family and friends apprised as to patient's condition.
- Be honest and forthright with them.
- Support family in their needs for sleep, meals, etc.

PART 3

- Use active listening skills to support family in expressing concerns and fears.
- Encourage questions.
- Establish a caring relationship with them and support time for immediate grief work.
- Seek clarity regarding the death rituals (religious specific) needed by patient and family.

Each organization has an extensive policy and procedure for preparation of the body after death and for completion of all the paperwork involved.

Source: Kübler-Ross, E. (1969). *On death and dying.* New York: MacMillan.

PART 4

Special Populations

PART 4

PART 4

Maternal–Infant Nursing

This section is an overview of concepts and skills needed to provide care to mothers and infants and their families through the pregnancy cycle. For in-depth information, see a maternal–child health textbook.

Preconceptual Counseling

Preconceptual counseling ranges from contraceptive options to preparation for pregnancy. Because women are frequently unaware or unsure of pregnancy until after eight weeks of gestation, they can be unaware of the many important issues affecting the developing fetus. Critical fetal development occurs between 17 and 56 days following fertilization. It is the timeframe during which inadequate folic acid in the mother can cause neural tube defects. For example, to lower the incidence of neurological anomalies, women in the childbearing age should take daily supplemental folic acid (present in most vitamin supplements). Women considering pregnancy need to focus on a healthy lifestyle, which can be discussed at a visit prior to pregnancy. Discussion and educational topics include:

Preconceptual care
Nutrition
Healthy diet (including folic acid)
Optimum weight
Exercise and rest (good physical condition)
Substances to be avoided (tobacco, alcohol, recreational
    drugs)
Substance abuse (treatment prior to pregnancy)
Safe sex practices

PART 4

Medical risk factor identification (to be addressed prior to pregnancy)

Chronic illness, such as diabetes mellitus (good glucose control reduces fetal abnormalities and complications)

Consider effects of any chronic medications

Identify carrier status for any inherited disease (e.g., sickle-cell, cystic fibrosis, etc.)

Infections (STDs and those which cause congenital problems)

Health hazards at work or home

Psychosocial preparation for pregnancy and parenting

Teaching and counseling around medical and general health issues as identified above

Confirmation of Pregnancy

Presumptive Signs   These could also be caused by other medical conditions; therefore do not confirm the diagnosis of pregnancy.

- Amenorrhea
- Nausea and vomiting (morning sickness)
- Excessive fatigue
- Urinary frequency (first trimester)
- Breast changes (enlargement/darkening of the areola)
- Quickening (first awareness of fetal movement)

Probable Signs   Physical signs of pregnancy documented by examination but could also be caused by other disease conditions.

- Uterine enlargement
- Goodell's sign (softening of the cervix)
- Chadwick's sign (change in color of vaginal, cervical, or vulvular mucus membranes from pink to bluish purple)
- Hegar's sign (softening of the lower uterine segment)

- Ballottement (occurring only when the fetus is small—4th and 5th month—fetus rebounds when pushed by examiner either vaginally or abdominally)

Positive Signs Physical findings confirming pregnancy:

- Fetal heart sounds
- Fetal movement
- Visualization of the fetus with ultrasonography

History Taking Specific to Pregnancy

This history is taken in conjunction with a normal adult history. Standard forms exist to structure the intake history and physical examination (e.g., American College of Obstetrics and Gynecology or Hollister Company).

Gynecologic History

Menstrual history
    Onset (age)
    Date of last menstruation (period)
    Date of last normal menstruation
    Cycle frequency
    Length of menstruation
    Amount of bleeding
Birth control history
    Type used
    Success vs. failure
    Level of satisfaction with method
History of gynecologic infections
    Sexually transmitted diseases (STD) (can also be referred to as sexually transmitted infections)
        - Trichomonas, gonorrhea, syphilis, HIV or AIDS, hepatitis (A, B, or C), group B streptococcus, chlamydia, herpes, pelvic inflammatory disease
Sexual preference(s) and number of partners

Obstetric History

Previous pregnancies, outcomes

    Gravida

    Para

    TPAL (documentation of prior pregnancies)

        T = Number of term neonates born after 37 weeks gestation

        P = Number of preterm neonates born prior to 37 weeks

        A = Number of pregnancies ending in spontaneous or therapeutic abortions

        L = Number of currently living children

Present pregnancy

    Last menstrual period

    Viral exposures (e.g., TORCH, parvovirus)

    Change in sexual activity

    Nausea

    Vomiting

    Fetal activity

    Concerns of patient/mother

Calculation of Estimated Date of Confinement (EDC)

Using Nagele's rule, calculate using the following:

First day of the last menstrual period + 7 days − 3 months

$$= EDC$$

For example: first day of last period: July 1, 2005

	Month	Day	Year
	7	1	2005
	− 3	+ 7	+ 1
EDC =	4	8	2006

Normal Antepartum Examination (Repeat Visits)

Antepartal Caregiver Visits (for Normal Pregnancy)

- Every 4 weeks from first visit thru 28 weeks gestation
- Every 2 weeks from 29 thru 36 weeks
- Weekly from 37 weeks until birth

Interview Questions

- What relevant events occurred since the last visit?
- How is your general physical status and emotional well-being?
- What personal and family needs do you have?
- How is your family reacting to your pregnancy?

Physical Examination at Each Visit (Documented in Chart)

- Pulse and respirations
- Blood pressure (use same arm and same position—usually sitting)
- Weight and weight gain
- Urine (for protein, ketones, and sugar)
- Presence of any edema
- Abdominal evaluation (bladder should be empty)
  - Fundal height
  - Fetal position, using Leopold's maneuvers (see Figure 4-1)
- Fetal evaluation:
  - Estimation of fetal size
  - Listening for fetal heart tones (with either fetoscope or Doppler)

Prenatal Education

Knowledge is critical to a successful pregnancy, labor, birth, postpartum, and parenting. Teaching/learning can occur in the office or clinic during prenatal visits or through structured prenatal/childbirth education classes. Most birthing units or clinics have

PART 4

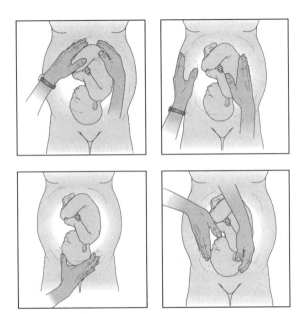

Figure 4-1   Leopold's maneuvers.

developed educational programs for patients. These encompass such content areas as labor and birth, childbirth preparation methods (e.g., Lamaze); VBAC (vaginal birth after cesarean); classes for new fathers, grandparents, siblings; care of the newborn; breast feeding; and classes on parenting the infant and toddler.

Prenatal Education Plan (For Use at the Prenatal Visits)

1. First trimester content areas
   a. Anatomy and physiology of pregnancy
   b. Maternal physical and emotional changes and adjustments
   c. Fetal growth and development

    d. Value of prenatal care
    e. Warning signs for any impending complications (see next section)
    f. Breast feeding and breast assessment
    g. Exercise, diet, and prenatal vitamins

2. Second trimester content areas (builds on previous teaching)
    a. Fetal development
    b. Assessment of fetal movement
    c. Signs of possible complications (review)
    d. Management of maternal physical and emotional changes (e.g., heartburn, back pain, comfort measures, hygiene, and body image)
    e. Enrollment in childbirth preparation classes
    f. Initiation of birth plan
    g. Preparation of siblings, home, and family for new infant
    h. Selection of pediatric care provider

3. Third trimester content areas (build on all previous teaching)
    a. Anatomy and physiology, and signs and symptoms of labor (review)
    b. Medication and anesthesia for labor
    c. Labor preparation
    d. Pack for the hospital trip
    e. Diet and exercise
    f. Comfort measures
    g. Antepartal risk factors and signs of labor
    h. Plan for help when bringing baby home

Antepartal Risk Factors for Impending Complications

The following conditions necessitate notification of the caregiver. Be sure the family also understands these symptoms.

- Repeated vomiting
- Fever greater than 101°F (38.3°C)

- Painful urination or decreased urine output
- Severe headache
- Dizziness, blurred vision, double vision, or spots before eyes
- Edema (swelling) of the hands, feet, or face
- Muscle cramps or convulsions/seizures
- Abdominal pain or cramping
- Epigastric pain (located between the xiphoid process and the umbilicus)
- Sudden rush of fluid or continuing leakage of fluid from the vagina
- Vaginal spotting of blood or any frank bleeding (red or brown)

Common Complications of Pregnancy

1. Abortion
- **Description:** Spontaneous abortion is a naturally occurring pregnancy termination that occurs in 20% of pregnancies, usually in the first trimester, and sometimes before the woman realizes she is pregnant. Fifty percent can be a result of chromosomal abnormalities.
- **Symptomatology**
  - Frank vaginal bleeding or a bloody discharge with or without cramping
- **Treatment**
  - Vaginal examination to determine dilatation of the cervix
  - If confirmed, the patient may be put on bedrest to await spontaneous delivery or a D & C may be performed.
  - Pain medication may be needed.

2. Ectopic pregnancy
- **Description:** The fertilized egg implants someplace other than the endometrial lining, most commonly in the fallopian tube. Occurrence is 19.7 per 1000 pregnancies, and it can be life threatening.

- **Symptomatology**
  - Severe abdominal pain and/or pelvic pain
  - Possible vaginal bleeding
  - Abdominal tenderness on palpation
- **Treatment**
  - Usually requires surgery
  - Mother can experience hemorrhaging into the abdomen.

3. Hyperemesis gravidarum
- **Description:** Severe vomiting leading to weight loss and dehydration, acidosis, alkalosis, and/or hypokalemia
- **Symptomatology**
  - Unrelieved nausea and vomiting extending into the second trimester
- **Treatment**
  - May require hospitalization
  - Intravenous fluids and electrolytes
  - Administration of antiemetics

4. Pregnancy-induced hypertension (PIH) (also known as pre-eclampsia or toxemia)
- **Description:** Hypertension, edema of face and extremities, and proteinuria, usually occurring after the 20th week of pregnancy. Etiology unknown.
- **Symptomatology**
  - Elevated blood pressure (30 mmHg systolic or 15 mmHg diastolic at two different readings) or a reading of 140/90 or higher
  - Edema unrelieved by bed rest
  - Headache
  - Protein in the urine
  - Excessive weight gain (more than 2 lb/week)
  - Visual disturbance
  - Epigastric pain
- **Treatment**
  - Bed rest with closely monitored blood pressures

- Daily protein check of urine, antihypertensives, daily weight
- Hospitalization required if symptoms are unresponsive.
- Close monitoring for intake and output, presence and location of edema, deep tendon reflexes, nausea, vomiting, and epigastric or right-upper quadrant pain in the mother.
- Close monitoring of the fetus.

5. Preterm labor

- **Description:** Spontaneous labor occurring prior to 37 weeks gestation and resulting in cervical dilation. Highest risk factor for preterm labor is a previous preterm labor; others include multiple gestation pregnancy, infections, previous spontaneous abortions, history of smoking, or maternal age.
- **Symptomatology**
  - Abdominal cramping (much like a period)
  - Backache
  - Vaginal bleeding
  - Change in vaginal discharge
  - Change in patterns of urination
  - Diarrhea
  - Pelvic pressure
  - Regular uterine contractions (could be painless)
- **Treatment**
  - The focus is on prolonging the pregnancy for the benefit of the growing fetus.
  - Tocolytic medications to stop labor
  - If tocolytics fail, corticosteroids are given to enhance fetal lung maturity.

6. Premature rupture of the membranes

- **Description:** Spontaneous rupture of the membranes prior to the onset of labor, regardless of gestational age. There is increased risk of infection in the mother and a risk to the fetus due to prematurity, sepsis, respiratory distress syndrome, and cord prolapse.

- **Symptomatology**
  - Reports of an uncontrollable gush of vaginal fluid
  - Determination of the time of the incident, color, and odor of the fluid.
  - Sterile pelvic examination may reveal fluid leaking from the uterine os
  - Vaginal secretions may be Nitrazine paper positive
  - Vaginal secretion smear may reveal ferning patterns (microscopic examination). These tests can confirm rupture of membranes.
- **Treatment**
  - Depends on the risk assessment
  - Proactive treatment, such as induction of labor and delivery either vaginally or by cesarean section
  - Close monitoring for amnionitis or fetal distress required with a failed induction.
  - Action delayed until infection or fetal distress appears.

7. **Placenta previa**
  - **Description:** There are three classes of placenta previa (see Figure 4-2):
    - **Complete previa:** Placenta completely covers the cervical os (third trimester of pregnancy).
    - **Marginal previa or partial previa:** Placenta is located within 2–3 cm of the os but does not completely cover it.
    - **Low-lying placenta:** Placental distance to the os is undetermined but is close because significant bleeding occurs during labor and cervical dilation. The incidence of placenta previa is estimated at 1 in 200 deliveries; previous cesarean section(s) or induced abortion seem to be related to an increased incidence of this complication.
  - **Symptomatology**
    - Mother presents with sudden, painless vaginal bleeding in the second or third trimester.
    - Amount of bleeding varies from a small amount (it can stop spontaneously) to severe bleeding.
    - Can hemorrhage and be life threatening.

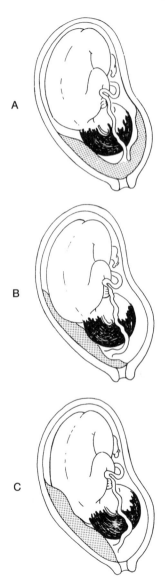

A

B

C

Figure 4-2   Placenta previa: A. complete; B. partial; C. marginal.

- **Treatment**
  - Hospitalization and bed rest to see if bleeding will stop
  - If unsuccessful and bleeding is severe, must deliver, regardless of fetal gestational age.
  - Usually performed by cesarean section
8. Abruptio placenta
- **Description:** Separation of the placenta from the site of implantation prior to delivery
  - Bleeding can be concealed behind the placenta (in about 10% of cases).
  - Bleeding can exit through the vagina.
  - Occurs once in 150 deliveries.
  - Associated with pregnancy-induced hypertension, premature rupture of the membranes, and maternal trauma (such as automobile accidents).
- **Symptomatology**
  - Vaginal bleeding
  - Abdominal tenderness, pain, and rigidity (boardlike abdomen).
  - Fetal heart tones may be absent or a nonreassuring fetal heart rate.
  - Mother may go into shock.
  - Most common cause of pregnancy-related disseminated intravascular coagulation (DIC)
- **Treatment**
  - Stabilize mother and minimize bleeding.
  - Plan is dictated by fetal gestational age.
  - Mother is hospitalized for close observation.
  - Severe bleeding requires cesarean section.

Signs and Symptoms of Prelabor

- Lightening (fetal presenting part settles low in the pelvis)
  - Primips: Occurs 2–3 weeks prior to onset of labor
  - Multips: Can occur with onset of labor
- Urinary frequency due to increased pressure on the bladder from the lower lying fetus

PART 4

Table 4-1 Differentiating True Versus False Labor

Contractions	Labor	
	True	**False**
Location	Back and abdomen	Lower abdomen
Frequency	Regular with decreased intervals	Irregular with no change or increase in intervals
Intensity	Increases over time or with walking	Remains the same; unaffected or decreased with walking
Pain	Becomes more painful	No change in pain
Effect on cervix	Dilation and effacement	No dilation or effacement
Membranes	Documented through fern test, Nitrazine paper, pooled fluid in the vagina	Cannot document; negative for each test

- Backache (due to pressure of low-lying fetus on the spine)
- Braxton Hicks' contractions (painless, irregular contractions that help prepare for labor)
- Cervical changes (softening, thinning, shortening, and increased pliability)
- Mucus plug expelled due to cervical changes
- Bloody show (resulting from cervical changes that rupture cervical capillaries)
- Weight loss of 1–3 pounds
- Membranes may rupture (12% of women prior to labor).
- GI upset (diarrhea, nausea, vomiting, and indigestion)

The 5 Ps of the Labor Process

Passenger   The fetus and placenta navigating the passageway is determined by:

- **Head size:**
  - Fetal skull bones united by membranous suture lines intersecting at the fontanels.
  - Soft suture lines allow for contraction and overlap (molding) so the fetal head adapts to the passageway. (See Figure 4-3.)
- **Fetal presentation:**
  - That part of the fetus that presents first into the passageway—cephalic, breech, shoulder, or compound (See Figures 4-4 and 4-5).
  - Breech, compound, and shoulder presentations are linked to cesarean births.
- **Fetal lie:**
  - Position of fetus as relates to mother's spinal cord (see Figure 4-6)
  - Cephalic and breech—the lie is longitudinal

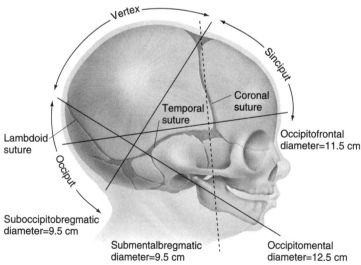

PART 4

Figure 4-3   The term fetal head.

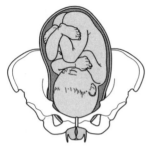

Left occiput posterior (LOP)

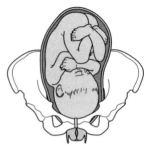

Right occiput posterior (ROP)

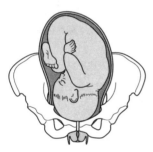

Left occiput transverse (LOT)

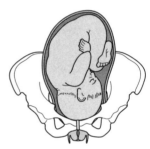

Right occiput transverse (ROT)

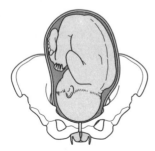

Left occiput anterior (LOA)

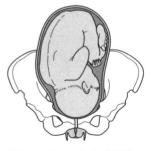

Right occiput anterior (ROA)

Figure 4-4 Positions of a vertex presentation.

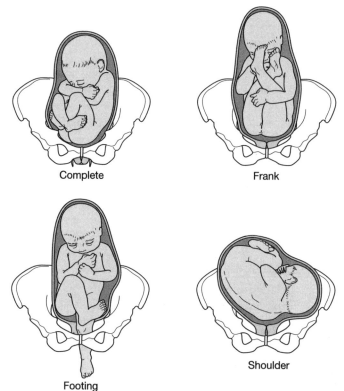

Complete

Frank

Footing

Shoulder

Figure 4-5   Breech presentations.

- Shoulder presentation—lie is transverse (to the mother's spinal cord)
- Oblique fetus is at 45° angle to mother's spine. Position usually converts to either longitudinal or transverse.

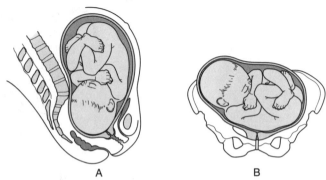

Figure 4-6 Fetal lie: A. longitudinal; B. transverse.

- **Fetal attitude:**
  - Relationship of fetal parts to each other
  - Fetal head: Flexes or extends from the fetal trunk
  - Head extends: Presents a broader diameter to the passageway—can necessitate C-section.

Passageway The birth canal:

- Composed of the bony pelvis: Ilium, ischial spines, pubis, sacrum, and coccyx
- Passageway (divided into two parts)
  - False pelvis: Shallow upper part of the pelvis
  - True pelvis: Lower, curved, bony part of the canal, includes inlet, cavity, and outlet
  - Station: Relationship of ischial spines to the presenting part of the fetus. Ischial spines = Station 0 (see Figure 4-7); narrowest part of the pelvis
  - Passageway: Adequate for passenger (regardless of fetal position)

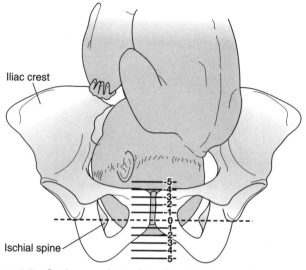

Iliac crest

Ischial spine

Figure 4-7   Station, or relationship of the fetal presenting part to the ischial spines. The station illustrated is +2.

Powers

- **Uterine contractions:**
  - Involuntary powers responsible for dilatation and effacement, descent, and delivery of the fetus.
  - Correct method for palpation of contractions shown in Figure 4-8.
  - Representation of phases of uterine contractions found in Figure 4-9.
- **Effacement:**
  - Shortening and thinning of cervix
  - Prior to the onset of labor in primigravida women, cervix is 2–3 cm long and 1 cm thick.
  - In multigravida women, the cervix begins to thin in the third trimester.

PART 4

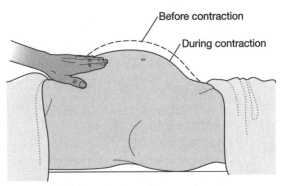

Figure 4-8   Method for palpation of contractions.

- **Dilatation:**
  - Cervix: Long and closed prior to the onset of labor
  - Labor: Cervix dilates to 10 cm and retracts into the lower uterine segment
  - Full dilation: Cervix is no longer palpable (see Figure 4-10.)

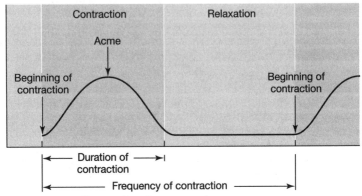

Figure 4-9   Phases of uterine contractions.

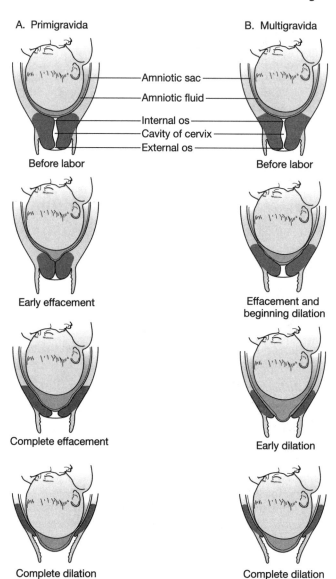

A. Primigravida

B. Multigravida

Amniotic sac
Amniotic fluid
Internal os
Cavity of cervix
External os

Before labor

Before labor

Early effacement

Effacement and
beginning dilation

Complete effacement

Early dilation

Complete dilation

Complete dilation

PART 4

Figure 4-10 Effacement and dilation of the cervix.

- **Bearing down:**
  - Mother's efforts to push fetus out
  - Pushing can be involuntary.
  - Intentional pushing—nurse encourages pushing.
  - Mother contracts abdominal muscles around the uterus and bears down.
  - Fetus propelled toward the pelvic floor.
  - Leads to eventual expulsion

Position

- Can affect the conduct of the labor; the perception of pain, and well-being of the fetus
- Find comfortable position:
  - Sitting in a chair
  - Using a birthing ball
  - Walking
- Avoid supine position (not comfortable).
- Monitor fetal well-being (monitoring equipment can be used with various positions).
- No single position works for everyone.
- Nurse support of mother and partner critical to decreasing maternal discomfort.

Psychological Response   The mother's responses affect labor. Influencing on response include:

- Culture: Beliefs, values, norms, and practices about childbirth influence childbearing behavior.
- Maternal role adaptation (described by Reva Rubin):
  - Knowledge acquisition
  - Transition into role of mother
  - Positive, safe labor and birth facilitate transition.
- Knowledge and support overcome fears and anxieties.
- Fear and anxiety impact labor progress, birth, recovery, and postpartum period.

- Quality care results from:
  - Positive and supportive environment
  - Respect for the mother and family
- Therapeutic communication and assessment of physical, psychological, social, and spiritual needs are essential.

Stages of Labor

The stages of labor consist of four stages beginning with the onset of true labor and are completed four hours after delivery of the placenta.

First Stage of Labor   The longest stage of labor, divided into phases.

1. **Latent phase**
   a. Onset of true labor beginning with regular contractions (can be 10–15 minutes apart)
   b. Contractions: Closer and stronger in intensity and duration
   c. Back pain and abdominal cramping
   d. Mother can remain at home.
   e. Bloody show or mucus plug occurs.
2. **Active phase**
   a. Cervix dilates
      - Primip: 1.2 cm per hour
      - Multip: 1.5 cm per hour
   b. Begins at about 4–5 cm; ends at 8 cm
   c. Contractions: Every 2–5 min, duration of 40–50 sec and of moderate intensity
   d. Descent of fetus continues (see Figure 4-11)
3. **Transition phase**
   a. Shortest phase
   b. Lasts until the cervix is completely dilated
      - Primip: No more than three hours
      - Multip: An hour

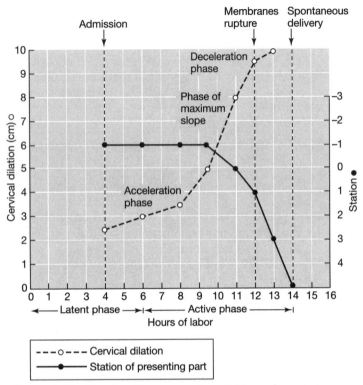

Figure 4-11 Charting the progression of labor of a primiparous woman using the Friedman graph.

   c. Contractions:
- Every 1½ to 2 mins
- 1 min duration
- Extremely intense

   d. Woman can experience:
- Discomfort
- Irritability
- Loss of control

- Difficulty with breathing techniques
- Nausea and vomiting

e. Nursing support to mother and support person is essential.

Second Stage of Labor   Complete cervical dilation ending with birth.

1. **Pushing:**
   a. Intense contractions
   b. Involuntary urge to push
2. **Duration:**
   a. Primip: 60–90 min
   b. Multip: Less than 30 min
   c. Greater than two hours is abnormal and requires assessment.
3. **Descent:**
   a. Through the birth canal and appears at the vulvar opening (crowning)
   b. Mechanisms of labor shown in Figure 4-12.
4. **Birth of the fetal head:**
   a. Should be slow, controlled
      i. Decreases perineal lacerations
      ii. Allows for suctioning the mouth and nasal pharynx of infant as head emerges
   b. Neck examined for umbilical cord
      i. If present, cord removed
      ii. If too tight, cord is clamped and cut prior to birth of shoulders
5. **After delivery of shoulders, body and extremities delivered without problem.**

Third Stage of Labor   Birth of the fetus to expulsion of placenta.

1. Contractions: Strong but less painful; occur every 5 min
2. Placenta emerges spontaneously 5–10 minutes after infant.

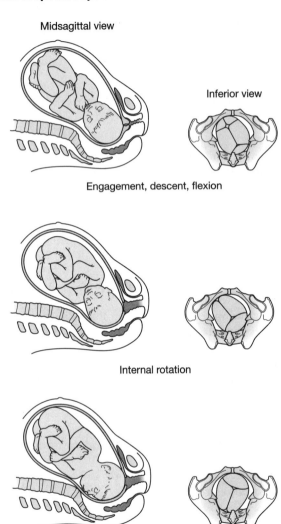

Midsagittal view

Inferior view

Engagement, descent, flexion

Internal rotation

Extension beginning, rotation complete

Figure 4-12   Mechanisms of labor.

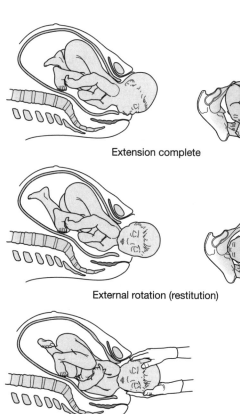

Extension complete

External rotation (restitution)

External rotation (shoulder rotation)

Expulsion

Figure 4-12 *Continued*

3. Placental separation results from forceful uterine contractions
   a. Contractions shrink size of placental site and uterine involution begins.
   b. Placenta separates from uterine wall.
   c. Placental site bleeding occurs prior to contraction of muscles and then decreases.
   d. Blood collects and is expelled through the vagina (one of the signs of separation), and as this separation occurs the umbilical cord lengthens (the second sign of separation).
4. Delivery of the placenta
   a. Shiny Shultze: Center of placenta separates first, folding on itself and expelling with the "shiny" fetal side appearing first.
   b. Dirty Duncan: Placental edges separate first and placenta rolls up on itself, is expelled sideways, maternal side first.
      • More likely to separate incompletely and leave placental fragments in uterus
      • Causes excessive bleeding or postpartum hemorrhage
      • Examine the placenta to determine if intact to avoid bleeding episodes.

Fourth Stage of Labor   Recovery stage; successful delivery of placenta.

1. Ends four hours later
2. Assessment and evaluation to assure normal physiologic adjustments
3. Uterus must remain firm.
4. Blood pressure stabilizes
5. Can be 500 cc of blood loss
6. Uterus begins transformation to normal size.

Mechanisms of Labor

During labor the position of the fetal head and body must change to accommodate the maternal pelvis. This process of movement through the birth canal is known as the *cardinal movements* or the *mechanism of labor* (see Figure 4-12). These movements consist of descent, flexion, internal rotation, extension, restitution, external rotation, and expulsion.

Nursing Care of the Laboring Mother and Her Family

Follow the policies and procedures of the individual facility in which the birth is taking place.

Maternal Assessment

- **Vital signs**—(blood pressure, temperature, pulse, and respirations) determined by stage of labor and level of risk to mother and infant
- **Hydration and nutrition**—Intake is limited to fluids and ice chips (maternal dehydration can occur)
- **Elimination**
  - Urinate every 2 hours (full bladder can impede the progress of labor)
  - Assess for recent bowel movement.
- **Labor assessment**
  - Uterine contractions (frequency, duration, and intensity)
  - Status of the membranes and fluid being expelled
  - Assessment of pain or pain relief
- **Activity**
  - Frequent position changes
  - Up walking in early labor
  - Use of birthing ball to alter positions
- **Comfort measures**
  - Anxiety assessment of woman, partner, or family
  - Coaching support people

Fetal Assessment

- According to policy and procedures
- Monitoring of the heart tones important (see next section).

Family Members   Assessment of family and their support of the mother.

Communication and Documentation   Documentation is done on a flow sheet or entered into the computer according to the policies of the facility. It should be:

- Timely
- Utilize guidelines
- Communicate with the primary care provider regarding change in status or progress of labor.

Monitoring the Fetus

Fetal Heart Rate Monitoring   The fetal heart rate (FHR) is the number of times the fetal heart beats in one minute. The rate is monitored by auscultation or by electronic monitoring.

Auscultation of Fetal Heart Tones (FHT)   Intermittent method of monitoring the FHR with OB stethoscope (fetoscope), or with small, handheld Doppler device.

- Listen to fetal heart tones during and immediately following a contraction.
- Assess and record every 30 minutes during the active phase of labor.
- Advantage: Method allows the mother mobility
- Disadvantage: Does not create a continuous printed record of heart tones, and does not show variability or other subtle changes.

Electronic Fetal Monitoring (EFM)

- Auditory and visual method of monitoring FHRs
- Frequency and duration of contractions recorded on paper printout.

- EFM can be done externally using an ultrasonic Doppler and tocotransducer to monitor intensity and duration of contractions.
- Internal monitoring uses a fetal scalp electrode applied to the fetal head to assess FHR and uses an intrauterine pressure catheter to assess contractions.
- Internal monitoring requires ruptured membranes.

Fetal Heart Rate Patterns

- **Baseline fetal heart rate**
  - Consistent rate occurring between contractions
  - Serves as a reference point for subsequent FHR activity
  - Normal baseline 120–160 beats/minute.
  - Strip evaluated for 10 minutes to determine base rate.
  - Rate is frequently charted as a range (eg., 130–140) due to the natural variation in rate.
- **Variability**
  - Beat-to-beat fluctuations in the heart rate
  - Occur due to the stimulation from the sympathetic and parasympathetic nervous systems
  - Assessed only with internal scalp electrode
  - **Long-term variability**
    - Long-term deviations above and below the baseline FHR
    - Normal variation is 5–20 beats/min, 3 to 5 times per minute.
  - **Short-term variability**
    - Instant fluctuations in the heart rate
    - Appear as difference in the R-R wave interval of the QRS cardiac cycle
    - Described as normal, increased, decreased, or absent
    - Most reliable indicator of fetal well-being.

- **Increased variability**
  - Fetal movement increases
  - Fetal heart rate and long-term variability can occur in beginning stages of mild hypoxia (hypoxia of second-stage labor)
- **Decreased variability**
  - Occurs when fetus is asleep
  - CNS depressant drugs (narcotics) cause decrease in variability.
  - Caused by fetal arrhythmias and needs to be corrected
- **Periodic changes:** Transient accelerations and decelerations that deviate from the baseline FHR; can be caused by uterine contractions or fetal movement and reflect normal fluctuations from resting fetal pulse.
  - **Accelerations:** Caused by uterine contractions or fetal movement; reflect normal fluctuations from the resting fetal pulse.
  - **Decelerations:** Periodic changes from normal FHR that vary in timing and wave form.
    - Early decelerations
      - Begin early in the contraction
      - Well tolerated by the fetus
      - Have no effect on FHR variability
      - Unaffected by position change or administration of maternal oxygen
      - Require no nursing intervention
    - Late decelerations
      - Start after beginning of contraction with lowest point of the deceleration occurring after the contraction ends
      - Both the descent and return are smooth and gradual
      - Wave form is U shaped
      - Nonreassuring decelerations indicating uteroplacental insufficiency

- Decreased blood flow leading to inadequate fetal oxygen exchange
- Some conditions respond to nursing interventions:
  - Maternal hypotension (turn mother to right side and increase the intravenous fluids)
  - Hyperstimulated uterus due to oxytocin (decrease or turn off the oxytocin)
- Variable decelerations
  - Can be mild, moderate, or severe
  - Can be dramatic and unpredictable
  - Vary in shape, duration, depth, and timing
  - Caused by fetal movements or umbilical cord compression
  - Can be alleviated by changing maternal position to alleviate cord compression
- Prolonged decelerations
  - Deceleration lasting 60–90 seconds
  - Response to a sudden vagal system stimulation
  - Can occur with vaginal examination or scalp electrode application or after drug administration
  - May persist for several minutes but variability remains normal
  - Could be an indicator of impending birth or prolapsed umbilical cord

The guidelines for monitoring FHR were developed by the Association of Women's Health, Obstetrics, and Neonatal Nursing (AWHONN).

Anesthesia and Analgesia

Nonpharmacologic Pain Control Minimal pharmacologic intervention in laboring women is optimal for delivery of a healthy infant. Various approaches have been developed to support women during labor. Most involve knowledge about the labor and birth process, relaxation so that the body can do the necessary work, visualization of the body working appropriately, and distraction from the discomfort of the process. An important aspect of labor and birth preparation is choice. Methods for nonpharmacologic pain control can be used alone or in combination, and include the following:

Childbirth preparation such as Lamaze, Grantly Dick-Reed, and Bradley
Relaxation breathing techniques
Music
Effleurage and counterpressure
Water therapy
Transcutaneous electrical nerve stimulation
Acupressure
Heat and cold application
Therapeutic touch
Hypnosis
Biofeedback
Aromatherapy

The mother and her partner need to have choices available to them. Flexibility is a critical aspect. If unforeseen events occur, such as problems with the fetus, the mother can make optional choices, even though her goal may have been to labor and birth her infant with no analgesia or anesthetic intervention.

Analgesia or Pharmacologic Pain Control Drugs (either intravenous or intramuscular route) provide some pain relief for labor. Opioids and sedatives are often coadministered (e.g., Phenergan with Demerol)

- **Advantages**
  - Minimally invasive pain relief
  - Administered by a registered nurse
- **Disadvantages**
  - Maternal—Inadequate pain relief; side effects including nausea, vomiting, drowsiness

- Fetal—CNS depressant; respiratory depression; decreased beat-to-beat variability

Anesthesia   Defined as the absence of sensation.

- **Local:** The loss of sensation at a small localized area of the body following infiltration either topically or through injection
  - Advantages
    - Minimal loss of function
    - No loss of maternal awareness
    - Minimal or no impact on the infant
    - Disadvantages: Pain relief may be inadequate
- **Regional:** The loss of sensation to a large area of the body due to blocking neural impulses. The most common examples for labor and birth include: spinal block and epidural block
  - **Advantages in epidural**
    - Effective pain relief for labor
    - Indefinite duration
    - Titratable
  - **Disadvantages in epidural**
    - Confined to bed (unless a walking epidural)
    - Possible interference with pushing
    - Possible postanesthesia headache
    - Possible slowing of labor
    - Possible increase in cesarean birth rate
  - **Advantages for spinal block for delivery**
    - Rapid onset
    - Less reaction, such as shivering
    - Less systemic medication
    - Less placental transfer (as opposed to general anesthesia)
    - Mother is awake
  - **Disadvantages of spinal block**
    - Limited duration
    - Possible severe hypotension

- Possible total spinal
- **General:** The loss of sensation for the entire body due to the loss of consciousness from either intravenous or inhaled anesthetic agents
  - **Advantages:** Is quick acting for emergency situations
  - **Disadvantages**
    - Mother is asleep
    - Possible aspiration
    - Infant can be depressed.

Apgar Score

A scoring mechanism to evaluate newborns at birth developed by Virginia Apgar. Five physiological parameters were chosen to evaluate the status of the newborn: heart rate, respiratory effort, muscle tone, reflex response (response to breath test, and to skin stimulation of the feet), and color. Each parameter is given a score of 0, 1, or 2 as shown in the table and the maximum score is 10. Scoring is done at 1 minute, 5 minutes, and 10 minutes. This assesses the physiological condition at each interval and the effectiveness of whatever interventions were performed.

Table 4-2 Apgar Score

Signs	0	1	2
Heart rate	Absent	Below 100	Over 100
Respiratory effort	Absent	Weak cry, hypoventilation	Good strong cry
Muscle tone	Limp	Some flexion of extremities	Well-flexed extremities
Reflex response	No response	Grimace	Cough or sneeze
Color	Blue, pale	Body pink, blue extremities	Completely pink

Source: Apgar, V. (1966). The newborn (Apgar) scoring system. *Pediatric Clinics of North America, 13*(3), 645. Reprinted with permission from Elsevier.

Table 4-3 Newborn Physical Assessment

Area Assessed	Procedure	Normal Variations	Etiology	Findings
Posture	Inspect prior to disturbing infant for examination Vertex: Presentations: Arms and legs flexed with resistance to having extremities extended	Infant usually assumes same position as had in utero. Vertex: Extremities flexed; fists clenched; Breech: Legs more straight	Intrauterine pressure on a particular part may cause temporary facial asymmetry or resistance to extension of extremities	Hypotonia from prematurity or maternal medications; or CNS disorder
Vital signs	Check heart rate	Visible heart pulsations in left midclavicular line; apical pulse in 4th intercostals space	100/min (sleeping) 160/min (crying); can have temporary irregularity with crying	Persistent tachycardia (greater than 160/min) can be respiratory distress syndrome (RDS) Persistent bradycardia (less than 120/min) can be congenital heart block

Table 4-3 (continued)

Area Assessed	Procedure	Normal Variations	Etiology	Findings
	Check femoral pulse	Femoral pulses equal and strong		Weak or absent can be hip dysplasia, coarctation of aorta, thrombophlebitis
Temperature (axillary)	Electronic thermometer probe	37°C or 98.6°F	Variation by ½ degree Heat loss or gain from evaporation, conduction, convection, or radiation	Subnormal from prematurity, environment, inadequate clothing, or dehydration Increased: Infection, environmental (too hot or too many clothes), drug addiction, or diarrhea

Respiratory rate	Observe respiration when infant is at rest; count for full minute. Listen for audible sounds without stethoscope; observe respiratory effort and count per minute	40/min. Tend to be shallow and irregular in rate, rhythm and depth when awake. No audible sound on inspiration or expiration	Apneic episodes of greater than 15 sec can indicate prematurity. Bradypnea: Less than 25/min can be maternal analgesics, anesthetics, or birth trauma. Distress: Nasal flaring, retractions, chin tug, labored breathing can be RDS or fluid in lungs.
Blood pressure	Assessed only for suspected problem	Range of 78/40 to 55/24	Can vary with sleep or awake. Hypotension: Sepsis, hypovolemia. Hypertension or variation between pressure in upper

PART 4

Table 4-3 (continued)

Area Assessed	Procedure	Normal Variations	Etiology	Findings
	Check with electronic cuff of 2.5 cm width and palpate radial pulse			and lower extremities: coarctation of aorta
Measurements				
Weight	Use protective liner with scale Weigh at same time each day Protect infant from heat loss	Female: 3400 gm Male: 3500 gm Regain birth wt. within 2 weeks	Range 2500–4000 gm Acceptable wt loss of 10% of birth wt. Second infant weighs more than first	Less than 2500 gm: Prematurity, small for gestational age, rubella syndrome More than 4000 gm: Large for gestational age, maternal diabetes, hereditary Wt. loss of more than 10%: Dehydration

Length	Measure from top of head to heel	50 cm	45–55 cm	Less than 45 cm or more than 55 cm: Chromosomal aberration or heredity
Head circumference	Measure at greatest diameter: Occipitofrontal circumference	33–35 cm; Circumference of head and chest nearly the same for day 1 & 2 after birth	32–36 cm	Less than 32 cm: Microcephaly (possible rubella, toxoplasmosis, cytomegalic inclusion disease); More than 37 cm: Hydrocephaly; Sutures widely separated & head circumference greater than chest by 4 cm; or increased intracranial pressure from hemorrhage; or lesion

PART 4

Table 4-3 (continued)

Area Assessed	Procedure	Normal Variations	Etiology	Findings
Chest circumference	Measure at nipple line	Within 2–3 cm of head circumference		Less than 30 cm: Prematurity
Skin	Check color: Inspect naked newborn in well-lit warm area with natural daylight; infant should be quiet	Generally pink; varying with ethnic origin; acrocyanosis, especially if chilled	Some mottling; harlequin sign; plethora telangiectasis (stork bite or capillary hemangiomas); erythema toxicum (newborn rash); milia	Dark red (prematurity, polycythemia); pallor (cardiovascular problem, CNS damage, blood dyscrasia, blood loss, nosocomial infection) Cyanosis (hypothermia, infection, hypoglycemia, cardiac disease; cardiac, neurologic, or respiratory malformations); petechiae over

			any other area: (clotting factor deficiency, infection); ecchymoses in any other area (hemorrhagic disease, traumatic birth)
Check for jaundice	None at birth	Physiologic jaundice in 50% of term infants after first 24 hr	Gray (hypotension, poor perfusion) jaundice within first 24 hr. (Rh isoimmunization)
Check for birthmarks	Transient hyperpigmentation of genitals, areolae, linea nigra / No skin edema / Opacity	Mongolian spotting	Hemangiomas / Port-wine stain / Strawberry mark / Cavernous hemangiomas
Check for general condition		Marked peeling; Meconium on the skin; jaundice prior to 24 hrs of age	Postmaturity

PART 4

Table 4-3 (continued)

Area Assessed	Procedure	Normal Variations	Etiology	Findings
	Assess hydration	Dehydration as assessed by weight loss	10% is normal	Loose wrinkled skin, no subcutaneous fat (prematurity, postmaturity, dehydration)
	Check voiding	First voiding within first 24 hrs; voiding 6–10 times per day		
	Check vernix caseosa		Variation in amount; usually more found in creases, skin folds	Absent or minimal (postmaturity); excessive (prematurity)
	Assess lanugo	Fine downy hair over shoulders, ears, forehead	Various amounts	Absent (postmaturity) excessive (prematurity); yellow color (Rh or ABO incompatibility); green color

Head	Palpate	Caput succedaneum; some ecchymosis	(meconium in utero; or bilirubin) Order (infection) Cephalhematoma
	Assess shape & size	Molding	Severe molding (birth trauma); indentation (fracture)
		Slight asymmetry from position in utero	
	Inspect fontanels	Anterior fontanel—diamond shaped; larger than posterior fontanel	Full, bulging (tumor, hemorrhage, infection); large, flat (malnutrition, hydrocephaly, hypothyroidism), depression (dehydration)
		Variations with amount of molding	
Eyes	Check placement on face	Space between eyes	Epicanthal folds; When present with other signs (chromosomal disorders such as Down's)
		Epicanthal folds; normal racial characteristic	

Table 4-3 *(continued)*

Area Assessed	Procedure	Normal Variations	Etiology	Findings
	Check for discharge	None	Some discharge if silver nitrate given	Purulent discharge (infection)
	Check pupils	Equal & react to light		Unequal, constricted, dilated, fixed (intracranial pressure, medications, tumors)
Nose	Assess shape, placement, patency, configuration of bridge of nose	Midline; some mucus without drainage; nose breather; sneezing to clear nose	Slightly misshapen due to birth process	Significant drainage without periods of cyanosis (choanal atresia, congenital syphilis) Malformed (congenital syphilis, chromosomal disorder); flaring nares (respiratory distress)

Ears	Assess shape, size, placement, auditory canal	Correct placement, well formed	Small or large, floppy	Agenesis; lack of cartilage (prematurity); low placement (chromosomal disorder, mental retardation, kidney problems); Overly large, prominent, or protruding
	Assess hearing	Responds to voice or other sounds, loud noise	State of alertness influences response	Deaf (no response to sound)
Mouth	Assess and palpate for placement, color, configuration, movement	Symmetry of movement	Transient circumoral cyanosis	Anomalies in placement, size, shape (cleft lip or palate); cyanosis (respiratory distress, hypothermia); asymmetry in movement

Table 4-3 *(continued)*

Area Assessed	Procedure	Normal Variations	Etiology	Findings
				(7th cranial nerve paralysis)
	Assess tongue for attachment, mobility	Freely movable; symmetric in shape		Macroglossia (prematurity, chromosomal disorder); Thrush (white plaques on cheeks or tongue, bleed when touched)
	Assess palate (hard and soft); arch and uvula	Palates intact; uvula in midline		Cleft in hard or soft palate
	Assess reflexes: rooting, sucking, extrusion	Present		Absent (prematurity)
Neck	Assess and palpate for length and mobility	Head held in midline, movement: Side to side, flexion, & extension		Absence of head control (prematurity, Down's); masses (enlarged

Chest	Inspect shape	Circular, barrel shaped		thyroid); distended veins (cardiopulmonary disorder) Bulging or unequal movement (pneumothorax)
	Assess respiratory movement	Symmetric movement	Occasional retractions when crying	Retractions with or without respiratory distress (prematurity; RDS)
	Assess clavicles	Intact		Fractured (birth trauma)
	Check nipples & breast tissue	Breast nodule 6 mm in size with prominent well-formed nipples		Lack of breast tissue (prematurity)
Lungs	Auscultate	Respiratory rate 30–60/min; abdominal breathing; bilateral bronchial sounds	Rhonchi shortly after birth; apneic periods up to 15 sec	Grunting (RDS); absence of bilateral breath sounds (pneumothorax)

Table 4-3 *(continued)*

Area Assessed	Procedure	Normal Variations	Etiology	Findings
Heart	Auscultate	Rate: 120–160; 5th intercostal space; Soft murmur during first few days of life		Loud murmur, displacement of PMI, thrill, sustained rate above or below limits (cardiac abnormalities)
Abdomen	Inspect, palpate	Cord: 2 arteries & 1 vein; cord drying, odorless, clamp in place		1 artery (renal anomalies); meconium stained (intrauterine stress); bleeding around cord (hemorrhagic disease); redness or drainage around cord (infection); hernia (omphalocele)

	Assess size and contour	Rounded, prominent, liver palpable		Gastroschisis (fissure of abdominal cavity); distended at birth (ruptured viscus, masses or tumors, transient overfeeding, partial intestinal obstruction, sepsis)
Genitalia: Female	Observation	Usually edematous	Blood tinged discharge	Ambiguous genitals (chromosomal disorder)
Male	Observation	Meatus at top of penis; prepuce covering glans penis and not retractable. Scrotum large, edematous with rugae. Testes palpable on each side	Wide variation in size	Urinary meatus not on tip of glans penis (hyperspadias) Scrotum smooth and testes undescended

Table 4-3 (continued)

Area Assessed	Procedure	Normal Variations	Etiology	Findings
				(prematurity) Hydrocele; Inguinal hernia
Extremities	Inspect and palpate flexion, ROM, symmetry, muscle tone	Attitude of general flexion, full ROM, spontaneous movements	Slight tremors, some acrocyanosis	Limited motion (malformations); poor muscle tone (prematurity, maternal medications, CNS anomalies); asymmetry of movement (fracture); palmar creases (Down's); unequal leg length or asymmetric gluteal folds (dislocated hip)
Gestational age	See charts			
Reflexes	See Table 4–4			

Table 4-4 Newborn Reflexes

Reflex	Eliciting Response	Characteristics	Observations
Sucking and rooting	Touch infant's lip, cheek, or mouth with nipple	Infant turns toward stimulus, opens mouth, takes hold and sucks	Cannot elicit after infant has been fed; if response is weak or absent consider neurologic defect or prematurity
			Avoid turning head by hand; wait for infant to root (disappears after 3–4 mos)
Swallowing	Swallowing follows sucking and taking fluids	Occurs with sucking and without gagging, coughing, or vomiting	Weak or absent response may indicate prematurity or neurologic defect. May be uncoordinated in premature infant
Grasp			
Palmar	Place finger in palm of hand	Infant's fingers curl around examiner's fingers; toes curl downward	Palmar response decreases by 3–4 mo. Plantar lessens by 8 mos.
Plantar	Place finger at base of toes		

PART 4

Table 4-4 *(continued)*

Reflex	Eliciting Response	Characteristics	Observations
Extrusion	Touch or depress tip of tongue	Newborn forces tongue outward	Response disappears after 4 mos.
Glabellar (Myerson's)	Tap forehead, bridge of nose, or maxilla of infant whose eyes are open	Newborn blinks for first 4 or 5 taps	Continued blinking with additional taps indicates a disorder
Tonic neck or "fencing"	When infant is falling asleep or is asleep, turn head quickly to one side	Infant on left side with left arm & leg extended, the right arm and leg flex when head is turned right	After 6 weeks, persistent response is sign of possible cerebral palsy. Normally response disappears after 3–4 mos.
Moro's	Infant in semisitting position to an angle of 30°, then place infant flat and strike the surface to create startle	Symmetric abduction & extension of arms seen; slight tremor is common; arms abduct in embracing motion & return to flexion; legs follow similar pattern	Response is present at birth and remains until 8 weeks; disappears by 6 mos. Asymmetric response may indicate injury to brachial plexus, clavicle, or humerus

		Persistent response after 6 mos. indicates possible brain damage
Stepping or walking	Hold infant in vertical position, allow one foot to touch table surface	Infant simulates walking, alternating flexion & extension of feet; term infants walk on soles & preterm infants walk on toes
		Response is present for 3–4 weeks
Crawling	Place infant on abdomen	Infant makes crawling motions with arms and legs
		Response disappears after age 6 weeks
Deep tendon	Infant must be quiet & relaxed. Use finger to elicit knee jerk reflex	Reflex is present & may be accompanied by overall reflexive reaction of limbs
Crossed extension	Place infant on its back (supine), extend one leg, press down on the knee, stimulate the bottom of the foot	Opposite leg flexes, adducts, and then extends
Startle	After 24 hrs. of age, perform large noise, e.g., sharp hand clap	Arms abduct with flexed elbows, hands clenched
		Response disappears after 4 mos. Startle is readily elicited in preterm infants

Table 4-4 (continued)

Reflex	Eliciting Response	Characteristics	Observations
Babinski's sign	Stroke upward along lateral aspect of the sole of one foot and across the ball of the foot, beginning at the heel	All toes hyperextend with dorsiflexion of the large toe	Absence of this response indicates a problem and requires neurologic evaluation. Sign disappears after 12 mos. of age
Pull to sit (traction)	Pull infant up by wrists from the supine position; head in the midline	Head will lag until infant is upright, then head will come to same plane as shoulders for a moment, then fall forward. Infant will attempt to hold head upright	Response depends on maturity and condition of the infant
Trunk incurvation (Galant)	Place infant in prone position, run finger down spine, 4–5 cm from back, first on one side and then on the other	Trunk flexes and pelvis swings toward stimulated side	Response disappears after 4th week of age Absence of response indicates general nervous system depression

Magnet	Place infant in supine position, partially flex both legs and press on the soles of the feet	Both legs should extend against the examiner's pressure
		May be depressed due to maternal analgesia, anesthesia, hypoxia, or infection
Responses such as yawning, stretching, burping, hiccupping, or sneezing	Spontaneous behaviors	Absence indicates damage to spinal cord; reflex may be weak or exaggerated after breech delivery
		Reassure parents that these behaviors are normal; sneeze is a result of lint, etc., in nose and not a "cold"; hiccups are not treated but sucking may help

Source: Ballard, J. L., Khoury, C., Wedig, L., Wang, L., Eilers-Walsman, B. L., & Lipp, R. (1991). New Ballard score, expanded to include extremely premature infants. Journal of Pediatrics, 119, 417. Reprinted with permission from Elsevier.

The Nurse's Role in a Precipitous Delivery

Occasionally, laboring women progress so rapidly that there is inadequate time to reach their health care facility or for their care provider to attend them. Police officers and even cab drivers have attended births in unusual places. There is no reason to panic. Fortunately, when birth occurs this rapidly, the infant is usually healthy. It is important for nurses to know what to do when such an incident occurs:

- Rapidly assess the imminence of delivery including taking the mother's clothes off from the waist down. Check the perineum to determine if the head is crowning. Grab a "precip pack" and open it.
- Instruct the mother to pant during contractions (telling her *not* to push isn't helpful).
- If you can see the baby's head, pull on a glove and apply gentle pressure against the head to maintain flexion and prevent the head from "popping" out quickly and tearing the perineum. Support the perineum with the other hand as it stretches.
- At the birth of the infant's head, tell the mother to pant; suction the infant's mouth and nose with the bulb syringe in the precip pack.
- Check for the umbilical cord by putting fingers along the back of the head and neck. If present, check for tension. If it is loose, pull the cord over the baby's head. If tight, clamp it twice with the clamps in the pack and cut between the clamps. Unwind the cord from the baby's neck.
- Next request the mother to push gently while you pull down gently to facilitate the birth of the anterior shoulder. Then pull upward gently, to support the birth of the posterior shoulder. Support the rest of the infant's body as it slides out of the introitus.
- Place the infant on the mother's abdomen and dry the baby with blankets or towels from the pack. Leave the in-

fant on the mother's uncovered abdomen so that the
mother's body keeps the infant warm. Keep the infant's
head and body covered.

- Check the firmness of the abdomen and the amount of
  bleeding.
- Watch for separation of the placenta. The placenta will
  deliver without intervention.
- If the mother seems to be bleeding excessively, find the
  fundus (the top of the uterus) and massage it gently but
  firmly.
- Proceed with normal postpartum care.

If there is no pack, improvise. The cord does not have to be
cut unless it is so tight around the neck, the infant's ability to
breathe will be obstructed. If there are no clamps, use string or
even a shoe lace. The mouth can be cleaned out with gauze or a
piece of cloth. The two most important things are to keep the infant warm and to be certain the mother isn't hemorrhaging.

Recovery

Labor and delivery are completed with the delivery of the placenta. However, the time immediately after (the 4th stage) is very
important for the physical safety of the mother, as well as the psychological role transition for the mother. The nurse is responsible for facilitating both aspects.

1. Maternal/family newborn attachment: During this period
   mother and family members are encouraged to see, touch,
   and hold the infant to begin the bonding process.
2. Close assessment of maternal physical status including:
   a. Check the uterus to be sure it is firm rather than
      boggy
   b. Check for the amount of bleeding or lochia noting the
      amount, color, and the presence of clots.

   c. Assess for excessive bleeding or soft fundus that can lead to hemorrhage. Predictors of possible hemorrhage include:
  - Rapid labor
  - Prolonged first and second stage
  - Forceps or vacuum-assisted birth
  - Overdistention of the uterus due to large fetus
  - Multiple gestation
  - Polyhydramnios
  - History of previous postpartum hemorrhage
  - Advanced maternal age
  - Multiparity of four or more
  - Abrupted placenta or placenta previa
  - Induction of labor
  - Preeclampsia or eclampsia

   d. Monitor episiotomy repairs for bleeding, hematoma, and edema.

   e. Check for the ability to urinate and for a distended bladder.

   f. Assess vital signs every 15 minutes until mother is stable

   g. Assess psychosocial status and plan accordingly: Mother may be both exhausted and excited or talkative; she may be hungry.

   h. Assess for pain
  - After pains or cramping
  - Massage the uterus to assure firmness.
  - Perineal repair may require an ice pack.

   i. Regional anesthesia requires postanesthesia monitoring; check for ability to move legs and walk with assistance.

Feeding

Breast-Feeding

Breast-feeding is influenced by culture and family. Factors such as general attitude toward maternal role, personality, self-concept, cultural beliefs, family history, genetic factors, response to the infant, family and partner support, interpersonal relationships, and previous pregnancy history influence the decision.

Supporting the breast-feeding mother includes the following:

1. Help the mother find a comfortable position and begin to relax.
2. Find a comfortable position for the infant.
3. Help the mother support the baby's head with one hand and then grasp her breast with the other placing four fingers underneath and the thumb on top without touching the areola.
4. Help the mother to stroke the baby's cheek with her nipple, eliciting the rooting reflex in the infant.
5. When the infant opens its mouth place the nipple in the mouth (latch-on).
6. Correct latch-on occurs when the infant takes the nipple and most of the areola into its mouth.
7. When the feeding is complete (start with just a few minutes on each side) be sure to take the infant off the breast by inserting a finger into the corner of the infant's mouth breaking the suction.
8. Sore maternal nipples come from:
   * Improper removal of the infant from the breast
   * Not having enough of the nipple and areola in the mouth
   * Infant sucking on the tip of the nipple
9. Infants may be burped between feedings at breasts and at the end of the feeding by:
   * Positioning the infant in an upright position resting on the mother's shoulder
   * Placing the infant face down on the mother's lap and gently rubbing or patting the back
   * Sitting the infant on the mother's lap, supporting the infant with a hand to the front of the chest, and patting or rubbing the baby's back

Breast feeding is a time of touching, giving, and cuddling an infant. Fathers can be included through such activities as changing diapers, getting the baby in the middle of the night for the mother, or burping the baby.

Bottle Feeding

1. The prepared formula (which has been prepared according to the specific directions and kept cold) should be at room temperature either sitting out for 30 minutes or running under warm water from the faucet.
2. Hold the infant in a comfortable position with the head raised.
3. Hold the bottle so that the formula fills the nipple and there is no air in the neck of the bottle.
4. Burp the infant at least twice during the feeding either upright on the shoulder or in a sitting position with one hand supporting the chin and the other rubbing the back.
5. Watch for regurgitation.
6. Resume feeding.

References

Littleton, L. Y., & Engerbretson, J. C. (2002). *Maternal, neonatal, and women's health nursing.* Clifton Park, NY: Delmar Thomson Learning.

Branden, P. S. (1998). *Maternity care* (2nd ed.). Springhouse, PA: Springhouse.

Lowdermilk, D. L., Perry, S. E., & Bobak, I. M. (2000). *Maternity and women's health care* (7th ed.). St. Louis, MO: Mosby/A. Harcourt Health Sciences System.

Pediatric Nursing

The care of children is a very special mission. Children are vulnerable and dependent on adults. They are not "little adults" but are a work in progress. They are a part of a family of caretakers. Thus they require special knowledge, understanding, and skills in physical, psychological, cognitive, and emotional development as well as family interactions.

Rights of Children (from the United Nations)

All children need the following:

To be free from discrimination

To develop physically and mentally in freedom and
dignity

To have a name and nationality

To have adequate nutrition, housing, recreation, and medical services

To receive special treatment if handicapped

To receive love, understanding, and material security

To receive an education and develop his or her abilities

To be the first to receive protection in disaster

To be protected from neglect, cruelty, and exploitation

To be brought up in a spirit of friendship among people

Elements of Family-Centered Care

The family is the constant human factor in a child's life while
caregivers and care systems change. Caregivers need to:

- Facilitate family/caregiver collaboration in home and
  community.
- Share relevant information between families and caregivers.
- Recognize and honor cultural diversity, strengths, and in-
  dividuality within families (including ethnic, racial, spiritual, social, economic, education, and geographic
  diversity).
- Encourage support within families and networking between families with similar situations.
- Ensure that home, hospital, and community services and
  support systems for special needs children and their families are flexible, accessible, and comprehensive.
- Appreciate children and families—their strengths, concerns, emotions, and aspirations as well as their specialized healthcare needs.

Families

As the family has such an overarching effect on social development of a child, it is important to clarify that families are present in several different types:

- **Single-parent:** Consisting of one parent who may or may not have been married and at least one child
- **Nuclear family:** Consisting of a father, mother, and their children
- **Extended family:** Consisting of one person, a possible mate, any children, and other relatives living in the household (grandparents, aunts or uncles, and other relatives living in close proximity)
- **Blended or reconstituted family:** Formed when a divorced or widowed parent (with or without children) remarries another person (with or without children). If either party has children they bring into the setting, a stepfamily is formed.
- **Binuclear family:** A family separated by divorce, now consisting of two nuclear families, one headed by the mother and one by the father. These two groups include whatever children were in the original family.
- **Communal family:** A group of people who live together and share various aspects of family living such as household chores, resources, and responsibilities
- **Homosexual family:** Adults of the same sex living together, who may or may not have children but who share sexual aspects of their lives and commitment
- **Cohabiting family:** Consists of two people of the opposite sex, living together with or without children, who are not legally married but share sexual aspects of their lives as well as commitment

Guidelines for Creating a Relationship Between Nurses and Children and Families

Empower Families by:

- Exploring strengths and needs and increasing family involvement in the care of the child
- Teaching families rather than doing everything for them
- Working with families to decrease their dependence on health care providers
- Separating family needs from caregiver needs

Strive to Empower Yourself As the Caregiver Through:

- Being aware of your emotional response to different people and situations
- Understanding how your own family experiences influence interactions with patients and families
- Developing a calming influence in stressful situations
- Developing interpersonal skills to balance knowledge of technical skills
- Learning about ethnic and religious family practices
- Communicating directly with the person with whom you are upset or have an issue; eliminating gossip and third-party conversations
- "Stepping back" and taking a deep breath during an emotional breakdown or upheaval, while choosing to remain engaged in the problem-solving process
- Taking care of yourself and creating balance in your life
- Maintaining clear, open communication
- Interviewing families, periodically assessing issues, feelings, attitudes, and wishes, then communicating these data to peers and recording the data
- Avoiding gossip, assumptions, and negative first impressions of families
- Assessing families who are not participating in care

- Providing encouragement and support to patients and families, as well as peers
- Maintaining positive communication channels between yourself and all the members of the team (physicians, nurses, allied health workers, and support personnel)

Questionable Interactions by the Nurse

- Having excessive involvement with children and their families
- Becoming overinvolved with children and underinvolved with parents or family
- Working overtime to care for the family
- Spending off-duty time with the family either in- or outside of the clinical area
- Buying toys, food, clothes, or other items for the child or the family
- Calling frequently to ask how the family is doing
- Showing favoritism toward certain patients
- Competing with other staff members for the affection of specific patients or their families
- Competing with parents for a child's affections
- Influencing family's decisions rather than facilitating their knowledgeable decision making
- Restricting family's access to the child
- Focusing on the technical aspect of care while losing sight of the human beings involved
- Criticizing when parents do not visit their children

Initiating Communication with Various Age Children and Young Adults

1. Take time and allow children to feel comfortable.
2. Avoid sudden rapid movements, broad smiles, or extended eye contact—any activity that could be interpreted as threatening.
3. Talk to the parents, particularly when the child seems shy.

4. Use toys such as dolls, puppets, or stuffed animals as a method of beginning interaction with the child.
5. Speak quietly and in a confident, unhurried tonality.
6. Use a position that allows eye-to-eye contact with the child (such as kneeling or being on the same level as the child).
7. Speak to the child in clear, simple words, using short sentences.
8. Be positive when providing suggestions or directions.
9. Offer choices *only* when there is one.
10. Be honest with children.
11. Support children to express concerns and fears.
12. Use a variety of techniques.
13. Provide older children with the opportunity to talk alone without parents.

Child-Focused Communication Techniques

I messages

- Avoid the use of *you*; speak in the first person by using *I*.
  - *You* messages are judgmental and can stimulate defensiveness.
- Relate feelings about self, others, and their behavior in terms of *I*, then describe the effect the behavior had on yourself or others.
  - Example of *you* message: "You are going to hurt yourself if you don't get down from that table."
  - Example of *I* message: "I get scared when I think you might get hurt. Please come down from the table."

Third-person technique

- Express feelings or ideas in third person (e.g., he, she, they).
  - It is less threatening than asking directly about feelings or ideas.

- Give the child an opportunity to respond or comment without attributing the response directly to themselves; this reduces "risk" to themselves and prevents a defensive response.
  - This allows children three choices: (1) to agree and express how they feel, (2) to disagree, or (3) to remain silent (meaning they may have feelings but are unable or unwilling to express them).
  - Example: "Sometimes when a person is sick a lot, she feels angry and sad and maybe a lot disappointed that she can't do what other kids can do." The caregiver can either wait until the child responds or follow up with "Did you ever feel that way?"

Facilitative responding with unconditional positive regard

- Using the model developed by Carl Rogers, this method involves careful listening and reflecting back to the child the feelings and content of their message.
- Reflection is done in an empathic and nonjudgmental way that legitimizes the child's statements and feelings.
  - Example: "I hear you saying that you are overwhelmed by all the surgeries and procedures done here in the hospital and you want to go home. That's an understandable wish."

Storytelling

- Ask that the child tell a story about being in the hospital.
- Telling a make-believe story allows the child to express fears and inhibitions without owning them.
- The story can be initiated by showing the child a picture of a child and his/her family in the hospital or clinic and having the child tell a story about the picture.

Using books as therapy

- The storybook allows the child to explore an event that is similar to his/her own yet "make believe," so the child's fears similar to his/her own are reduced and he/she feels in control.
- Guidelines:
  - Read the book with the child.
  - Explore the message of the book with the child:
    - Have the child retell the story.
    - Read a special section with caregiver or parents.
    - Draw a picture about the story and talk about the picture.
    - Talk about the people in the story.
    - Summarize the meaning of the story. Assess the emotional and cognitive development in terms of readiness to understand the book's message.
    - Be familiar with the book's message and whether it is age appropriate.

Dreams

- Ask a child to talk about a dream or a nightmare (which may reveal unconscious or repressed feelings).
- Explore possible meanings of the dream.

"What if" questions

- Encourage the child to explore potential situations and consider optional solutions.
- Example: "What if you got sick and had to go see the doctor or go to the hospital?" The response indicates what a child knows already and what he/she has concerns about. This discussion could help examine coping skills, especially in scary situations.

Games and Exercises to Facilitate Exploring the Child's Feelings

Three Wishes

Ask the child "If you could have three wishes, anything in the world, what would you want?" Encourage specifics. Have the child discuss what made him/her choose those three.

Rating Game

- In this game, use some type of scale, 1–10 or sad to happy faces, to rate feelings or events.
- Example: Ask how the child's day has gone on a scale of 1–10, with 10 being the best.

Word Association Game

- The caregiver states key words and asks the child to say the first word he/she thinks of in association with the word.
- Begin with neutral words (e.g., snow, beach, leaves, pet) and progress to more anxiety-producing words (e.g., doctor, hospital, operation, tests)
- Select key words with which the child can relate.
- Encourage the child to talk about word choices.

Sentence Completion

- Present a partial sentence and have the child complete the sentence:
  - What I like best (least) about school is _____.
  - The best (worse) age to be is _____.
  - The most (least) fun I ever had was _____.
  - The one thing I would change about my family is _____.

Pros and Cons

- Select a topic and have the child list "the five best things and the five worst things about it," such as being in the hospital.

- This can also be used about relationships or family members, as in what the child likes or dislikes about his/her sibling.

Children's Drawing

1. One of most valuable forms of communication with children
   - Verbal: What the child tells the caregiver about the drawing
   - Nonverbal: What the caregiver understands from examining the drawing
2. Drawings convey a great deal about the children as they are projections of the children's inner selves. Two types of drawings:
   - Spontaneous: Provide the child with art supplies and the opportunity to draw, then observe.
   - Directed drawing: Child is given direction such as "Draw a person or a family"; or make three observations about the child and ask the child to draw one of them.
3. Evaluation of drawings includes:
   - Use spontaneous drawings, preferably more than one.
   - Be certain that the drawings are used only as one piece of family information.
   - Examine the whole drawing versus one specific aspect of it.
4. Elements of the drawings that may be significant include:
   - Gender of first figure drawn usually relates to the child's self perception.
   - Size of individual figures conveys importance, power, or authority.
   - Order in which figures are drawn can convey order of importance.
   - Position of drawn figures and relationship to one another can express child's feelings of status or alliances.
   - Missing members can denote feelings of exclusion or not belonging.

- Accentuated parts can express issues or concerns (e.g., large hands may be sign of aggression).
- Absence of parts can indicate timidity, immaturity or passivity; tiny feet can express insecurity; hidden hands can indicate guilt.
- Page placement: Free use of paper and strong, dark, firm strokes indicate security; insecurity can be depicted by a small area of the paper, lightly drawn figures or broken or wavy lines
- Use of many eraser marks, shading or cross-hatch marks may indicate ambivalence, concern, or anxiety.

Magic

- Caregiver can use simple magic tricks to help establish rapport with the child and encourage adoption and participation with health interventions.
- Tricks can provide distraction during painful procedures.
- Magician/caregiver can talk and the child need not respond.

Play

- This is the work of children and serves as a universal language.
- Children project their inner selves during play and reveal what they think or believe:
  - Spontaneous play: Child is given play materials and given opportunity to play.
  - Directed play: More specific toys are given to child (medical equipment or a doll house) to explore fears such as health care situation concerns or relationships within the family.

Writing
Can be an alternative communication tool for older children and adults and employs these strategies:

Keep a journal or diary.
Write down feelings or thoughts that are difficult to express.

Write letters (to people with whom you have issues or concerns) that are never mailed.

Keep an account (parents could do this) of a child's progress, both physical and emotional.

Children and Discipline: Guides for Parents
Minimizing Misbehavior

1. Set realistic goals for behavior.
2. Create opportunities for small successes so that feelings of inadequacy are decreased.
3. Praise children for desirable behavior (e.g., attention and verbal approval).
4. Teach desirable behavior through example such as speaking in a calm quiet voice instead of yelling.
5. Set clear and reasonable rules, and expect the same behavior regardless of circumstances. If exceptions are made, clarify it is for one time only.
6. Structure the environment to prevent problems (e.g., place fragile objects in inaccessible areas and childproof electrical outlets and cabinets).
7. Review expected behavior prior to special events such as visiting someone else's home or going to a restaurant.
8. Phrase requests for behavior in the positive such as "Put the dish down" rather than "Don't touch the dish."
9. Give advanced notice or "reminders" such as "When the TV program is over, it is time for dinner."
10. Call attention to misbehavior as soon as it begins:
    - Use distraction to shift behavior.
    - Redirect child into another activity.
    - Exchange quiet toys for noisy ones.
11. Be attentive to situations that increase the likelihood of misbehaving (e.g., overexcitement or fatigue).
12. Give sympathetic reasons for denying a request (e.g., "I'm sorry I can't play with you now, I have to finish cooking dinner. I'll read with you after dinner.").

13. Keep any promises made (e.g., be sure to read with the child later).
14. Avoid outright conflict or arguments with statements such as "Let's discuss it and see what we can decide together" or "I'll have to think about that request."
15. Provide children with opportunities to make decisions; give them some control over situations.

Implementing Discipline

1. Be consistent. Implement discipline exactly as agreed upon and for each and every infraction.
2. Be timely. Initiate discipline as soon as misbehavior begins. If delays are necessary (such as embarrassment) quietly verbally disapprove and state that the disciplinary action will be enacted and when it will.
3. Be committed. Pay attention to the details of the discipline. Time the minutes and avoid distractions such as phone calls (e.g., use something like a kitchen timer).
4. Be united. All parental figures must agree on the plan and know enough of the details to prevent confusion and making alliances with one parental figure against the other.
5. Be flexible. Choose strategies that are in keeping with the severity of the infraction and are age appropriate.
6. Create a plan. Plan strategies ahead of time and be sure the child knows and understands. For unanticipated problems, do your best to remain calm.
7. Focus on behavior. Criticize the behavior *not* the child. Make statements such as "I am unhappy when I see behavior like that."
8. Choose privacy. Administer discipline in private; never in front of friends or family. Refrain from using shame.
9. Choose a short memory. Once discipline is administered, the child now has a "clean slate." Do not bring the incident up again. Avoid lecturing.

Time Out as a Disciplinary Strategy

1. Determine with your partner what behaviors merit time out.
2. Select a time-out space in the home that is:
   - Safe
   - Convenient
   - Unstimulating
   - Easily monitored
     - Examples: hallway, bathroom, laundry room
     - *Do not use* closed or dark spaces.
3. Children must understand the "rules" for time-out.
   - Explain the time-out process.
   - When they misbehave, they will receive one warning.
   - For the second incident, they will be sent to time-out place.
   - They must stay for a specified period of time.
   - If they cry, refuse or are disruptive, the time-out begins after they have quieted.
   - When they are quiet for the designated time, they may leave the time-out area.
4. Other time-out guidelines:
   - Use one minute of time out for each year of age.
   - Use a timer with a bell or buzzer.
   - If a suitable place is found when away from home, implement time out in conjunction with the misbehavior.
   - Consistency is important. If no suitable place is available, implement as soon as you return home.
   - It is important to remember the disciplinary measure to institute consistency.

Well-Child Assessment

Visits with children require more time than those with adults. Perform the exam in an appropriate, nonthreatening area which includes:

   - A room that is warm and well lit

PART 4

- Placing all equipment out of sight
- Availability of toys, dolls, or stuffed toys and games
- Privacy, particularly for school-age children and adolescents

Provide "get acquainted" time through play. Watch for signs of child's readiness to cooperate:

- Talks to caregiver
- Makes eye contact
- Accepts toys or exam tools
- Allows physical touching
- Sits on exam table willingly rather than parent's lap

If child is not ready, additional strategies include:

- Talk to parent while "ignoring" child
- Shift focus to child gradually, perhaps with use of toy
- Compliment child's appearance, dress, or favorite object (e.g., toy, blanket, etc., that the child has brought to visit).
- Tell a story or do a simple magic trick.
- Use a doll or stuffed animal as a "friend" that can talk to the child who is afraid or had a difficult previous experience.

If child refuses:

- Assess reason for refusal (may have had a previous negative experience).
- Involve child and parent in the process (examine child on parent's lap).
- Avoid prolonged explanations about procedures.
- Use firm direct approach.
- Perform exam as quickly as possible.
- Have attendant assist by gently restraining child.
- Perform exam/procedure quickly.
- Minimize disruptions and stimuli, including number of people.

Begin exam in nonthreatening way

- Use parts of the exam that can be used as games, e.g., cranial nerve or developmental screening tests.
- Use a game such as "Simon Says" to encourage child to make a face, squeeze your hand, stand on one foot, etc.
- Use "paper-doll" game:
  - Lay child on paper on the floor in supine position.
  - Trace around child's body outline.
  - Use the paper and tracing to demonstrate what will be examined (e.g., draw a heart, and listen with the stethoscope prior to doing it with child)

If several children in the family will be examined, begin with the most cooperative, providing modeling for remaining children.

Involve the child in the examination:

- Provide choices, such as sitting on parent's lap or exam table.
- Encourage child to hold equipment.
- Encourage child to use equipment on a doll or stuffed animal.
- Explain each step in plain language.
- Perform most invasive parts last.

Proceed with exam in logical order (usually head to toe) except for:

- Alter sequence to accommodate different age groups
- Examine painful areas last
- **In emergencies,** examine vital functions first (airway, breathing, circulation) and the injury second. Other parts of exam follow.

Reassure child as exam progresses.
Discuss findings with parents.
Acknowledge child for cooperation during exam and give a reward such as a sticker or a small toy.

PART 4

Table 4-5   Physical Assessment of the Child and Probable Findings

Assessment	Normal Findings	Abnormal Findings
Head		
Circumference (measured above eyebrow)	Between 5th and 95th% on standard growth chart	Below 5th and above 95th%
	Exceeds chest circumference by 1–2 cms until 18 months	
Anterior fontanel	3–4 cm in length and 2–3 cm in width until 9–12 mos. of age	Unusually large fontanel: possible hydrocephaly
		Unusually small fontanel: possible craniosynostosis
	Soft, flat, or bulges while crying	Sunken or bulges while at rest
	Closes between 9–18 mos.	Early or delayed closure
Posterior fontanel	0.5–1 cm across; may be closed at birth or by 3 mos.	Delayed closing may indicate hydrocephaly
Eyes	Infants follow objects with eyes; smile in response to smiles from adults	Does not follow objects or smile
	Young children reach for objects	
	Child who doesn't know alphabet and can follow directions can respond to Blackbird or Snellen E eye chart	

	Less than 20/20 is normal until age 5–7 yrs. 20/30 or 20/40 acceptable in younger.	
Ears	Top of pinna is in line with inner canthus of eye	Top of pinna below inner canthus
		Low-set ears associated with Trisomy 21 or Down's syndrome
	3 yrs and older: Tympanic membrane is red when child is crying	Red tympanic membrane when child is not crying may be otitis media (infection)
	Infant startles to loud noise	Does not turn toward noise
	6 mos. or older turns head to noise	
	Older children follow simple directions	
Nose	Symmetrical with patent nares	Asymmetrical; non-patent nares
	Child can identify common odors with eyes closed	Unable to identify odors
	Septum is straight & intact	Septum has deviation, perforation
	Mucosa is moist and pink	Yellow/green mucosa indicates infection
Mouth (examine at end)	Pharyngeal tonsils are normally large in toddler	Tonsils very red or with white patches (thrush or bacterial infection)
Neck	Supple and head flexes easily	Neck stiff with signs of pain (possible meningitis)
	Lymph nodes: firm,	

PART 4

Table 4-5   (*continued*)

Assessment	Normal Findings	Abnormal Findings
Neck cont.	movable; nodes are pea-sized Torticollis Intercostal retractions	Tender and enlarged nodes (may indicate infection)
Chest & lungs	Infant thorax: round Usual adult shapes evolves at about 6 yrs. Respirations are abdominal until age 6	Retractions during inspiration
Cardiac	Pulse is irregular and varies with respiratory rate PMI visible in thin child Innocent murmur, always systolic, in 30% of children; may disappear with position change	Diastolic murmur
Abdomen	Young child has "potbelly" Both spleen and liver can be palpable below the left and right costal margin, respectively	Enlarged spleen (more than 2 cm below the left costal margin) may indicate mononucleosis or sickle-cell crisis Enlarged liver (more than 2 cm below the right costal margin) may indicate CHF
	Umbilical hernia: soft bulge normal until 4 yrs.	Hernia persists after 4 yrs. or is nonreducible (could be an emergency, e.g., strangulated tissue)

Genitalia: male	Urinary meatus slightly ventral	Meatus displaced
	Testicles palpable by age 3 yrs.	Testicles nonpalpable by age 3 yrs.
	Presence of small amount of fluid in scrotal sac prior to 1 yr.	Fluid in scrotal sac after 1 yr.
		Bulge in femoral or inguinal area (hernia)
	Onset of sexual maturation (secondary sex characteristics appear) between ages 10–14 yrs.	Varies outside normal parameters
Genitalia: female	Onset of sexual maturation between ages 9–14 yrs.	Onset of maturation outside of parameters
	Irregular menses during 1st year	Prolonged irregularity of menstrual periods
	One breast larger than other	
Spine	Lateral spine curve that disappears when child bends forward	Lateral spine curve that does not correct with position change
	Small dimple at lower end of spine with normal leg movement	Small dimple without movement of lower leg (indicate underlying neurologic defect)
Extremities	Equal leg lengths	Unequal leg lengths
	Symmetric gluteal folds	Asymmetric gluteal folds
		Limited leg abduction
	Hips symmetric	One hip prominent (possible dislocation)
	Knock knees normal until age 7	Knock knees that persist past 7 yrs. (should be evaluated)

PART 4

Table 4-5 *(continued)*

Assessment	Normal Findings	Abnormal Findings
Extremities cont.	Bow legs throughout toddler period	Investigate if persist after age 7 yrs.
	Feet in anatomic alignment	Foot turned in or out (should be investigated)
	Arch of foot commonly flat until age 4 yrs.	Persistent flat arch may be problematic
	Toe walking until several mos. post walking	Prolonged toe walking (may indicate cerebral palsy)

Vital Signs

Table 4-6 Heart and Respiratory Rate

Heart rate: Average at rest by age

Age	Average Rate
Birth	140
1–6 mo	130
6–12 mo	110
1–2 yrs	110
2–4 yrs	105
6–10 yrs	95
10–14 yrs	85
14–18 yrs	82

Respiratory rate: Variation by age

Age	Rate per Minute
Premature	40–90
Newborn	30–80
1 yr	20–40
2 yr	20–30
3 yr	20–30
5 yr	20–25
10 yr	17–22
15 yr	15–20
20 yr	15–20

Blood Pressure   Blood pressures should be taken annually after 3 years old.

Techniques for measuring blood pressure:

1. Use an appropriately sized cuff.
2. Use same position, preferably sitting.
3. Alternate sites can be used, such as thigh or calf.
4. Position extremity level with heart
5. If using manual blood pressure equipment:
   - Rapidly inflate cuff to 20 points above when pulse disappears.
   - Release cuff pressure at a rate of 2–3 mmHg/second.
   - Read mercury gravity manometer at eye level.
   - Record systolic value as onset of a clear tapping sound.
   - Record diastolic value:
     Children up to age 12 yrs.—the low muffled sound
     Children 12 to 18 yrs.—disappearance of all sounds
   - Record extremity, position, cuff size, and method of measurement

PART 4

Table 4-7   Average Blood Pressure Ranges for Girls and Boys

	Girls			Boys		
Age	**5th%**	**50th%**	**95th%**	**5th%**	**50th%**	**95th%**
Newborn	46/38	65/55	72/84	54/38	73/55	92/72
1 mo	65/35	84/52	102/69	67/35	86/52	105/68
6 mo	72/36	91/53	110/69	72/36	90/53	109/70
1 yr	72/38	91/54	110/71	71/39	90/56	109/73
3 yr	72/40	91/56	110/73	73/39	92/55	111/72
6 yr	72/40	96/57	115/74	77/41	96/57	115/74
10 yr	83/46	102/62	121/79	84/45	102/62	121/79
14 yr	92/49	110/67	129/85	93/46	112/64	131/82
18 yr	94/48	112/66	131/84	102/52	121/70	140/88

6. If using electronic monitor, follow manufacturer's instructions.
   - Can be used on any extremity.
   - Be sure to stabilize the extremity, or reading could be inaccurate.

Immunizations (see Medications)

Children and Eating

Introducing Solid Foods

1. Introduce rice cereal first (4–6 mos.); it is easily digestible, low in potential allergic reactions, and contains iron.
2. Include fruits and vegetables (6–8 mos.); they provide needed vitamins.
3. Add meats (8–10 mos.); meats are more difficult to digest, are high in protein, and should not be added to diet early.
4. Avoid "combined food" baby foods; they have more sugar, salt, and fillers.
5. Introduce one food at a time; a food allergy may be easier to identify.

6. Feed mashed table food (e.g., carrots, rice, and potatoes); this is less expensive than purchased baby food.
7. Do not add sugar, salt or spices; infants don't need these and could receive too much sodium.
8. Avoid honey until at least 1 year.
9. Delay eggs until after 9 months.

Table 4-8 Eating Patterns

First Year	
Birth to 1 month	Eats every 2–3 hours; breast or bottle Eats 2–3 oz. per feeding
2–4 months	Eats every 3–4 hours; 3–4 oz.
4–6 months	Eats 4–5 times daily; takes 4–5 oz.; begins rice cereal
6–8 months	Eats 4 times daily; has cereal, fruits, & vegetables; drinks 6–8 oz./feeding
8–10 months	Eats soft finger foods, eats 4 times/day; drinks 6 oz./feeding
10–12 months	Eats soft finger foods with family; uses cup with lid; attempts use of spoon; eats 4 times per day; drinks 6–8 oz. per feeding
Toddler Years	Often food intake declines; finger foods are good, but fast foods with high sodium and fat are not. Healthy snacks: yogurt, cheese, milk, peanut butter with bread, fruits slices, and soft vegetables
Preschool	Food jags are common: child only wants certain foods for several days. Eating at specific times with family is important. Children who don't eat at these times should not be fed in between. Three meal times with 2–3 snack times/day are normal. Limit fruit juice to 8–12 oz.

10. Wait three days between any new foods to rule out allergic reactions.
11. Read food labels.

Safety for Children by Age

The leading cause of death in children from age 1–19 is *injuries.* This is also the leading cause of morbidity in children. Injuries are categorized as injuries from aspiration of foreign objects, suffocation, motor vehicle injuries, falls, poisoning, burns, drowning, and bodily damage (such as sharp objects being poked or jabbed into the body, physical abuse, or from broken bones, etc., acquired in play or sports).

Making the Home Safe for Young Children

Approximately 2½ million children are injured or killed by hazards in the home each year. The following list is from the US Consumer Product Safety Commission.

1. Use **safety latches and locks** for cabinets and drawers in kitchens, bathrooms, and other areas to help prevent poisonings and other injuries. Safety latches and locks help prevent children from gaining access to medicines, household cleaners, knives, and other sharp objects.
2. Use **safety gates** at stairs or other hazardous areas in the home. For stairs, gates that are screwed into the woodwork are more effective than "pressure gates."
3. Use **door knob covers and door locks** to prevent children from entering rooms that contain anything posing danger to children (including swimming pools).
4. Use **antiscald devices** for faucets and shower heads so that water cannot be turned on hot enough to scald children. Also set water heater temperature at 120°.
5. Have **smoke detectors** on every level of your home, especially near bedrooms to alert you to fires. Check detectors to be certain they are working properly and change batteries regularly (e.g., when the time changes in the spring or fall)

6. Install **window guards and safety netting** to help prevent falls from windows, balconies, decks, and landings. Guards are important if windows are low enough for the child to climb onto, but one window must be available for escape in case of fire.

7. Use **corner and edge bumpers** to help prevent injuries from falls against sharp edges of furniture and fireplaces.

8. Install **outlet covers and outlet plates** to help prevent electrocution. Be sure the protectors cannot be easily removed by children and are large enough that children cannot choke on them.

9. Install **carbon monoxide detector (CO)** outside of bedrooms to help prevent CO poisoning. These are particularly important in homes that use gas or oil heat or have attached garages.

10. Cut **window blind cords and use safety tassels and inner cord stops** to prevent children from strangling in blind cord loops.

11. Use **door stops and door holders** to help prevent injuries to fingers and hands. These can help prevent small fingers and hands from being pinched or crushed in doors and door hinges.

12. Use **cordless phone** to make it easier to continuously watch young children, especially when they are in bathtubs, swimming pools, or other potentially dangerous areas. Parents don't have to leave a potentially dangerous area to answer the phone.

Checklist for Home Safety

The following lists are from the US Consumer Product Safety Commission.

Fire, Electrical, and Burns Safety

___ Guards in front of or around heating appliances, fireplaces, or furnace

___ Electrical wires hidden or out of reach

PART 4

___ No frayed or broken wires or overloaded sockets
___ Plastic guards or caps over electrical outlets
___ No hanging tablecloths when hot items are on them
___ Smoke detectors tested and operating properly
___ Kitchen matches stored out of child's reach
___ No smoking in the home preferred, but if smoking, use large deep ashtrays
___ Small stoves, heaters, coffee pots, and other hot objects (coffee pots, candles, and slow cookers) placed where they cannot be reached or tipped over by children.
___ Cords never hang over the edge of counter or table.
___ Hot water heater temperature set at 120°F or lower
___ Pot handles turned toward back of stove; never set on table with handles out
___ No cooking hot foods or liquids with child standing nearby or being held in arms
___ All small appliances such as irons, curling irons, etc., turned off after use and disconnected, placed out of reach of child
___ Fire extinguisher available on each floor and checked periodically
___ Electrical fuse box and gas shutoff accessible
___ Escape route for fire planned and practiced with fire escape ladder available for upper stories of house
___ Telephone number (usually 911) available with cross streets nearest the house posted near phone

Suffocation or Aspiration Safety

___ Small objects stored out of reach
___ Toys inspected for small removable parts or long strings
___ Hanging crib toys and mobiles placed out of reach
___ Plastic bags stored away from child's reach; large plastic garment bags discarded or tied in knots
___ No mattresses or pillows covered in plastic

___ Crib slats no more than 2½ inches apart with a mattress that fits snugly

___ Crib positioned away from windows and other furniture

___ Crib sides up at all times when in use

___ *No* accordion type gates used in home

___ Bathroom door kept closed and toilet lid in down position

___ Faucets turned off firmly

___ Pool fenced with a locked gate

___ Proper safety equipment at poolside

___ Electric garage door openers stored safety and garage door set to rise when door strikes object

___ Doors of ovens, trunks, dishwasher, refrigerators, and front loading clothes washers and dryers kept closed

___ Unused appliances, such as refrigerator, locked or door removed

___ Food served in small, noncylindrical pieces

___ Toy chests without lids or with lids that securely lock in open position

___ Buckets and wading pools kept empty when not in use

___ Clothesline above head level

___ At least one member of household trained in basic life support (CPR), including first aid for choking

Poisoning Safety

National Poison Control: 1-800-222-1222. Always call whenever there is an incident.

___ Toxic substances, including batteries, placed on a high shelf and preferably locked in cabinet

___ Toxic plants placed or hung out of reach

___ Excess quantities of cleaning fluids, paints, pesticides, drugs, and other toxic substances stored outside the home

___ Used containers of poisonous substances placed where children will have no access. Discard as soon as possible.

___ Local poison control center phone number placed near phone with nearest cross streets

___ Syrup of ipecac in home (two doses per child). *Do not administer before* calling National Poison Control or the primary care provider.
___ Medicines clearly labeled and kept in childproof containers
___ Household cleaners, disinfectants, and insecticides kept in original containers and separated from food and out of reach
___ Any smoking done away from children

Fall Safety

___ Nonskid mats, strips, or surfaces in tubs and showers
___ All exit halls and passageways kept clear of toys, boxes, and furniture or other obstructions
___ All stairs and halls well lighted with switches at top and bottom
___ Steps and stairways with handrails
___ Nothing stored on stairways
___ Carpeting, treads, and risers of stairs in good repair
___ Glass doors and glass walls marked with decals
___ Safety glass used in doors, windows, and walls
___ Gates on top and bottom of stairs and elevated areas (e.g., porch and fire escape)
___ Locks on windows that limit heights of opening and access to areas such as fire escape
___ Crib side rails raised to full height and mattress lower as child grows
___ Restraints used in high chairs, walkers, or other baby furniture
___ Preferable not to use walkers
___ Scatter rugs secured in place or used with nonskid backing
___ Walks, patios, and driveways in good repair

Bodily Injury Safety

___ Knives, power tools, and firearms stored safely or placed in locked cabinets

___ Garden tools returned to appropriate racks (placed high and away from children) after use
___ Pets properly trained or restrained and vaccinated for rabies
___ Swings, slides, and other outdoor play equipment kept in good repair
___ Yard free of broken glass, boards with nails, and other litter
___ Cement birdbaths situated so that a child cannot turn them over

Toilet Training

The nurse's role is to help parents identify the readiness signs in children, to give some helpful hints, and to discourage use of negative feedback to the child.

Techniques

- Involve child in selection of a potty chair or the use of the adult toilet.
- Feet firmly on the floor or on a step stool (if using the adult toilet) facilitates defecation.
- Keep potty chair in the bathroom.
- Allow child to see excrement flushed down the toilet.
- Child may sit on the toilet facing the tank (gives greater sense of security).
- Boys may begin standing (imitating their father).
- Sessions should be limited to 5–10 minutes.
- Children should be praised for cooperative behavior as well as successful evacuation.
- Dress children in clothes that are easily removed.
- Use training pants, pull-on diapers, or underpants.
- Encourage imitation by watching other children.

Avoid using the following techniques:

- Forcing children to sit on the potty for long periods of time
- Spanking them for accidents
- Other negative methods

PART 4

Table 4-9 Guidelines for Assessing Toilet Training Readiness

Physical Readiness	Mental Readiness	Psychological Readiness	Parental Readiness
Voluntary control of sphincters (18–24 mos.)	Recognizes urge to defecate or urinate	Expresses willingness to please parent	Recognizes child's level of readiness
Ability to stay dry for 2 hrs; decreased # of wet diapers; waking dry from nap	Verbal or nonverbal communication skills to indicate wet diapers or the urge	Able to sit on toilet for 5–10 min. without fussing or getting off	Willing to invest the time required for toilet training
Regular bowel movements	Cognitive skills to imitate appropriate behavior and follow directions	Curiosity about adults' or older sibling's toilet habits	Absence of family stress or change (e.g., divorce, moving, new sibling, or imminent vacation)
Able to sit, walk, squat (gross motor skills)		Impatience with soiled or wet diapers; desire to be changed immediately	
Able to remove clothing (fine motor skills)			

Factors Influencing Abuse of Children

The definition of abuse of children has expanded over the past decade to include:

- Physical abuse and neglect
- Emotional abuse
- Verbal abuse
- Sexual abuse

Between 10–20% of children from ages 3–17 years are physically abused each year, which equals 2.8 million children.

The exact cause of child abuse is unknown. The interaction of three factors seems to increase the chances of children being abused: parental characteristics, children's characteristics, and environmental factors.

Parental Characteristics

- Not all abusive parents were abused as children.
- As children, harsh physical punishment was used and is recalled as unfair and severe.
- Negative relationships existed with their parents.
- Significant difficulty managing anger and coping with stress
- Spouse abusers often also abuse their children.
- Families are more isolated with few supportive relationships.
- Being an adolescent mother
- Low self-esteem and less adequate maternal functioning
- Inadequate childrearing knowledge

Children's Characteristics

- Temperament, position in the family, additional physical needs (ill or disabled), activity level, or degree of sensitivity to parental needs
- Is not an "easy child"

PART 4

- Lack of fit between the child's temperament and the parents ability to deal with the behavioral style
- Illegitimate, unwanted, brain damaged, hyperactive, or physically disabled
- Reminds the parents of someone they dislike
- Failure of parent–child bonding during early infancy or hospitalization (occurs with prematurity)
- Mistreatment results from a family in distress
- Usually only one child is abused: "the family scapegoat."
- If abused child is removed, the remaining children are at risk. There must be a scapegoat in these families.

Environmental Characteristics

- Usually one of chronic stress, including divorce, poverty, unemployment, poor housing, frequent relocation, alcoholism, and drug addiction
- Is present in all educational, social, and economic levels
- Reporting increases in lower socioeconomic families and more often concealed in wealthy families (e.g., undergoing stress, or care giving performed by substitute care takers)

All abuse must be reported to the authorities!

Warning Signs of Abuse

1. Physical evidence of abuse or neglect, including previous injuries
2. Conflicting stories about the accident or injury from parents, child, or others
3. Cause of injury blamed on sibling or other child
4. Injury inconsistent with the history (e.g., concussion or broken arm from falling off the bed)
5. Story inconsistent with child's developmental level (e.g., 6-mo.-old turns on the hot water and is burned)

Table 4-10 Guidelines for Assessment of Child Maltreatment

Physical Neglect

Physical Findings

Failure to thrive

Signs of malnutrition (thin extremities, abdominal distention, lack of subcutaneous fat)

Poor personal hygiene, particularly teeth

Poor health care (e.g., no immunizations, untreated infections, frequent colds)

Frequent injuries from lack of supervision

Behavioral Findings

Dull and inactive, or excessive passivity or sleeping

Self-stimulation behaviors such as finger sucking or rocking

Older children begging or stealing food, absenteeism from school, drug or alcohol addiction, vandalism, or shoplifting

Emotional Abuse and Neglect

Physical Findings

Failure to thrive

Feeding disorders (e.g., rumination)

Enuresis

Sleep disorders

Behavioral Findings

Self-stimulating behavior (e.g., biting, sucking, rocking)

Lack of social smile and stranger anxiety in infants

Withdrawal

Unusual fearfulness

Antisocial behavior (e.g., destructiveness, stealing, cruelty)

Extremes of behavior (e.g., over-compliant and passive or aggressive and demanding)

Lags in emotional and intellectual development, especially language

Suicide attempts

Table 4-10 *(continued)*

Physical Abuse

Physical Findings

Bruises and welts:
* Face, lips, mouth, back, buttocks, thighs, or torso

Regular patterns suggestive of object use: belt buckle, hand, wire hanger, chain, wooden spoon, squeeze, or pinch marks

(May be present in various stages of healing)

Burns
  On soles of feet, palms of hands, back or buttocks
  Patterns descriptive of object used such as round cigar or cigarette burns, rope burns on wrists or ankles, burns shaped like an iron, radiator, or electric stove burner
  Symmetric burns
    Stun gun injury: circular uniform lesions, paired about 5 cm apart
* Fractures and dislocations
  Skull, nose, or facial structures

Behavioral Findings

Wary of physical contact with adults

Apparent fear of parents or going home

Lying very still while surveying environment

Inappropriate reaction to injury such as failure to cry from pain

Lack of reaction to frightening events

Apprehensive when hearing other children cry

Indiscriminate friendliness and displays of affection

Superficial relationships

Acting-out behavior (aggressive) to seek attention

Withdrawal behavior

Physical Findings	**Behavioral Findings**
Injury may denote type of abuse, such as spiral fracture or dislocation from twisting an extremity or whiplash from shaking	
Multiple new or old fractures in various stages of healing	
• Lacerations and abrasions	
On backs of arms, legs, torso, face, or external genitalia	
• Unusual symptoms (e.g., abdominal swelling, pain, and vomiting from punching)	
• Descriptive marks (e.g., human bites or pulling hair out)	
• Chemical	
Unexplained repeated poisoning, especially drug overdose	
Unexplained sudden illness such as hypoglycemia from insulin administration	

Sexual Abuse

Definitions

Incest	Any physical sexual behavior between family members
Molestation	Indecent liberties such as touching, fondling, kissing, masturbation, oral-genital contact

Table 4-10   (*continued*)

Sexual Abuse

Definitions

Exhibitionism	Indecent exposure, usually genitals by an adult male to children or women
Child pornography	Photographing (or any media) of sexual acts involving children regardless of consent from guardian
Child prostitution	Involving children in sex acts for profit, often with varying partners
Pedophilia	Adult preference for children as a means of sexual excitement

Physical Findings

- Bruises, bleeding, lacerations, or irritation of external genitalia, anus, mouth, or throat
- Torn, stained, or bloody underclothing
- Pain on urination; pain, swelling, or itching in genital area
- Penile discharge
- Sexually transmitted disease, nonspecific vaginitis, or warts
- Difficulty walking or sitting
- Genital odor

Behavioral Findings

Sudden emergence of sexually related problems (e.g., public masturbation, promiscuity, or overt sexual behavior)

Withdrawn

Excessive daydreaming or fantasies

Poor relations with peers

Anxiety, clinging behavior or sudden weight change

With incest, excessive anger at mother

Sudden phobias or fears (e.g., dark, men, strangers, leaving the house, or going to daycare or sitter's house)

Running away from home

Physical Findings	Behavioral Findings
• Recurrent urinary tract infections	Substance abuse (alcohol or drugs)
	Decline in school performance
• Presence of sperm	Personality changes (e.g., extreme
• Pregnancy in early adolescence	depression, hostility, aggression, or suicide attempts)

6. Chief complaint is different from the physical signs (e.g., presents with "a cold" when signs of severe burns are evident).
7. Caregiver is inappropriate in his/her response (e.g., an exaggerated emotional response or no response at all; refusal to permit additional tests or treatment; excessive delay in seeking treatment or absence of the parent with child).
8. Inappropriate response in the child (e.g., little or no response to pain, fear of being touched, excessive or lack of separation anxiety, indiscriminate friendliness to strangers)
9. Child's report of physical or sexual abuse
10. Previous reports of abuse in the family
11. Repeated visits to the emergency room with injuries

Behaviors of the Hospitalized Child

Young children are particularly vulnerable to the crisis of hospitalization due to the stress of illness as compared to their normal state of activity and the difficulty in coping with the stressors imposed: separation, loss of control, bodily injury, and pain. See Tables 4-11 and 4-12.

Children and Death

There are three aspects which are essential to children and death. First there are issues and concerns related to the terminally ill child, there are issues related to the loss and bereavement experienced by the child whose sibling or close family member dies, and there are the issues faced by the parents in coping with the loss of a child. The nurse has a significant role in support and intervention in all three of these situations.

PART 4

Table 4-11   Separation Anxiety in Young Children

Phase I: Protest	Behaviors: Crying, screaming, searching for parent with eyes, clinging to parent, and rejecting contact with strangers
	Toddler's behaviors include verbal attacks (e.g., "Go away"), physical attacks (kicks, bites, and hits), attempts escape (to search for parent)
	Time period: Lasts for hours or even days; protests such as crying can be continuous, ceasing from exhaustion
	Strangers approaching can increase protest
Phase II: Despair	Behaviors: Withdrawn from others, inactive, sad and depressed, uninterested and does not communicate
	Regresses to earlier developmental behaviors (e.g., thumb sucking, pacifier, or bed wetting)
	May refuse to eat, drink, or move causing physical deterioration
Phase III: Detachment	Behaviors: Increased interest in surroundings, interacts with caregivers and surroundings, appears "happy"
	Represents a superficial adjustment to loss

Table 4-12 Most Frequently Seen Conditions (Nonchronic) in Children

Condition	Manifestation	Intervention
Asthma (reactive airway disease)	Airway inflammation, obstruction or narrowing with airway hyperactivity. Breathing difficulty, nasal flaring & intercostal retractions. Possible productive cough & expiratory wheezing	Maintain airway patency, promote rest and stress reduction, meet fluid needs, teach family how to manage acute episodes and ongoing needs
Bronchitis	Dry, hacking and nonproductive cough that is worse at night and becomes productive in 2–3 days	Adequate fluids and cough suppressants as needed
Croup (laryngotracheobronchitis, which is most common form of croup)	Usually preceded by an upper respiratory infection; gradual onset of low-grade fever. Inflammation of the larynx & tracheal mucosal lining causing narrowing of the airway. The greater the narrowing the more difficult for	High humidity with cool air mist. If the respiratory distress is more pronounced (lower rib and soft neck tissue retraction, labored respiration and use of accessory muscles to breath) medical attention should be sought.

Table 4-12 (*continued*)

Condition	Manifestation	Intervention
Croup cont.	the child to inhale, producing stridor and sternal retraction and thus the seallike cough or bark. Can proceed to respiratory failure	In hospital, hoods and tents are used to increase humidity and provide supplemental O_2. Medications to reduce swelling are also given.
Diarrhea	Sudden increase in frequency and change in consistency of stools, often caused by infectious agent in GI tract. Lasts less than 14 days. Spread through food or water and from person to person. Pathogens include rotavirus, salmonella, shigella, and campylobacter	Rehydration, maintenance of fluid therapy, and reintroduction of an adequate diet
Dehydration	Common body fluid disturbance in children where total output exceeds total fluid intake. May result from diseases causing insensible fluid losses through	Assessment of extent of fluid and electrolyte imbalance Rehydration Maintenance fluid therapy Reintroduction of adequate diet

	skin, respiratory, and GI tract	
Failure to thrive Organic	Resulting from a physical cause such as congenital heart disease, chronic renal failure, malabsorption syndrome, cystic fibrosis, or AIDS	Treatment of primary cause
	Insufficient breast milk due to fatigue, maternal illness, insufficient glandular tissue, or lack of maternal confidence	Increased education and support. Supplemental feedings
Nonorganic	Definable cause unrelated to any disease process. Results from psychosocial factors such as deficiency in maternal care or disturbance in maternal-child attachment. Etiologies include: poverty, health, and child-rearing beliefs; inadequate nutritional knowledge; or family stress	Psychosocial intervention Social workers facilitate acquisition of food Education and support
Idiopathic failure to thrive	Unexplained by usual organic or nonorganic causes	

Table 4-12   *(continued)*

Condition	Manifestation	Intervention
Fevers	• Dehydration • Increased body temperature • Uncomfortable • Little or no appetite • Irritable • Restless • Fitful sleep • General muscle pain Observe for • Seizures • Toxic appearance (lethargy, poor profusion, very rapid or slowed respirations, cyanosis)	Supportive therapy Fever can be a beneficial physiologic response Helps to eradicate organisms which thrive at a lower temperature Mobilizes immune response May enhance effects of antibiotics Testing for organism causing fever: skin, pharynx, blood, urine, cerebrospinal fluid, feces Fevers are treated with antibiotics only when indicated by culture & sensitivity
Fever and communicable disease	Communicable diseases, particularly chickenpox, diphtheria, measles (both rubeola & rubella), mumps, and whooping cough (pertussis) all manifest with some	Supportive therapy with antibiotics for most of them.

level of fever and most have an accompanying rash. These diseases are all vaccine preventable, and if encountered must be reported to the state health department.

Otitis media (inflammation of the middle ear) Otitis media with effusion (inflammation of the middle ear with a collection of fluid)	Caused by infectious organisms or by blocked eustachian tubes resulting from the edema of allergic rhinitis or hypertrophic adenoids. Passive smoke can be a significant factor.	Antibiotics used sparingly Pain relief is important Facilitate drainage from middle ear, prevent complications or recurrence, educate the family in care of the child, and provide emotional support of the child and family.
Meningitis (common infection of the central nervous system caused by bacterial, tubercular, or viral organism)	Diagnosed with lumbar puncture and findings of elevated CNS fluid pressure, and culture and stain of the fluid to determine what organism is involved and to which drugs it is sensitive.	Child is hospitalized with isolation precautions, antibiotic therapy, maintenance of hydration, appropriate ventilation, reduction of intercranial pressure, management of bacterial shock, control of seizures, body temperature

Table 4-12	*(continued)*	
Condition	**Manifestation**	**Intervention**
		control, correction of anemia, and treatment of any complications
Pneumococcal infection	Organism causes otitis media, sinusitis, pharyngitis, laryngotracheobronchitis, pneumonia, meningitis, and bacteremia With the accompanying fever and all the related symptoms (see fever)	Supportive therapy and antibiotics
Roseola (also known as baby measles)	Sudden high fever (as much as 105°F for 3–8 days but maintains normal appetite and behavior) Fever is followed by rash of 1–2 days	The disease is self-limiting and supportive therapy is all that is required.
Streptococcus	Abrupt onset, sore throat, malaise, high fever, chills, headache, abdominal pain, anorexia, and vomiting. Characteristic erythematous rash 12–48 hrs after onset of symptoms	Prompt antibiotic treatment is effective: Penicillin

The Terminally Ill Child

1. Children need honest and accurate information regarding their illness, treatment, and prognosis. Honesty creates trust.
2. Information must be given in clear, concise, and simple language that is age appropriate.
3. Providing an atmosphere of open communication from the beginning makes it is easier to answer tough questions as the child's condition worsens.
4. Involving children in decision making needs to be individualized, age appropriate, and developmentally appropriate (e.g., do they want to receive end-of-life care in the hospital or at home).
5. Children will often indicate how much they want to know about their disease and its process. Use questions such as, "If someone were not getting better, do you think they would want to know?" "Do you want to know everything, even if the news is not good?" This approach helps the child set guidelines about the amount of truth he or she can tolerate or handle.
6. Children need time to process and assimilate both information and feelings.
7. The child and the family often fear pain and suffering, dying alone, and the actual death itself. The nurse can facilitate pain control, arrange schedules for family and friends to be with the child, and offer support through education and using the family's spiritual belief systems, about death itself.
8. In most communities, hospice care is available to support children choosing to die at home.

Loss and Bereavement in Children

1. Generally, the process of bereavement occurs in three phases:
   a. Acute grief work that includes intense somatic distress such as crying, sadness, and feelings of emptiness; a preoccupation with the image of the deceased person (sibling or family member); feelings of guilt and anger; and disruption of usual patterns of daily living.

PART 4

b. Disintegration when the above feelings continue after the death and accompanying services (funeral and memorial).

c. Reintegration when the above symptoms and behaviors gradually subside and life continues and an adjustment is made in which the deceased person is integrated and new relationships can be established.

2. Surviving children need to be able to talk about the dead sibling with their parents and to discuss their feelings. Many children ages 3–7 years feel they somehow were the cause of the death (they fantasized something happening to the sibling when they were fighting or had a disagreement or were jealous). This is a reflection of the normal egocentric development in children.

3. Behaviors indicating bereavement problems in children include:

a. Persistent blame and guilt

b. Patterns of overactivity including aggressive or destructive outbursts

c. Compulsive caregiving of parents or other siblings

d. Persistent anxieties (fears of another family member's death)

e. Excessive clinging to the parent

f. Difficulty forming new relationships

g. Problems at school

h. Delinquent behaviors such as stealing, drugs, etc.

Parents and Coping with Terminal Illness and Death

Terminal Illness

1. Parents require support from nurses to cope with their own feelings as well as telling the child about the diagnosis. They may want to conceal the diagnosis, or feel the child is too young to know, will be unable to cope, or will lose hope

and the will to live. Often these feelings and concerns are the parent's issues and are projected onto the child.

2. Approach the issue of sharing information with the child in a positive way by asking "How will you tell your child about the diagnosis?"

3. Support parents in understanding the disadvantages of withholding information (e.g., decreases opportunities to discuss their feelings or ask questions of the child, increases the risk of the child learning the truth from an outside less tactful source, and may decrease the child's trust and confidence in the parent).

4. Help parents to see the potential problems associated with a conspiracy "of not telling."

5. Support parents with guidelines and examples of what to tell children about death based on age and developmental level.

6. Discussing the name of the illness and the treatment actually can instill hope in the child and serve as the basis for explaining and understanding subsequent events.

7. Acknowledge that honesty is not always the easy way because it may prompt children to ask difficult questions such as "Am I going to die?" However, the nurse can prepare the parents for such questions that must be answered.

Death

1. Educate parents to understand the feelings associated with death of a child and the process of bereavement (see also end-of-life care).

2. Support parents to think through how they will work with their other children while acknowledging their own feelings.

3. Support them in thinking through the immediate issues of funerals, memorials, and notification of other family members.

References

Ball, J. W., & Bindler, R. C. (2003). *Pediatric nursing: Caring for children* (3rd ed.). Upper Saddle River, NJ: Prentice Hall.

Mott, S. R., James, S. B. & Sperhac, A. M. (1990). *Nursing care of children and families.* Redwood City, CA: Addison-Wesley.

US Consumer Product Safety Commission. (n.d.). *Childproofing Your Home—12 Safety Devices to Protect Your Children.* Retrieved February 21, 2006, from http://www.cpsc.gov/CPSCPUB/PUBS/GRAND/12steps/12steps.html

Wong, D. L., & Hockenberry-Eaton, M. (2001). *Wong's essentials of pediatric nursing* (6th ed.). St. Louis: Mosby.

Psychiatric and Mental Health Nursing

This specialty field is complex; it is one that frequently coexists with other clinical areas. The information presented here is a general approach to common clinical issues. Readers are referred to comprehensive psychiatric/mental health (PMH) nursing texts for any intense or prolonged work with this client population. The following sections focus on commonly experienced situations and strategies.

Prioritizing Needs

Because psychological issues are so complex and challenging, having some framework to prioritize needs is important. The most common way of considering patients' needs is using Maslow's Hierarchy of Needs. From most emergent to least, the needs are as follows: physiological, safety, love and belonging, self-esteem, and self-actualization. When a patient's condition prevents him or her from self-managing needs, the nurse needs to intervene, especially at the two most basic levels. Remember that needs at lower levels (i.e., physiological and safety) must be met before needs of higher levels can be met. So, if a care goal is to promote self-esteem, the nurse needs to be sure that the needs at the lower levels are not concerns.

Therapeutic Relationships

In most interpersonal relationships, the most effective tool available is the self. In some cases, it is the only tool available. So, knowing how to communicate is critical (see also Part 2, Communication). Thinking through how another person wants and deserves to be treated with respect, even when the behavior seems bizarre, is an important consideration before engaging with any patient, and especially one with PMH issues. This person-to-person relationship varies with each dyad that forms. Unlike personal or nontherapeutic relationships, therapeutic ones are goal-oriented and the goal often relates to altering the behavior and gaining greater understanding of the other person. While setting such goals is always better when the goals are set mutually, in some situations where PMH issues prevail, it may be necessary to move toward such goals without the patient's participation in setting the goals.

In order to be therapeutic, the nurse must first understand him- or herself. Self-insight is important so the nurse is acutely aware of avoiding manipulating the other person. Knowing what one's personal values and beliefs are and how they are shaped by one's culture helps in understanding and accepting another person's values and beliefs and his or her cultural context. Establishing a rapport or special relationship helps both persons in a relationship to value the other person.

To establish and maintain a therapeutic relationship, common human interaction elements need to be present. These elements include empathy, honesty, respect, and trust. Empathy is especially important to understanding how another person sees a situation. Honesty not only includes not being devious in communication or in purpose of the relationship, but also includes truth-telling. What this means is that if a patient says to the nurse, "All you want to do is stop me from killing myself," the nurse should honestly reply, "I do want you to live," or "Yes, I hope to be able to stop you from taking such action." Respect may seem strange in the above example, yet we can value each other as human beings with needs and desires. Showing respect might include such simple strategies as looking at the patient, using the person's preferred name, and accepting the angst the person is expressing that he or she is experiencing. Finally, trust is important in order to have the relationship be meaningful. Trust has to be earned through prior statements and actions of truth. If it is impossible to guarantee something, don't suggest that it is possible to do so. Being truthful leads to trust. Following through with any promise further creates the foundation for trust.

Critical Communication

Basic communication skills are essential (see Part 2 for basic information), but they are insufficient by themselves to work effectively with clients who have PMH issues. Any prior statements such as "being honest" and "listening actively" are magnified when working with an individual with a PMH need. Very often the only tool readily available is the nurse's ability to relate to the individual or group. Thus, the phrase *therapeutic use of self* means the way in which the nurse (you) interacts in positive ways with others.

Use of Silence

One of the most effective communication tools is that of silence. In other words, when the patient says something, sit quietly. Often this break in the conversation precipitates the opportunity for the person speaking to reshape an existing conversation or totally redirect the conversation. This is especially effective if the caregiver has posed a question that causes the other person to think. If the caregiver provides the answer, the individual need not exert the thinking required to self-discover information. Because society has reinforced the way communication occurs, people frequently have difficulty remembering to use this technique.

Some additional common communication approaches are listed in Table 4-13.

Table 4-13   Common Communication Approaches

Approach	General Description	Example
Amplifying	Getting the details, such as when something happened or how a person felt about something	How did that make you feel? Would you describe that in more detail?
Clarifying	Eliminating misperceptions and verifying accuracy of perceptions	So, it was X not Y?
Focusing	Centering on a single idea, statement, or word to elicit clarification or validation	You just said your neighbor to the south, is that right?
Open-ended questions	Questioning that cannot be responded to with a yes or no response and therefore leads to details or clarification	How was that event different from the previous time?
Reality testing	Clarification of facts to determine client's response	If Mr. Smith went to the store, that must have left Mrs. Smith at home. (If this is the fact)
Reflecting	Using the same words, typically in an unfinished sentence	You thought that wasn't right? (Said as a question, not as a statement)
Restating	Using different words to validate prior information	So you say this neighbor is in the red brick home, the one to the south?

Assessing an individual's thoughts as expressed through oral communication is critical. Specifically, the nurse needs to listen for rational and irrational thoughts and beliefs. For example, if Tiger Woods said he could drive a golf ball 300 yards, that would be a rational statement. For most casual golfers and even many professionals, that becomes an irrational statement.

One final point to consider in communication is the importance of nonverbal aspects. This topic is discussed in Part 2. Remember, however, that it is how one "attends" to an interchange that helps the other person determine whether the exchange is sincere and how to interpret the oral communication. Looking distressed while saying, "I am calm," loses the communication; it is unbelievable. Nonverbal communication is read by people who are experiencing PMH issues. Use of hands, posture, facial expressions, and proximity all convey messages about the relationship and its meaning to the nurse.

Cultural Considerations

Although culture is an important element of any health condition, it is critical within PMH situations. Behavior that may look bizarre to someone may be considered normal behavior in another. This does not mean that we should tolerate behaviors that are harmful to self or others. Rather, we should be able to acknowledge the importance or value of a behavior within a certain context and simultaneously limit or prohibit its use in a different cultural context. Nurses therefore become cultural liaisons, explaining why some behavior is unacceptable and reinforcing the appropriate behavior to be exhibited in the current context. One example might be preventing a patient who is homeless and often digs through garbage containers from digging through waste containers in a hospital setting. Another example might be prohibiting a teenager from cutting his body, a part of the ritual in his community. Nurses can (and should) explain why both practices outside of the hospital are unsafe, while not condemning the practices.

Additionally, some cultures believe that someone with a mental illness is a disgrace to the family or is possessed by an evil demon. Recognizing that overlay of psychodrama on the basic condition of a patient is important. The significant others who hold and reinforce these perceptions of mental illness are not likely to change because we can explain various disorders and their treatments. However, they should not be supported in conveying those negative messages to the patient.

Process Recordings

A common strategy for students and nurses to increase their perceptive abilities is to use process recordings. These typically comprise two key elements: conversation and analysis. The conversation is typically a dyad (nurse and patient), but could be a group situation too. The conversation part consists of as much detail as possible about what the nurse and the patient each said (think about how play scripts are developed; name: [words said] followed by name of the second person: [words said]). The analysis section consists of what the nurse was thinking about the meaning of the conversation and then a conclusion about the effectiveness of the conversation. For example, was a statement therapeutic or did the conversation slip to and remain at a social level?

Sample Process Recording

Patient: I really hated my mother.

Nurse: Do you have an idea why that might have been the case?

. . . etc.

Analysis: This response prompted the patient to respond further about the feeling of hatred. I tried to avoid asking why, but found that I used the word indirectly.

Table 4-14   Common Defense Mechanisms

Mechanism	Definition
Denial	Refusing to accept reality or truth
Displacement	Placing cause or blame on another, frequently someone of less authority
Identification	Emulating characteristics or attributes of another who is admired
Intellectualization	Distancing self from emotions of situation by using logic and reasoning
Projection	Attributing personal feelings to another. Sometimes used by referring to what another's motivation is
Rationalization	Creating rationale (excuses) for behavior or feelings
Reaction formation	Exaggerating opposite feelings to prevent recognition of real feelings
Regression	Moving backward to an earlier level of development to gain comfort
Repression	Blocking unacceptable feelings involuntarily
Sublimation	Refocusing unacceptable impulses into other acceptable activities
Suppression	Restricting feelings from entering awareness
Undoing	Canceling a feeling symbolically. Frequently tied to ritualistic practices learned in childhood

Common Psychiatric Disorders

Many disorders exist other than those listed in Table 4-15; however, these are the most common ones. Readers are referred to psychiatric medicine and nursing texts and Web sites for further details.

Table 4-15 Common Psychiatric Disorders

Disorder Category	Types	Basic Description/Key Action
Abuse (see Part 3)	Child	Physical or emotional injury or neglect to a minor. Behavioral signs depend on type of abuse/neglect and may include fear of parent or caretaker, rage, apprehension, withdrawal, low achievement, regression, sleep disorders, self-destructive behavior, or seductive behaviors. *Report suspected condition immediately through established procedures.* Offer comfort to child.
	Elder	Physical or emotional injury or neglect to an older adult. Behavioral signs depend on type of abuse/neglect and may include depression, anxiety, confusion, agitation, or inappropriate dress. *Report suspected condition immediately through established procedures.* Offer comfort to the victim.
	Sexual	Physical or emotional injury involving any sexual act that is not consensual. This abuse category includes date rape, marital rape, and statutory rape (victim is under a state-defined age

Table 4-15 (*continued*)

Disorder Category	Types	Basic Description/Key Action
		limit). *Report suspected condition immediately through established procedures.* Offer comfort to the victim.
	Spouse	Physical or emotional injury or neglect to a spouse. This may include sexual abuse. A key characteristic is a cycle of a triggering event, leading to battering, and then to a "make up" phase, and finally to a tolerance awaiting the next triggering event. *Report suspected condition immediately through established procedures.* Offer comfort to the victim. Remember not to condemn the fact that the victim usually stays in this type of relationship through several cycles.
	Substance	A syndrome resulting from ingestion or exposure to various substances. These substances include alcohol, psychoactive substances (legal and illegal), and caffeine and nicotine, although the latter are often not treated in the same manner as the other substances. The Substances Abuse and Mental Health Administration Web site

		(🖱 www.samhsa.gov) is useful in determining specific signs and symptoms, emerging substances of abuse, and therapeutic interventions.
Anxiety	Mild	Lowest level, causes one to focus on situation, often beneficial
	Moderate	Difficulty focusing on situation
	Severe	Physical symptoms appear and focusing is extremely limited
	Panic	Extreme anxiety, acts terrorized
	Generalized	Overly anxious for an extended period of time
	Obsessive-compulsive	Presence of recurring thoughts that distract from ongoing events; also presence of repetitive behavior such as washing hands.
	Posttraumatic stress	Condition subsequent to specific, intense event (war, death, assault). This often includes flashbacks to precipitating event. Includes anniversary reaction (yearly reaction that typically diminishes over years)
Delirium, dementia		Disturbance of consciousness (see index for more details)
Dissociation		A general category representing disruption in normal consciousness. Includes amnesia, fugue, identity disorder, and depersonalization disorder
Eating	Anorexia	Characterized by abnormal fear of being obese. Includes distortion

PART 4

Table 4-15	(continued)	
Disorder Category	**Types**	**Basic Description/Key Action**
		of body perception, preoccupation with food, and refusal to eat. The person usually is underweight and describes self as fat. Amenor-rhea accompanies this condition.
	Bulimia	Compulsive ingestion of large amounts of food (binging) followed by behaviors (often purging) to rid the body of what was ingested
Impulse control		Inappropriate responses to stressful situation characterized by atypical functioning and compulsive acts that may be harmful to self or others
Mental retardation		Characterized by significant limitations in intellectual ability and adaptation. Demonstrated in conceptual, social, and practical skills. Includes levels based on degree of compromise ranging from mild (higher intellectual level) to profound, which requires total care. For further information, visit ⌐🖱 www.aamr.org.
Mood disorders		A set of conditions related to the affective state and demonstration through behaviors

	Depression	Characterized by persistent lack of interest in normal life; unipolar
	Bipolar	Characterized by swings between depression and mania
	Mania	Characterized by persistent, high intensity elevated mood; unipolar
	Postpartum depression	Characterized by depressive behavior. Occurs within 3 months post delivery
Personality disorders		Maladaption classification applying to multiple disorders including paranoia, schizoid, borderline personality, antisocial personality, and dependent personality
Psychotic	Schizophrenia	Includes other diagnoses, but schizophrenia is most prevalent. Characterized by disconnections from reality, including hallucinations (auditory and visual), delusions, and disorganization of speech, thought, and behavior
Sleeping Disorders	Insomnia	Difficulty initiating or maintaining sleep with resultant impairment in personal functioning
	Hypersomnia	Excessive sleep; narcolepsy is similar
	Parasomnias	Abnormal sleep behaviors including nightmares, sleepwalking

Typical Therapies

The following therapies are listed in alphabetical order. It is not uncommon to find that more than one therapeutic approach is used for a patient. This information is to help recall the strategy focus of the therapy. A PMH text should be used before using these approaches with patients.

Table 4-16   Typical Therapies

Therapy	Description
Assertiveness training	Specific ways to express self without being combative or retiring. Allows for expression of needs and what the person believes he or she wants to satisfy those needs. Specific techniques include using the word "I," a verb that tells what is desired (e.g., "need" or "want"), and specific detail that produces an expectation on the part of the other to respond or to fulfill a request. For example, "I want you to call me by my first name." The nurse responds by saying, "I will, [name]," or explaining why that is not possible.
Behavior	Modification of behavior through such techniques as modeling (exhibiting desired behavior), shaping (rewards for increasing approximation to desired behavior), aversion (unpleasant consequences associated with undesirable behavior)
Cognitive	Goal-oriented, problem-oriented approach using educational techniques to learn new approaches to dysfunctions; focus is on creating new ways of thinking and acting

Complementary therapies	Use of such strategies as art, dance, music therapy, or biofeedback. Intent is to help person express emotions and gain greater insight into personal expressions and responses
Electroconvulsive (ECT)	Production of grand mal seizures via electrical current to the brain (somewhat controversial)
Family	Treatment of the family unit in terms of their relationships with each other; can focus on communication, role relationships, or specific situations
Group	Creation of common approaches to general issues frequently associated with a specific diagnosis or interrelationship issue; frequently seen as support groups (people with common concerns who desire to learn from each other to prevent complications or deal with a current condition in a better manner in the future) or self-help groups (people with experience with a diagnosis who have found successful coping strategies or desire to find such)
Milieu	Creation or modification of an environment that is designed to produce positive results for the individuals in therapy
Pharmacological	Use of medications in the primary categories of antianxiety agents, antidepressants, antimanic agents, antipsychotics, CNS stimulants, hypnotics, sedatives
Prayer	Use of religious beliefs to aid patient in expressing concerns and seeking wellness

PART 4

Common Nursing Interventions

Anger Management

Although most people have experienced what they would describe as anger, some people are extreme in their intensity, duration, or response. Because the expression of anger can be controlled, anger management strategies are commonly used by nurses to help patients respond within more defined parameters. The goal of anger management is to help the patient identify anger when it occurs and to divert the increasing tension that builds up into a constructive activity. The goal is to help the person self-identify anger before some more aggressive expression occurs and to divert the energy in some personally productive way. For example, for some people, being able to tense and relax muscles is helpful. For others, using some form of distraction therapy is useful. Because violence is a fairly common event in society, getting anger under control can avert or diminish violent behavior.

Key strategies nurses use to help people control their anger are:

- Remaining calm (for example, don't escalate the situation by speaking louder or using more physical gestures)
- Observing for any indication of escalation of anger (for example, note any increased intensity of words, increased swearing, or greater physical gesturing or movement)
- Role-modeling appropriate responses; for example, acknowledge that this event (or behavior or statement) would be distressing and how that could precipitate a need to analyze what precipitated the event (behavior or statement)
- Setting limits on verbal and physical behaviors (for example, say "If you continue to swear, I will need to leave" and then be prepared to do so)
- Helping to define what the precipitator of an anger event is (for example, offer insight as to possible precipitating events, behaviors, or words)
- Defining and encouraging the use of acceptable options for anger (exercise, deep breathing, specific messages); for example, tell the person to take a deep breath

It is also wise to avoid physical contact, even comforting gestures, during any anger outbursts. However, if it becomes necessary to physically restrain someone, the least restrictive approaches should be used first. One of the early actions needed is to notify another staff member that assistance may be necessary. Walking a patient is better than carrying, although both may be necessary strategies. *Remember: protect yourself.* Keep an appropriate distance between yourself and the person until it is necessary to have physical contact, as in the need to restrain. Be clear about an escape route. Don't try to be a hero! Many health care organizations have specific protocols for working in such situations—use them!

Crisis Intervention

Crisis refers to an increasing state of psychological instability that an individual cannot address through normal coping strategies. A patient may describe a crisis as feeling "out of control," have a sense of pending doom, or demonstrate an increased state of agitation. Although the crisis is fairly short lived (usually less than 2–3 days), the intensity of the crisis disrupts logical thinking. Decision making is impaired and sometimes the situation is life threatening. If the patient is at risk to self or others, seek help immediately (see Suicide Intervention later in this section).

Follow the key communication techniques: be honest, avoid judging behaviors, provide facts, remain calm, listen actively. Remember to set limits on verbal and physical behaviors. If true, assure the patient that the response is typical to others (for instance when a family is told that someone suddenly died). Believe what the patient tells you in terms of planned actions, especially destructive behavior. Help the patient as much as possible through a problem-solving process.

Suicide Intervention

Suicide is more common in older and younger people (50 plus and under 20). It is also more common among men. In general, the following behaviors are indicative of a high suicide risk: panic (or at least a high intensity of anxiety), extreme feelings of hopelessness and inability to help self, few reliable coping strategies, access to few resources, dramatic hostility, irrational thought patterns and speech, frequent reference to a plan to "end it all" (usually more concerning when there are specific details), disruption of activities of daily living, and general unstable lifestyle and frequent substance abuse.

This patient should *not be left alone*. Most healthcare organizations have some protocol for suicide precautions that should be instituted immediately. Alert other staff and attempt to get the patient's assurance not to commit suicide or to implement the ideas of suicide in any physical activities such as carrying weapons or cutting any part of the body.

A common approach to assess the potential for suicide is the SAD PERSONS scale (see Table 4-17). The more factors that are

Table 4-17   SAD PERSONS Scale

Factor	Relevance of Risk
Sex	Women
Age	Under 25 and over 45
Depression	Acute depressive episode
Previous attempt	More likely to repeat
Ethanol (alcohol)	More likely to attempt (all substances count)
Rational thinking	Lost or diminished
Social support	Loss through death or isolation by family or friends
Organized plan	More likely to attempt when a specific plan exists
No significant other	More likely to attempt
Sickness	More likely to attempt, especially if serious or terminal

Source: Adapted from Patterson, H. H., Dohn, J., Patterson, C. A. (1983). Evaluation of suicidal patients: The SAD PERSONS scale. *Psychosomatics, 24,* 343–349. Summarized reference for this table is available at http://webits3.appstate.edu/apples/counsel/Suicide/warnings.htm

present, the more likely suicide might be attempted. A score of 3–4 suggests help is needed, and a score of 7–10 indicates the person will need a suicide precaution plan. (Count one for each factor present.)

Relaxation Intervention

A common set of strategies that nurses use are relaxation techniques. Each technique is described in a step-by-step manner so that it can be used readily.

Deep Breathing This technique can be done in any position in any situation. However, the more relaxed a person is (lie instead of sit, sit instead of stand), the more easily accomplished this technique is. Remember that most people know how to do this, they may merely need to be reminded.

1. Assume a comfortable position (as much as possible depending on the setting and situation).
2. Loosen any tight clothing (as much as possible depending on the setting and situation).
3. Place one hand on the abdomen.
4. Close eyes, if possible.
5. Think: in through your nose, out through your mouth.
6. Inhale slowly and deeply (hand should move, chest should move only slightly) through nose.
7. Hold breath for a few seconds.
8. Exhale slowly through mouth; if possible, purse lips (hand should move back down).
9. Repeat for several minutes as situation and setting permit.

Progressive Relaxation This technique is designed to relax muscles to alleviate the physical tension people may feel in difficult situations. Again, this technique can be accomplished in various situations and settings, but the more effective way to achieve results is to be as physically relaxed as possible. (Think lie instead of sit and sit instead of stand.) The basic technique is to start at the bottom and work up and to contract and then relax various

PART 4

muscle groups. The basic steps are tighten, hold, release/relax, and think.

1. Assume a comfortable position. (If sitting, both feet should be flat on floor.)
2. Close eyes if possible.
3. Take a few slow, deep breaths (see prior).
4. Point toes toward head, hold for a count of 5, release and think about the release of tension and the warmth that is present in the muscles.
5. Tighten thigh and gluteal muscles, hold, release, and think.
6. Tighten abdominal muscles, hold, release, and think.
7. Tighten lower back muscles, hold, release, and think.
8. Tighten upper back and chest muscles, hold, release, and think.
9. Tighten hands (make fists), hold, release, and think.
10. Tighten arm muscles, hold, release, and think.
11. Tighten shoulder and neck muscles, hold, release, and think.
12. Tighten facial muscles (squint eyes, frown, purse lips), hold, release, and think.
13. Relax entire body and think about the relaxation and warmth.
14. Take a few slow, deep breaths (see prior).
15. Slowly open eyes and refocus on the current situation.

Key Nursing Actions Based on Major Classifications of Psychiatric/Mental Health Disorders

Table 4-18 below identifies the key types of PMH issues nurses deal with whether as the primary diagnosis or a dual diagnosis. This is a broad-based guide that should be supplemented by appropriate specialty literature. Education is a key nursing action with each of the diagnostic categories.

Table 4-18 Categories and Treatments of Major Psychiatric/Mental Health Disorders

Category	Typical Symptoms	Types	Treatment	Nursing Actions
Anxiety	Increased vital signs, diaphoresis, vertigo, headache, urgency and frequency of urination, insomnia, crying, anger, forgetfulness, decreased concentration and productivity	Panic disorder, phobias, obsessive-compulsive, post-traumatic stress	Visual imagery, exercise, massage, meditation, biofeedback, therapeutic touch, hypnosis, medications	Stay with patient during acute phase Remain calm Speak simply Prevent harm to self and others Provide for therapy Administer medications
Depression	Anorexia or overeating, insomnia or excessive sleeping, fatigue, generalized pain or discomfort, decreased personal hygiene, decreased mental and physical activities	Bipolar (manic depressive), mood disorders	Medications, psychotherapy, phototherapy (seasonal affective disorder), electroconvulsive therapy	Positive interaction techniques Patience Assuring activities of daily living (ADL) accomplishment

Table 4-18 *(continued)*

Category	Typical Symptoms	Types	Treatment	Nursing Actions
Psychoses	Disorganized thinking and speech, delusions, hallucinations, diminished affect	Schizophrenia, paranoia, catatonia, delusional disorder	Medications, psychotherapy	Assistance with eating, physical activity, and sleeping Positive interaction techniques Focused communication about reality Avoid reinforcing delusions or touching patient Control environment to minimize stimuli and promote safety

Substance abuse: alcohol	Increased anxiety or depression, social drinking that escalates, possibility of blackouts, possible excuses for drinking, antisocial, drinks alone		Detoxification program if needed, psychotherapy including aversion therapy	Monitor for violent behavior Provide or assist with ADL Fluid and electrolyte replacement as needed Assistance with goals related to therapy Positive interaction techniques Avoid reinforcing delusions
Substance abuse: drugs	Varies depending on the medication abused	Amphetamines, cannabis, opioids, sedatives, hypnotics, anxiolytics	Detoxification program if needed; psychotherapy including aversion therapy	Positive interaction techniques Fluid and electrolyte replacement as needed

PART 4

Table 4-19 Quick Reference for Patient Behaviors and Nursing Actions

Patient Behavior	Nursing Action
Aggressive	Avoid harm, set limits
Anxious	Reduce stimuli
Delusional	Avoid harm, reinforce reality
Depressed	Avoid self-harm, assist as needed
Hyperactivity	Direct energy to physical activity
Manipulation	Set limits
Obsessive-compulsive	Attempt to distract; don't interrupt ritual
Suicidal	Stay with; get agreement to do no harm

Gerontological Nursing

This section is designed to address problems and conditions common to the elderly and the key strategies nurses take to prevent or correct those problems. Basic developmental content appears in the developmental section (Part 5) of this text. Because individuals age at different rates, there is not a "magic" number when certain characteristics are evident. Thus, the following information is a general guideline. In general, it is safe to say that older patients are more compromised in their recovery than a younger person with a similar condition. In general, older patients have a greater likelihood of having two or more coexisting diseases than a younger person. And, it is not uncommon for an older person to have multiple medication prescriptions. That said, it is also possible to encounter an older person in excellent health and physical condition and taking no prescription medications. The key is to be alert to the characteristics of and situations commonly encountered by older people so that a point of reference is possible.

Due to the fact that people over 65 years old are increasing in number and that they are often the main patient population in many institutional (e.g., hospitals and nursing homes) and com-

munity (e.g., home care) settings, a significant number of resources have been developed to provide readily available information for the public and for healthcare professionals. Remember
that a large number of individuals over 55 years old (the age
requirement) join the American Association of Retired Persons (AARP). AARP provides up-to-date information that
many older persons rely on for their health care decisions
(www.aarp.org/health). The Web site GeronurseOnline
(www.geronurseonline.com) is extremely useful in securing
answers to specific questions about the care of the elderly. In addition to providing essential information, this Web site permits
users to select specific geriatric condition information and also to
seek instant help through the "need help stat" drop-down menu.
Additionally, many of the tools are downloadable to personal digital assistants (PDAs).

Key Characteristics of Aging

- Abstract thinking powers diminish.
- Accessory muscles are more likely to be used in
  breathing.
- Awareness of temperature and pressure is lessened.
- Balance is less dependable.
- Bladder tone diminishes.
- Body shape changes.
- Body weight tends to decrease with increasing age.
- Bone mass decreases.
- Caloric intake decreases with increasing age.
- Chest diameter increases in anterior-posterior dimension.
- Chest "tightens" due to decreased rib mobility.
- Collagen and subcutaneous tissue decrease.
- Defecation sensation diminishes.
- Dietary absorption of various elements decreases.
- Dietary issues relate to poor oral health, especially peri-
  odontal disease.

- Esophageal sphincter tone decreases.
- Eye lens becomes less elastic and more dense.
- Gastric acid production diminishes.
- Hearing acuity decreases, especially for high frequencies.
- Hair thins and loses color.
- Hip and knee flexion increase.
- Hormone levels decrease.
- Insulin sensitivity (circulating) decreases.
- Kidney function decreases.
- Ligaments and tendons tighten.
- Medications are often consumed in large quantities (polypharmacy).
- Metabolism decreases as aging occurs.
- Muscle mass decreases.
- Nails thicken.
- Nerve transmission slows.
- Nocturnal urine production increases.
- Peripheral vascular resistance increases.
- Posture changes to "stooped" position (kyphosis).
- Pupil size decreases.
- Range of movements becomes more limited with increasing age.
- Respirations diminish.
- Saliva production diminishes.
- Scaly, raised areas on skin darken.
- Short term memory lessens.
- Skin "thins" as aging occurs so it is more susceptible to problems such as tears, pressure, and infections.
- Small intestine and large intestine motility diminishes.
- Smell sense deteriorates.
- Social isolation is possible due to decreased hearing.
- Spatial awareness diminishes.
- Strength and tone decrease.
- T lymphocytes decrease in number.

- Tactile sensation diminishes.
- Taste bud numbers diminish.
- Tear production decreases.
- Tissue elasticity diminishes.
- Urinary sphincter tone diminishes.
- Vascularity decreases as aging occurs.
- Vital capacity decreases.
- White blood cell production slows.

Critical Communication

Assume that an older person has an intact communication system before using any special strategies. As with other patients, stand (or sit) in front of the person, speak clearly. People who speak quickly may find it necessary to slow down, especially if a person lip-reads. Generational differences may affect the choice of words (for example, *cool* may mean *temperature*, not *a great idea*), the manner of interaction (for example, using formal titles rather than first names), and personal issues (for example, modesty, independence, or gender differences).

The initial nursing assessment should indicate what, if any, communication devices are used or problems exist. Common problems that may interfere with normal communication include issues with vision, hearing, and speaking.

Vision

Cataracts (clouded vision) and glaucoma (peripheral vision affected) are common issues of older people. Both can distort vision. Macular degeneration (central vision affected) is the leading cause of blindness in older people. Diabetic retinopathy causes spotty vision. Performing a simple eye test upon an initial encounter and when a patient complains of diminished vision can provide beginning data about vision loss. Patients with limited vision depend on oral communication to understand information presented.

Hearing

For older persons, in addition to general hearing loss, specific sounds are difficult to hear and can be confused with other sounds. The most common are high-pitched sounds such as those produced by the letters *s*, *z*, *sh*, and *ch*. Hearing is more challenging when background noises are more intense. (Remember this point in situations such as emergency rooms or large clinics. If the patient misunderstands the questions or points being made, he or she might provide incorrect information in response.) Hearing losses are a common cause of social isolation due to limited ability to "follow" conversations. Additionally, persons with hearing loss often feel others shout at them or ignore them. Hearing loss can be conduction loss, sensorineural loss, or both. Some patients may lip read to obscure the fact that they cannot hear clearly and they may need to be touched to gain initial attention.

Speaking

If a person wears dentures, they may not fit well. This is especially true for people who have worn them for a long time (and now aging changes affect their fit) and who do not have sufficient income to replace them. Although these people do well in private, they may be reluctant to speak in a public situation or when strangers are present. Mumbling or lisping may be signs of poor fitting dentures. Listening actively is even more important in such situations.

Common Health Concerns of Aging

Although most health concerns of older persons relate to medical diagnoses such as congestive heart failure or cancer, nurses are also concerned with the ongoing concerns that are often not addressed. The most common ones appear below.

Confusion

Merely putting someone in a different setting can cause confusion. For example, hospitalization can trigger confusion. The presence of an infection or serious illness, dehydration, vision impairment, and alcoholism can also contribute to confusion. Confusion can be manifested by misunderstanding questions asked. In more dramatic situations, rambling or incoherent speaking may be evident. The person may be lethargic or difficult to arouse. Confusion about new medical regimens is not a cause of alarm. Confusion about well-known information (such as name of spouse, address, or month) must be explored further. Orientation (person, place, time) is the minimum assessment that should occur. More sophisticated determinations can be made by testing executive functioning (a level of cognitive functioning) by using the Clox test, the Controlled Oral Word Association, or the Trailmaking Test (see www.geronurseonline.com under the topic "dementia"). Some of the most simplistic interventions are to decrease environmental stimuli, to emulate the person's regular daily schedule as much as possible to promote sleep (avoiding medications if possible), or to limit fluids several hours before going to bed.

Incontinence

Urinary incontinence is common among older persons. Some causes may be related to physiological changes, but others can be caused by inattention to physiological signals. Specific products are designed to assist with this health problem; however, people use numerous other strategies, such as using a wad of toilet tissue, rags, or sanitary napkins, to prevent embarrassing leakage. Although it is most common for this leakage to occur during such episodes as coughing, laughing, sneezing, bending, or lifting, some people experience leakage at other times. Asking a person to keep a record of frequency and precipitating events is important. In addition to personal protection, bladder training programs have been very successful.

Nutrition and Hydration

Multiple factors affect whether a patient consumes appropriate quantities and qualities of foods and fluids. Many factors are those

PART 4

of physiological changes normal for aging. Others have to do with such psychological factors as confusion, loss, and loneliness. Others may also relate to the condition of dentition, numbers and types of medications taken, cognitive status, availability of nutritious foods and fluids, and overall concern for one's health. The Web site for the food pyramid can be useful in working with patients with nutrition issues (www.mypyramid.gov). Monitoring weight and doing nutrition recording helps patients participate in their care.

Hydration is another important issue to attend to. Like nutrition, it is related to normal aging changes as well as other factors such as effects of medications. Some people merely need to be reminded to drink a beverage. Others may drink sufficient quantities, but not necessarily the right kind of fluids.

Another common consideration is that older people with problems of continence often limit or withhold fluids during certain public activities so they are sure to prevent urinary leakage. If laboratory tests suggest inadequate hydration and no condition contraindicates consuming fluids, patients should be encouraged to drink more fluids, especially water. The recommended amount for healthy adults is 8 glasses. For patients in nursing homes, the Web sites www.cdhcf.org/hcfa/index.htm and www.ltcnutrition.org offer suggestions to promote eating and managing a group of patients during mealtimes. For patients at home and who need nutritional support, programs such as Meals on Wheels can provide important services.

For some patients, using anthropometry to determine nutritional status may be important. This measure of the basal metabolic rate can determine over and under weights.

Specific diets may be used in conjunction with specific disease conditions. Part 5 of this text contains a description of common therapeutic diets.

Sleep and Rest

Sleep disturbances are a common complaint of many people, especially older adults. Some causes relate to normal aging processes and medication regimens. Other relate to medical conditions or to psychological issues. Disturbances range from difficulty falling asleep, to awakening during the night, from nocturia to difficulty breathing in a prostrate position, or from distraction of pain to physical exhaustion. Helping patients understand their particular pattern can be useful to determining an intervention. The American Academy of Sleep Medicine (⌐ www.aasmnet.org) recommends basic strategies such as trying to sleep only when drowsy, maintaining a regular sleep schedule, avoiding other activities (e.g., watching TV, doing work) in the bedroom, avoiding napping, using distraction, avoiding caffeine and alcohol before going to bed, and creating a relaxed atmosphere in the bedroom. As much as possible, distractions should be removed from patient care environments so that sleep is not disrupted.

Common Nursing Interventions

Table 4-20 uses the systematic approach illustrated in the Assessment section of this text. This table includes examples of common strategies, which may be direct care or patient counseling/education.

Major Clinical Nursing Care Concerns
Aspiration/Choking

Due to decreased muscular tone and dryness of the mouth and throat, sometimes older people choke or aspirate more quickly than younger persons. To prevent these complications, encourage fluids, especially before medications and meals. Be prepared to institute the Heimlich maneuver and remove any obstructions from the oral cavity. If aspiration occurs, request an X-ray and observe for any respiratory distress or signs of infection.

Chronic Illness and Multiple Diagnoses

Two of the most challenging aspects in working with elderly patients is the fact that they tend to have more than one diagnosis

PART 4

Table 4-20   Common Nursing Interventions for Aged Patients

System	Change	Examples of Common Strategies
Hair	Thinning or major loss	Sun protection for head: solid hat (not mesh); sun protective products with high SPF
Skin	Thinning and drying, decreased sweating	Protect from pressure (turn frequently if immobile), cracking (cleanliness and moisturizing), abrasions (lift, don't drag), infections (prevention and immediate attention to breaks in the integrity of the skin); prevent heat stroke
	Decreased sweating	Diminish pruritus (cleanliness, extra rinsing of clothes and sheets)
	Wrinkling	Dry skin folds
	Thickened nails	Trim and oil nails (soak first in warm water)
	Discolorations	Assess for abnormal changes
Head	Diminished range of motion	Prevent hyperextension of neck, especially when standing on stools or ladders (for example, when replacing ceiling light bulbs)
Eyes	Decreased visual acuity and visual fields; diminished light adaptation; increased	Use corrective lenses; prevent disorientation; encourage deliberative head movement to increase visual scan; create sharp color contrasts (light and dark) at

	intraocular pressure (potential for glaucoma); dryness	critical movement areas (for example steps), use low placed lights to illuminate areas of typical night movement; fall prevention assessment; use artificial tear products
Ears	Decreased sound discrimination; presbycusis	Use hearing aids (as appropriate); speak directly and slowly; keep socially connected (may feel isolated due to inability to follow conversations)
	Elongated ears	No action needed.
Nose	Diminished sense of smell	Use auditory odor alerts (smoke detectors); cleanliness; encourage adequate nutrition (related to diminished olfactory stimulation from food)
	Dry nasal passages	Prevent infections
Mouth/throat	Difficulty chewing related to condition of teeth or presence of dentures	Create menus with easily chewed food; cut into small sizes
	Dry mouth/ nausea (related to certain medications)	Monitor use of medications, encourage fluids sufficient to swallow without difficulty

Table 4-20 (*continued*)

System	Change	Examples of Common Strategies
	Periodontal disease	Floss; maintain regular dental examination schedule
Neck	Decreased flexibility	Prevent/treat pain; use range of motion exercises
Breasts	Decreased muscular support	Use of adequate breast support
Respiratory	Decreased lung elasticity; decreased chest muscle strength; thickening of chest	Deep breathe; prevent infections; increase attention to auscultation and palpation
Cardiovascular	Decreased cardiac output; decreased elasticity; fewer pacemaker cells; calcification; decreased response in stretch receptors	Use stress-reduction activities; monitor heart rate and blood pressure and pulse points (especially in extremities); prevent falls; maintain soft stools to prevent undue strain on defecation
Gastrointestinal	Decreased peristalsis; decreased gastric acid; decreased absorption of vitamins and	Prevent discomfort after meals; prevent constipation and other related conditions; prevent malnutrition; monitor response to any medications

	minerals; decreased size of liver	
Genitourinary	Decreased renal function; increased BUN; increased concentration of urine; decreased bladder tone	Monitor response to any medications; consume fluids (primarily before evening); remind to urinate before bedtime to prevent frequent urination at night
	Decline in fertility; decreased elasticity of vaginal wall	Evaluate concerns of sexual function including dyspareunia and need for lubrication
	Increased size of prostate	Monitor GU functioning
Musculoskeletal	Decreased muscle mass; deterioration of cartilage	Adjust physical activity to maintain range of motion without excessive demand; accommodate to slower response time; prevent/treat pain; monitor loss of height; monitor osteoporosis symptoms
	Decreased height	Adjust long clothing so it is not a safety hazard
Neurological	Changes in spinal cord and functioning of nerves; plaques; delayed reaction time	Monitor potential for leg weakness; prevent/treat pain; monitor cognitive functioning; conduct fall assessment

PART 4

Table 4-20 (*continued*)		
System	**Change**	**Examples of Common Strategies**
Endocrine	Decreased hormone production; alterations in thermoregulation; decreased BMR	Minimize stress responses; monitor body response to temperature changes; monitor weight gain

Table 4-21   Common Laboratory Variations Associated with Aging

Test	General Variation
Albumin	Decrease (slight)
Alkaline phosphatase	Increase (slight)
BUN	Increase
Calcium	Decrease (slight)
Creatinine	Increase
Glucose	Increase (slight)
Hematocrit	Decrease (slight)
Hemoglobin	Decrease (slight)
pCO_2	Increase (slight)
pO_2	Decrease
Potassium	Increase (slight)
Sedimentation rate	Increase (slight)
Thyroid stimulation hormone	Increase
Uric acid	Increase (slight)

Source: Lueckenotte, A. G. (2000). *Textbook of gerontologic nursing* (2nd ed.). St Louis: Mosby.

and many have had at least one diagnosis for many years. Thus, managing care overall is challenging. For example, a well-managed disease may suddenly become a challenge or a complicating factor due to the emergence of another condition. An example of this is the number of elderly with coexisting diabetes and cardiovascular disease. Refer to ⬧ www.geronurseonline.com for specific conditions.

End of Life

This topic is covered in greater depth in Part 3. Although younger people may also be faced with the issues of end of life (EOL), it is clear that older people will be. This aspect of care has numerous considerations. The key ones are making certain that the person has the appropriate legal documents executed while the person is legally able to make decisions. The key documents are wills (for distribution of the estate and authority for business transactions after death), living wills (for limiting use of extraordinary measures), and health care durable power of attorney (to designate who may act on behalf of an individual who is deemed no longer capable of making sound decisions). Other documents can enact a person's specific wishes.

Another key concern is the management of pain. Nurses are expected to be advocates for assuring sufficient strategies, including medications, to alleviate pain. Be sure that a pain scale is used so that comparisons regarding the effectiveness of various strategies is clear. (See the section on pain.)

Many people want to discuss key life events or to say goodbye to family or friends. For this to happen, if the person is in a formal institution, it may be necessary to make exceptions to practices and policies. If the person is at home, it may be necessary to create a schedule for some of these events so that the person is not excessively strained as a result of the intensity of activities.

Falls

Falls occur for a variety of reasons. For example, some people use rugs that aren't skidproof; some have orthopedic/arthritic changes that result in an altered center of gravity; some have limited visual acuity and are unable to see obstructions in their paths or have difficulty distinguishing colors that lack contrasts; some use inadequate clothing (such as loose shoes or baggy pants); and some are affected by necessary medications. Irrespective of the reason for falls, a falls assessment should be used to determine the risk of falling. Factors that can be eliminated or altered (remove the rugs or use a skidproof mat underneath; create contrast in colors; maintain exercise) should be addressed. If the patient falls, a thorough assessment should be done to determine skin breaks or abrasions, bruising, swelling, and pain. An X-ray may be needed to determine the potential damage to bone structures. Remember that if an older person falls once, he or she is likely to fall again. (See the falls inventory.)

Table 4-22   Categories and Factors in Fall Assessment

Category	Factors Indicative of Fall Potential
Age	Falls more common in elderly
Elimination	Increases as incontinence requires catheter or ostomy
Mental status	Increases with increasing confusion/disorientation
History of falls	Increases with increased reported times of falling
Activity	Increases with increased confinement
Gait	Increases with difficulty of gait
Balance	Increases with diminishing abilities of balance
Medications	Increases with the increasing of numbers of medications

Immunizations

The Centers for Disease Control and Prevention (🖱 www.cdc.gov/aging/health) specifies two immunizations that are based on age-related conditions: influenza and pneumonia. Influenza immunization is required each year. Pneumonia immunization is a one-time schedule and is particularly important for patients with chronic conditions. A third immunization, a tetanus/diphtheria booster, is required every ten years. (See 🖱 www.aarp.org for further information.) Additionally, in some situations, vaccinations for measles, mumps, and rubella (MMR), varicella (chicken pox), meningitis, and hepatitis A and B may also be recommended. For older adults who travel internationally, there may be additional requirements based on specific travel destinations.

Pain

Part 3 contains more detailed information about pain management. Because many older people have chronic pain, assessing this condition in a consistent manner is important. Two common strategies are the faces scale and the numeric scale. The faces scale shows faces ranging from a neutral position to a very pinched expression with corresponding numbers. The numeric scale usually ranges from 0 or 1 to 10 with words representing no pain to worst pain possible. Both can be shown as visuals. The numeric scale can be used orally also. Quality, duration, and frequency are also important.

Pain is a culturally influenced subjective experience. It is influenced by physiological and psychological factors. Unfortunately, it is often underassessed and poorly managed. Pain can be classified as acute or chronic. These classifications relate to time limitations; chronic is generally any pain that persists for several months. Nociceptive pain is usually localized and is the response of specific peripheral or visceral pain receptors. Neuropathic pain is typically diffuse and is related to the peripheral or central nervous systems.

PART 4

Pain assessment is a requirement of accreditation and is considered the fifth vital sign. Therefore, it holds major importance for nurses. Timing is a factor that is often overlooked. Anticipating or being on time for administration of pain medication helps control the intensity of pain. Using medication before painful events may help the patient to be better able to tolerate the event. Using nonpharmacological pain reduction treatments, such as relaxation exercises, distraction, music therapy, visualization, and heat and cold, may also be effective. Exercising, meditation, muscle relaxation, massage, guided imagery, and hypnosis are other forms of nonpharmacological pain management. They may be used singly or in combination with pharmacological agents. Evaluating the effectiveness of pain management is as important as assessing the presence of pain.

Polypharmacy

Because our society is so focused on simple and quick relief of any symptom or discomfort, the use of medications has proliferated. Many medications are beneficial. Often, however, medications have difficult side effects and thus another medication is consumed to alleviate the reaction to a prior one. This combination of multiple medications is known as *polypharmacy*. Because it is also common for older people to have multiple diagnoses, it is common to find they use multiple medications for the different conditions. Thus, the complexity of determining which medication is effective and which is precipitating untoward responses can be challenging. Additionally, multiple prescribers may provide medication regimens without knowing what other medications are being used. A medication assessment should include prescription medications, over-the-counter medications, and herbal preparations in order to determine the basic interactions among the medications.

Psychiatric and Mental Health

One of the most important aspects to successful aging is to keep mentally active. In addition to the usual thoughts such as social interaction, many strategies such as reading the newspaper, doing crossword puzzles, and doing mental exercises (such as number puzzles) have positive effects. These positive strategies are in contrast to the common problems associated with aging.

Depression   Loss is one of the developmental tasks of older adults and the intensity of loss (such as with the death of a spouse or a move from independence to dependence) or response to some medications or health conditions may precipitate depression. It is characterized by loss of interest in many activities. See the Psychiatric and Mental Health section previous to this section.

Delirium   This major state of disorientation is associated with serious conditions such as alcohol withdrawal, severe fever, or exhaustion. The treatment depends on the condition that precipitated the delirium; in the meantime, monitoring is critical.

Dementia   This term encompasses many conditions related to diminished cognitive capacity. It may be long term in onset, such as with Alzheimer's, or short term in onset, such as with a head injury. This condition seldom improves.

Restraints

As much as possible, restraints are avoided in today's practice. When they are used, they must be checked regularly and patients need to be monitored so that the minimal level of restraint is used if any is needed. Because this is such a major issue for the elderly population, although it clearly applies to other populations, most healthcare organizations have detailed policies about using, monitoring, and removing restraints. A variety of conditions are associated with the use of restraints. They include fall-proneness, confusion, pain, drug toxicity, mobility issues, and orthostatic hypotension. Therefore, when working with patients with these conditions, it is important to monitor them more closely to avoid the use of restraints.

Bed monitors (alarms that are sounded when a patient moves off of the surface) are a common strategy to prevent the use of restraints. These, however, do not prevent falls or protect patients from such. They are merely an alert system. Soft restraints take the form of cloth vests, limb or body straps, and mitts. Leather restraints may be applied, but should be avoided if possible.

If the physician order for restraints exceeds 24 hours, the physician must see the patient. Because restraints are designated for specific times (no more than 2 hours without release of the restraint), documentation must include the presence and release of the restraints. Refer to Standards of Medicare (Centers for Medicare and Medicaid) and JCAHO (Joint Commission on Accreditation of Healthcare Organizations) for details about expectations for restraints.

The most effective practice nurses can perform is managing behaviors, including wandering. These might include correcting problems that are the basis for disruptive or unsafe behavior. Maintaining fluid and electrolyte balances is an example, as is promoting sleep. Attempting to maintain a calm, relaxed environment is also important. Limit stimuli that promote disruptive or unsafe behavior. Paid sitters may also be needed.

Wandering is a special consideration associated with restraints. Healthcare facilities do not want to risk losing a patient and those who wander are at high risk for becoming lost. If the condition is preexisting prior to a hospitalization, being in a strange environment with strange sounds and people only adds to the potential for wandering. Again, limiting the stimuli in the environment is a positive strategy, as is using most of the items cited above that are not restraints. Additionally, an electronic tracking device is a strategy that can alert nurses to when a patient is leaving a room.

Safety Risks

Several risks result from the normal aging process, such as those listed here.

Table 4-23   Safety Risks for Aged Patients

Change	Potential Risk
Decreased ability of short-term memory	Possible injury, inconsistent use of medications and treatment
Decreased depth perception and visual acuity	Possible injury
Decreased tear production	Increased chance for eye infections
Diminished hearing acuity	Possible injury, possible reduction in social activities
Increased threshold for pain and touch	Possible injury and infection
Increased skin fragility and wrinkles/folds	Possible infections, dryness, cracking
Delayed reaction time	Increased potential for accidents and injury
Reduced income	Risk for basic nutrition, shelter, health care, and safety
Bone demineralization	Increased risk for fractures and for mobility
Decreased intracellular fluid	Potential for dehydration

PART 4

Skin Care

Because of all of the changes associated with aging skin, special consideration is given to nursing actions.

Hydration   Keep adequate fluid levels. Remember to consider if any fluid restrictions are necessary due to other diagnoses.

Cleanliness   Keep skin clean, dry, and moisturized. Note that it is not necessary to bathe every day. Rinse well, pat skin dry (don't rub) and apply a moisturizing lotion or cream. Avoid contact with materials that hold in moisture such as plastics and tapes.

Pressure   Prevent prolonged periods of pressure on same body structures. If the person is immobilized, turn at least every

2 hours (use lifting devices if possible; don't drag) and be sure the area is cleared of any element that could cause pressure, such as utensils, pencils, books, and food crumbs. Use supportive devices (such as special mattresses).

Circulation   Encourage activity or provide range of motion. Apply lotions in a gentle, nonvigorous massage manner.

Decubiti   Measure size, describe color, odor, drainage, and pain. Keep clean. Notify nurse manager/physician of increase in size, intensity of odor, drainage or pain.

Thermoregulation

Body temperatures of elderly people tend to be lower than younger people's. Due to decreased circulation, older people have greater difficulty responding to cold temperatures than do younger people. Hats, gloves, and warm, dry socks are especially helpful in maintaining body temperature. Additionally, decreased circulation results in drier extremities and thus the potential for drying and cracking skin is prevalent.

Older people are more susceptible to hypothermia than younger people. Encouraging them to wear warm clothes, especially socks, gloves, and a head covering, is important to prevent heat loss. In the summer, older people are also more susceptible to hyperthermia events, including heat exhaustion and heat stroke. Heat exhaustion is gradual and is evidenced by thirst, fatigue, oliguria, and confusion. Rest and fluids with salt replacement are required. Heat stroke results in extremely high body temperatures and is life-threatening. Heat stroke is evidenced by dryness and unconsciousness. Rapid cooling (preferably with a cooling blanket and without reaching a stage of shivering) is critical. In community settings, cold water and ice packs should be used, and as much clothing as possible should be removed. Fanning is also useful.

PART 5

Resources—Clinical

PART 5

Anatomy and Physiology

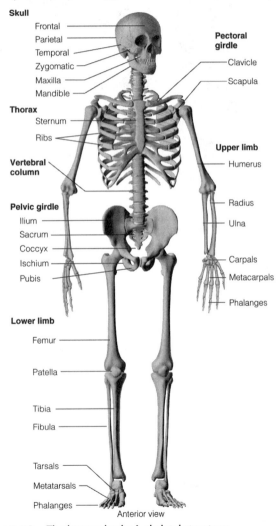

Skull
 Frontal
 Parietal
 Temporal
 Zygomatic
 Maxilla
 Mandible

Pectoral girdle
 Clavicle
 Scapula

Thorax
 Sternum
 Ribs

Vertebral column

Upper limb
 Humerus
 Radius
 Ulna

Pelvic girdle
 Ilium
 Sacrum
 Coccyx
 Ischium
 Pubis

 Carpals
 Metacarpals
 Phalanges

Lower limb
 Femur
 Patella
 Tibia
 Fibula
 Tarsals
 Metatarsals
 Phalanges

Anterior view

Figure 5-1A   The human body: A. skeletal structure.

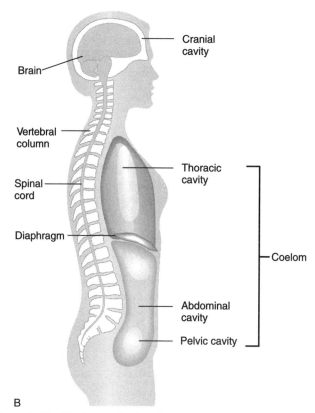

B

Figure 5-1B The human body: B. body cavities.

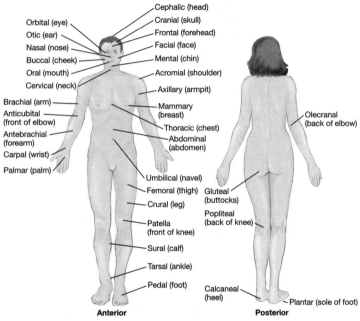

Figure 5-2 Body regions.

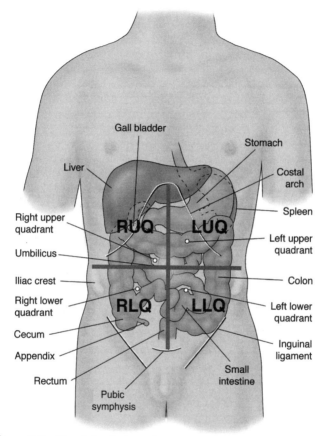

Figure 5-3   The abdominal quadrants.

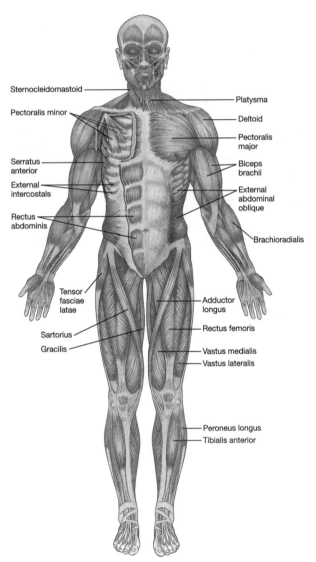

Figure 5-4 The anterior superficial muscles.

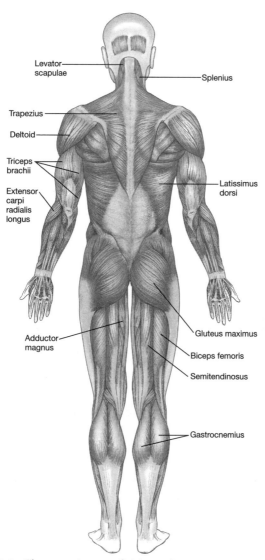

Figure 5-5 The posterior superficial muscles.

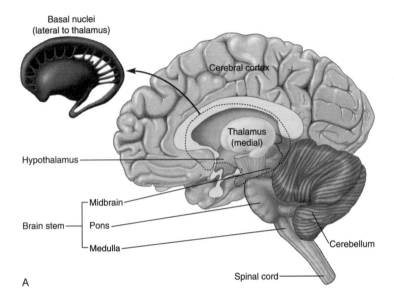

A

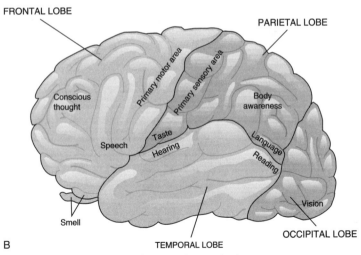

B

Figure 5-6   A. The human brain; B. the cerebral cortex.

Nerves

Cranial Nerves

(Acronym: On Old Olympus Tiny Tops a Finn and German View Some Hops)

I. Olfactory: smell. (Test by having patient close eyes and identify common odors [coffee, spices] through each nostril.)

II. Optic: vision. (Test by using standard vision screening devices for both near and far viewing.)

III. Oculomotor: eye movements. (Test by shining light directly into pupil . . . pupil constricts. Opposite pupil should constrict too. [Test by holding finger about 24 inches from the patient's nose and move the finger toward the nose . . . eyes converge and pupils constrict. See IV.])

IV. Trochlear: eye movements. (Test by holding finger about 24 inches from the patient's nose. Ask the patient to hold head still and move eyes only. Move finger horizontally, then diagonally left to right and right to left . . . smooth, symmetrical movement of eyes.)

V. Trigeminal: sensation of face, scalp, teeth and chewing. (Test by lightly touching cornea . . . blinking occurs.)

VI. Abducens: turning eyes outward. (See IV.)

VII. Facial: taste, control of facial expressions. (Test by having patient close eyes and identify the four tastes bilaterally: sweet, sour, salt and bitter . . . distinctions are made and are symmetrical.)

VIII. Auditory: hearing, sense of balance. (Test by whispering in ear about 24 inches from the ear . . . patient repeats what was said.)

IX. Glossopharyngeal: sensation of throat, taste, swallowing, secretion of saliva. (Test: Have patient stick out tongue and say "Ah" . . . symmetrical movement of soft palate and uvula. Stimulate gag reflex . . . gagging occurs. See VII.)

X. Vagus: sensations of throat and larynx, swallowing, peristalsis, heart contractions. (See IX.)

XI. Spinal Accessory: shoulder movements, turning head. (Test by having patient shrug shoulders while examiner holds hand on shoulders and presses down . . . able to shrug symmetrically. Test by having patient turn head side to side against resistance of examiner's hand . . . contraction of opposite sternomastoid muscle.)

XII. Hypoglossal: tongue movements. (Test: have patient stick out tongue . . . symmetrical response.)

Spinal Nerves

There are 31 pairs of spinal nerves:

- Cervical: 8 pairs
- Thoracic: 12 pairs
- Lumbar: 5 pairs
- Sacral: 5 pairs
- Coxygeal: 1 pair

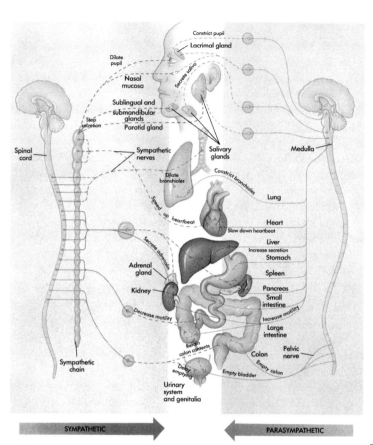

Figure 5-7 The autonomic nervous system.

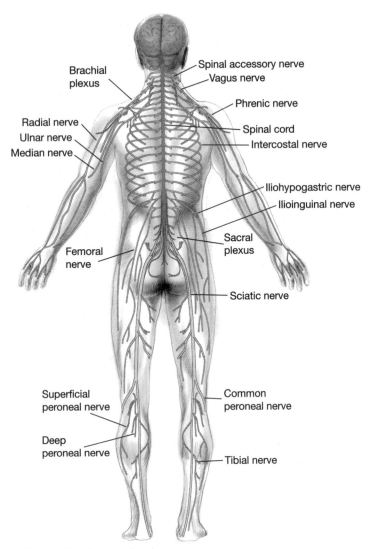

Figure 5-8   The peripheral nervous system.

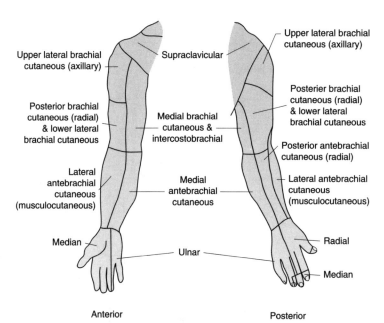

Figure 5-9 Cutaneous nerve distribution: upper limb.

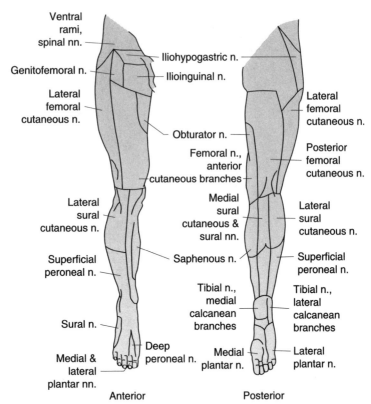

Figure 5-10 Cutaneous nerve distribution: lower limb.

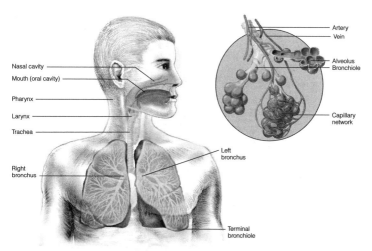

Figure 5-11a The upper and lower divisions of the respiratory system. The inset shows magnification of the alveoli, where oxygen and carbon dioxide exchange occurs.

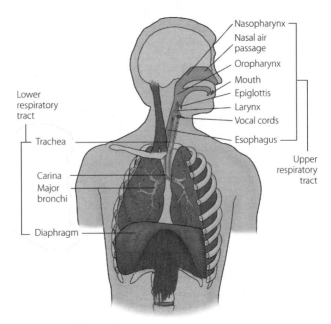

Figure 5-11b   The respiratory system.

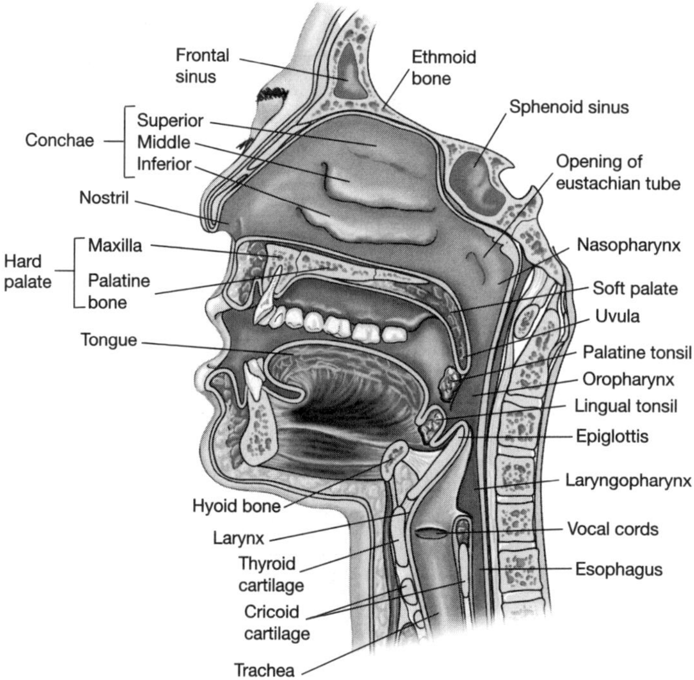

Figure 5-11c Midsagittal section of the head and neck showing the structures of the upper respiratory tract.

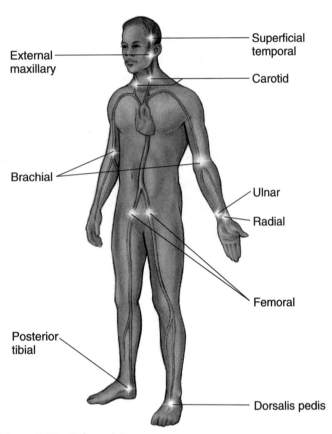

Figure 5-12   Pulse points.

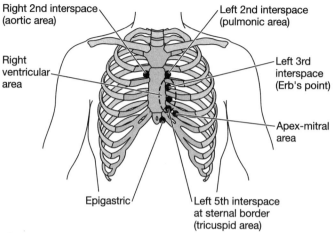

Figure 5-13 Cardiac auscultation sites.

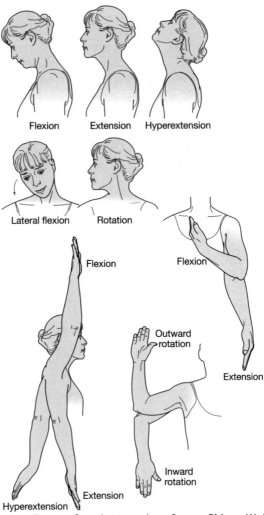

Figure 5-14   Range-of-motion exercises. *Source:* Phipps, W. J., Long, B. C., & Woods, N. F. (1995). *Medical–surgical nursing: Concepts and clinical practice* (5th ed.). St. Louis, MO: Mosby.

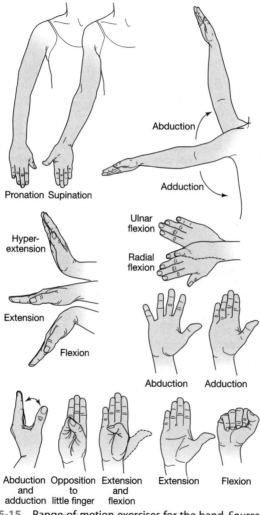

Pronation   Supination

Abduction

Adduction

Hyper-
extension

Extension

Flexion

Ulnar
flexion

Radial
flexion

Abduction   Adduction

Abduction   Opposition   Extension   Extension   Flexion
and   to   and
adduction   little finger   flexion

Figure 5-15   Range-of-motion exercises for the hand. *Source:* Phipps,
W. J., Long, B. C., & Woods, N. F. (1995). *Medical–surgical nursing: Concepts
and clinical practice* (5th ed.). St. Louis, MO: Mosby.

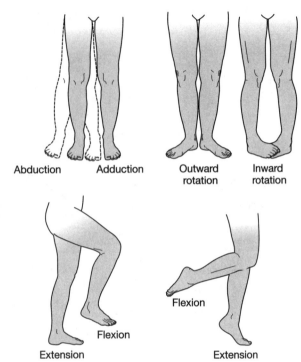

Figure 5-16   Range-of-motion exercises for the legs. *Source:* Phipps, W. J., Long, B. C., & Woods, N. F. (1995). *Medical–surgical nursing: Concepts and clinical practice* (5th ed.). St. Louis, MO: Mosby.

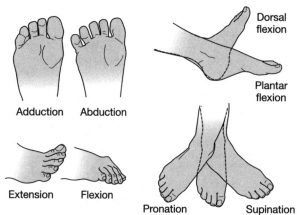

Figure 5-17 Range-of-motion exercises for the feet. *Source:* Phipps, W. J., Long, B. C., & Woods, N. F. (1995). *Medical–surgical nursing: Concepts and clinical practice* (5th ed.). St. Louis, MO: Mosby.

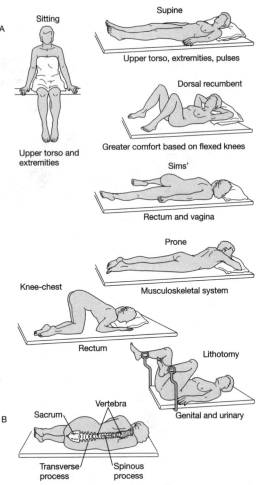

Figure 5-18   A. Examination positions; B. assessment area. *Source:* **A.** Phipps, W. J., Long, B. C., & Woods, N. F. (1995). *Medical–surgical nursing: Concepts and clinical practice* (5th ed.). St. Louis, MO: Mosby. **B.** Littleton, L. Y., & Engebretson, J. C. (2002). *Maternal, neonatal, and women's health nursing.* Clifton Park, NY: Thomson Delmar Learning.

Measurements, Calculations, Equivalents, and Conversions

Caution: Abbreviations can lead to errors. Avoid their use.

Table 5-1   Measurement Abbreviatons

Unit	Symbol	Usage
Cup	c	Volume: liquid or dry
Cubic	cc	Volume: liquid or dry
Centimeter	cm	Measure: length; circumference
Deciliter	dl	Volume: liquid or dry
Foot	ft	Measure: length; circumference
Gram	g (gm)	Weight or volume: dry
Grain	gr	Weight: dry
Drop	gtt	Measure: liquid
Inch	in	Measure: length; circumference
Kilogram	kg	Weight or volume: dry
Liter	L	Measure or volume: liquid or dry or gaseous
Pound	lb	Weight or measure: dry or liquid
Minim	m	Volume: liquid
Meter	M	Measure: length
Micrograms	mcg	Weight: dry or liquid
Milligram	mg	Weight or measure: liquid or dry
Milliliter	mm	Measure: length
Ounce	oz	Volume or measure: liquid or dry
Pint	pt	Volume or measure: liquid or dry
Quart	qt	Volume or measure: liquid or dry
Tablespoon	T (tbsp)	Volume or measure: liquid or dry
Teaspoon	t (tsp)	Volume or measure: liquid or dry
Yard	yd	Measure: length

PART 5

Table 5-2   Arabic and Roman Numerals

Arabic	Roman
1	I
2	II
3	III
4	IV
5	V
6	VI
7	VII
8	VIII
9	IX
10	X
11	XI
12	XII
13	XIII
14	XIV
15	XV
16	XVI
17	XVII
18	XVIII
19	XIX
20	XX
30	XXX
40	XL
50	L
60	LX
70	LXX
80	LXXX
90	XC
100	C

Table 5-3   Liquid Equivalents (approximate)

1 m (minim) = 1 gtt = 0.07 ml
1 ml = 1 cc = 15 m = 15 gtt = 1 g
1 dl = 100 ml = 0.1 L
4 mL = 1 dr = 60 gr
1 L = 1000 ml = 2 pt = 1 qt = 1 kg
1 t = 5 ml
1 T = 15 ml = 3 t = ½ oz
1 oz = 30 ml = 8 dr = 6 t = 2 T
1 c = 240 ml = 8 oz = ½ pt
1 pt = 480 ml = 16 oz = ½ qt
1 qt = 950 ml = 32 oz = 2 pt = 1 L

Table 5-4   Common Household Measures and Weights and Equivalents

1 teaspoon = 5 ml = 60 grains = 1 dram = ⅛ oz
1 teaspoon = ⅛ fluid oz = 1 dram
3 teaspoons = 1 Tablespoon
1 Tablespoon = ½ fluid oz = 4 drams
16 Tablespoons (liquid) = 1 cup
16 Tablespoons (dry) = 1 cup
1 cup = 8 fluid oz = ½ pint

Table 5-5   Weight Equivalents (approximate)

1 mcg = 0.001 mg
1 mg = 1000 mcg = 0.001 g = 0.017 gr
1 gr = 60 mg = 0.06 g
1 gm = 1000 mg = 15 gr
1 dr = 60 gr
1 oz = 31 gr = 0.06 lb = 0.03 kg
1 kg = 1000 gm = 2.2 lb = 34 oz

PART 5

Table 5-6 Length Equivalents (approximate)

1 mm = 0.1 cm = 0.04 in
1 cm = 10 mm = 0.4 in
1 in = 25 mm = 2.54 cm
1 ft = 305 mm = 30.5 cm = 12 in
1 M = 1000 mm = 100 cm = 39.37 in = 3.2 ft
1 yd = 91.44 cm = 36 in = 3 ft

Table 5-7 Temperature Equivalents (approximate)

Fahrenheit	Centigrade
212	100 (water boils)
105	40.56
104	40
103	39.44
102	38.89
100	37.78
99	37.22
98.6	37
98	36.67
97	36.11
96	35.56
32	0.0 (water freezes)

Table 5-8 Approximate Equivalents for Grains and Milligrams

Grains	Milligrams
$1/300$	0.2
$1/200$	0.3
$1/150$	0.4
$1/120$	0.5
$1/100$	0.6
$1/60$	1.0
$1/4$	15.0
$1/2$	30.0
1	60.0

Table 5-9 Fraction and Decimal Equivalents

$1/100 = 0.01$
$1/10 = 0.1$
$1/5 = 0.2$
$1/4 = 0.25$
$1/2 = 0.5$
$3/4 = 0.75$
$1/3 = 0.33$
$2/3 = 0.66$

Table 5-10   Time Conversions

12-Hour Time	24-Hour Time
12:00 a.m. (midnight)	2400
12:01 a.m.	0001
12:59 a.m.	0059
1:00 a.m.	0100
2:00 a.m.	0200
3:00 a.m.	0300
4:00 a.m.	0400
9:00 a.m.	0900
10:00 a.m.	1000
11:00 a.m.	1100
12:00 noon	1200
1:00 p.m.	1300
2:00 p.m.	1400
3:00 p.m.	1500
4:00 p.m.	1600
5:00 p.m.	1700
6:00 p.m.	1800
7:00 p.m.	1900
8:00 p.m.	2000
9:00 p.m.	2100
10:00 p.m.	2200
11:00 p.m.	2300
12:00 midnight	2400

Note: To change 12-hour time to 24-hour time, add 12 to the p.m. time.

Table 5-11   The Metric System

Linear Measure

 1 millimeter = 0.1 centimeter
10 millimeters = 1 centimeter
10 centimeters = 1 decimeter
10 decimeters = 1 meter
10 meters = 1 dekameter
10 dekameters = 1 hectometer
10 hectometers = 1 kilometer

Liquid Measure

 1 milliliter = 0.001 liter
10 milliliters = 1 centiliter
10 centiliters = 1 deciliter
10 deciliters = 1 liter
10 liters = 1 dekaliter
10 dekaliters = 1 hecoliter
10 hecoliters = 1 kiloliter

Weights

10 milligrams = 1 centigram
10 centigrams = 1 decigram
10 decigrams = 1 gram
10 grams = 1 dekagram
10 dekagrams = 1 hectogram
10 hectograms = 1 kilogram
100 kilograms = 1 quintal
10 quintals = 1 metric ton

Table 5-12   Making Conversions

Conversion Needed	Quick Strategy
c to ml	Multiply c by 240
cm to mm	Multiply cm by 10
cm to in	Multiply cm by 0.394
dr to ml	Multiply dr by 4
g to gr	Multiply g by 15
g to lb	Divide g by 454
g to mg	Multiply g by 1000
gr to g	Multiply gr by 0.06
gr to mg	Multiply gr by 60
in to cm	Multiply in by 2.54
in to mm	Multiply in by 25.4
kg to g	Multiply kg by 1000
kg to lb	Multiply kg by 2.2
L to ml	Multiply L by 1000
lb to kg	Multiply lb by 0.45; or divide lb by 2.2
lb to oz	Multiply lb by 16
m (minim) to ml	Multiply m by 15
mcg to mg	Divide mcg by 1000
mg to mcg	Multiply mg by 1000
ml to m	Multiply ml by 15
ml to oz	Divide ml by 30
ml to dr	Divide ml by 4
ml to t	Divide ml by 5
mm to cm	Divide mm by 10
oz to ml	Multiply oz by 30
t to ml	Multiply t by 5
T to ml	Multiply T by 15

Diagnostic and Laboratory Tests and Values

The complete evaluation of a patient often requires efficient diagnostic testing. Such tests can confirm or eliminate aspects of a differential diagnosis. Tests also allow for effective monitoring of both a disease process and the effectiveness of treatment. The normal values for various tests can vary from institution to institution, and the values for the specific institution in which the test is done should be used in evaluating the information.

Aspects of Testing

1. Standard precautions: All blood and body fluids are considered potentially infectious and the guidelines from the Centers for Disease Control and Prevention (see the reminder section in the front of this handbook) must be followed.
2. Sequencing and scheduling: When multiple tests are performed, be certain to follow the guidelines of the respective institution for the order of tests (e.g., radiographic tests that do not require contrast material should precede those that do).
3. Patient preparation: Adherence to the prescribed guidelines is critical so that tests do not have to be repeated. It is also important to counsel patients at risk for complications, address patient's fears, and educate the patient about the test. Pretest instructions should be reviewed orally, and written instructions should also be provided.
4. Proper identification: A key safety factor is verification of proper patient identification (e.g., ID band in the hospital). All specimens must have proper labeling.
5. Variables that affect tests:
   a. Age (pediatric and geriatric values may vary from adults)
   b. Gender (values may differ between the sexes)
   c. Race (this is especially true for genetic diseases)
   d. Pregnancy (significantly different values for endocrine, blood, and biochemical tests)

e. Food ingestion (several serum values are affected by food)
f. Posture (body position can affect the concentrations in the peripheral bloodstream and should be noted on the requisition slip)

Major Types of Studies

Blood   Common blood studies assess the quantity of red and white blood cells, enzymes, lipids, clotting factors, hormones, and metabolic waste products such as urea nitrogen. The results are used to diagnose multiple disorders and to assess body processes and functions.

Three methods used to obtain blood samples are:

1. Venous: Venipuncture is used to draw blood from a superficial vein (most often the antecubital fossa of the arm).
2. Arterial: This is used to measure oxygen, carbon dioxide, and pH (referred to as arterial blood gases or ABGs). Brachial or radial arteries are used if a heart catheter is not in place through which a sample may be drawn from the IV.
3. Skin punctures: Fingertips, earlobes, and heels are common sites. The heel is the most common site used for pediatric patients, especially infants, but can also be used for adults when small amounts of blood are required.

Microscopic   These examinations are used to diagnose and treat numerous diseases and infectious processes. Microbiologic specimens can be collected from tissue and organs (biopsy samples), blood, urine, wound drainage, cervical secretions, and sputum. Microscopic examinations are performed to evaluate the histology and cytology of tissues and to identify bacteria and other infecting organisms. Culture and sensitivity are important for identifying and treating infectious organisms.

Ultrasound   These tests send harmless, high-frequency sound waves into the body and record the pattern of the echo as sound waves bounce back to the transducer. These waves are converted into visual or auditory images and recorded on photographs or videotapes. Key advantages of ultrasonography include:

Noninvasive
No ionizing radiation
No risk with multiple images and repeated studies
Less expensive than CT or MRI
No contrast medium is required for testing

Stool   The waste products of digested food includes bile, mucus, shed epithelial cells, bacteria, and inorganic salts. These studies evaluate the function and integrity of the bowel. They are primarily used to evaluate patients experiencing intestinal bleeding, infections, infestations, inflammation, malabsorption, and diarrhea.

Only a small amount of stool is needed for most tests. Stool from a rectal examination may be used. The specimen does not need to be kept warm or examined immediately. Urine in the specimen can affect some tests.

Urine   Composed of water and a small percentage of solutes, urine is mostly end products of metabolism and any potentially harmful materials. Kidneys and thus urine are used to maintain normal acid/base ratio and fluid and electrolyte balance in the body. Urine specimens are painless to obtain, quick, and economic in providing significant amounts of information. A 24-hour specimen can reflect homeostasis and disease better than one random blood specimen as some products are rapidly cleared by the kidneys and may not be apparent in the blood. Many urine tests are less expensive to perform than blood tests (for example, a reagent strip or dipstick may be used to estimate glucose, albumin, hemoglobin, bile concentrations, pH, specific gravity, protein, ketone bodies, nitrates, and leukocyte esterase). Dipsticks are small strips of paper containing a chemical that reacts to products in the urine by changing color.

PART 5

Some tests (usually those for culture and sensitivity) require a "clean" specimen and this is accomplished through a midstream collection (see your institution's procedure book). Occasionally, a sterile specimen is needed and is obtained through catheterization.

Radiographic   These studies provide a picture of bodily structures because the X-rays penetrate body structures. As they pass through the structures, images are formed on photographic film which is positioned on the other side of the body. Due to radiation exposure risks, X-rays should not be performed more often than absolutely necessary.

Table 5-13 Tests and Values

Tests	Normal Range	Critical Values	Comments
Serum Chemistry Electrolytes:			
Sodium (Na)	136–145 mEq/L	**Critical:** < 120 or > 160 mEq/L	Hi: Increased diet or IV sodium in fluids, hyperaldosteronism, water loss due to vomiting or NG suction; or from sweating, burns, DI, osmotic diuresis, or use of diuretics Low: Low diet or IV intake, Addison's disease, diarrhea, vomiting, NG suction, third spacing, diuretics, chronic renal insufficiency, large volume pleural or peritoneal fluid, increased free water intake, CHF, ascites, edema
Potassium (K)	3.5–5 mEq/L	**Critical:** < 2.5 or > 6.5 mEq/L	Hi: Excess diet or IV fluids, acute or chronic renal failure, Addison's disease, hypoaldosteronism, aldosterone-inhibiting diuretics,

Table 5-13 *(continued)*

Tests	Normal Range	Critical Values	Comments
			crash injury, hemolysis, transfusion of hemolyzed blood, infection, acidosis, dehydration
			Low: Low diet or IV fluids, burns, diarrhea, emesis, diuretics, hyperaldosteronism, Cushing's syndrome, renal tubular acidosis, licorice ingestion, alkalosis, insulin, glucose, ascites, renal artery stenosis, cystic fibrosis, trauma/surgery/burns
Chloride (Cl)	90–110 mEq/L	**Critical:** < 80 or > 115 mEq/L	Hi: Dehydration, excess IV saline, metabolic acidosis, renal tubular acidosis, Cushing's syndrome, kidney failure, hyperparathyroidism, eclampsia, renal acidosis
			Low: Overhydration, CHF, emesis or GI suction, chronic diarrhea, high output GI fistula, chronic renal acidosis, metabolic acidosis, salt-

Test	Normal Value	Critical Value	Causes
			losing nephritis, Addison's disease, diuretics, low K, aldosteronism, burns
CO_2 combining power (CO_2)	24–30 mEq/L	**Critical:** < 6 mEq/L (equivalent to arterial HCO_3)	Hi: Emesis, GI suction, aldosteronism, mercurial diuretics, COPD, metabolic alkalosis Low: Chronic diarrhea, loop diuretics, renal failure, DKA, starvation, metabolic acidosis, shock (lactic acidosis)
Magnesium (Mg)	1.5–2.0 mEq/L	**Critical:** < 0.5 or > 3.0 mEq/L	Hi: Renal insufficiency, Addison's disease, MG antacids or salts, hypothyroidism Low: Malnutrition, malabsorption, hypoparathyroidism, alcoholism, chronic renal tubular disease, DKA; also associated with cardiac disease by unclear mechanism
Calcium (Ca)	Total 9.0–10.5 mg/dl Ionized 4.5–5.6 mg/dl	**Critical:** Total < 6.0 or > 13 mg/dl (½ is bound to albumin so will	Hi: Hyperparathyroidism, nonparathyroid PTH-producing tumor, metastatic tumor to bone, Paget's disease of bone, prolonged

Table 5-13 (continued)

Tests	Normal Range	Critical Values	Comments
		be low if albumin low.) Ionized is free Ca, not bound to albumin. Total Ca decreases 0.8 mg for each 1 gm decrease in albumin.	immobilization, milk-alkali syndrome, Vitamin D intoxication, lymphoma, Addison's disease, acromegaly, hyperthyroidism Low: Hypoparathyroidism, renal failure, hyperphosphatemia from renal failure, poor nutrition, Vitamin D deficiency, osteomalacia, poor absorption, pancreatitis, fat embolism, alkalosis
Kidney: Blood urea nitrogen (BUN)	10–30 mg/dl	**Critical:** > 100 mg/dl (Indicator of patient response/symptoms of renal failure. Not best indication of renal tubule function.)	Hi: Prerenal: Low volume, shock, burns, dehydration, CHF, MI, GI bleed, high-protein diet, high-protein catabolism, starvation, sepsis Renal: Renal disease/failure, nephrotoxic drug Postrenal: Azotemia, stone obstruction, bladder obstruction (BPH, tumor)

Creatinine, serum	0.5–1.5 mg/dl (most accurate indicator of renal tubule function)	Low: Liver failure, overhydration, malnutrition/malabsorption causing negative nitrogen balance, pregnancy, nephritic syndrome Hi: Glomerulonephritis, pyelonephritis, ATN, UTI, shock, dehydration, CHF, diabetic nephropathy, nephritis, rhabdomyolysis, acromegaly, gigantism Low: Debilitation, low muscle mass (MS, MG)
Liver: Ammonia (NH$_3$)	30–70 µg/dl	Hi: Primary hepatocellular disease, Reye's syndrome, asparagines intoxication, portal hypertension, severe cardiac cirrhosis, hemolytic disease of newborn, GI bleed or obstruction with mild liver disease, hepatic encephalopathy/coma, genetic metabolic disorder of urea cycle Low: Essential or malignant hypertension, hypermethionemia

Table 5-13   *(continued)*

Tests	Normal Range	Critical Values	Comments
Albumin, serum, and total protein	3.8–4.5 g/dl 6–8 g/dl (takes 1–2 weeks after insult or therapy to show changes in values)		Hi: Dehydration Low: Liver disease, protein-losing enteropathies and nephropathies, third spacing, malnutrition, SLE, overhydration, inflammatory disease, familial idiopathic dysproteinemia
Bilirubin	Total: 0.2–1.3 mg/dl Indirect: 0.1–1 mg/dl Direct: 0.1–0.3 mg/dl	**Critical:** > 12 mg/dl	Hi direct: Gallstones, hepatic duct occlusion, cholestasis from drugs, congenital defects Hi indirect: Erythroblastosis fetalis, transfusion reaction, sickle cell anemia, hemolytic jaundice or anemia, pernicious anemia, large-volume blood transfusion, resolution of large hematoma, hepatitis, cirrhosis, sepsis, neonatal, congenital defects of conjugation Low: Not significant

Test	Values	Significance
Alanine aminotransferase (ALT), formerly serum glutamic pyruvic transaminase (SGPT)	5–35 IU/L or 8–20 U/L; slightly higher in elders, men, African-Americans; up to 70 IU/L in infants	Hi: Hepatitis, hepatic necrosis or ischemia, cirrhosis, cholestasis, hepatic tumor, hepatotoxic drugs, bile duct obstruction, severe burns and trauma, myositis, pancreatitis, MI, mononucleosis, shock Low: Not significant
Aspartate aminotransferase (AST), formerly serum glutamic oxaloacetic transaminase (SGOT)	7–40 U/L; slightly higher for infants, females, elders	Hi: MI, cardiac surgery, hepatitis, hepatic metastasis, hepatic necrosis, hepatic cirrhosis, drug-induced liver damage, hepatic surgery, trauma, burns, muscular dystrophy, recent seizures, heat stroke, myopathy, myositis, acute hemolytic anemia, acute pancreatitis Low: Acute renal disease, beriberi, DKA, pregnancy, chronic hemodialysis
Alkaline phosphatase (ALP)	30–120 U/L; slightly higher for elders. Up to	Hi: Cirrhosis, biliary obstruction, liver tumor, third trimester pregnancy, bone tumor, healing fracture,

Table 5-13 *(continued)*

Tests	Normal Range	Critical Values	Comments
	300 ImU/ml for children and teens.		hyperparathyroidism, Paget's disease, rheumatoid arthritis, intestinal ischemia or infarction, MI, sarcoidosis
			Low: Hypophosphatemia, malnutrition, milk-alkali syndrome, pernicious anemia, scurvy
Lactic dehydrogenase (LDH)	45–90 U/Lm LDH-1: 17–27% LDH-2: 27–37% LDH-3: 18–25% LDH-4: 3–8% LDH-5: 0–5%		Hi total: Neoplasm, shock, heat stroke, collagen disease Hi LDH-1 & slight LDH-2: MI Hi LDH-2 & LDH-3: Pulmonary disease or renal parenchymal disease, or lymphoma or RES disease Hi LDH-5: Hepatic disease or skeletal muscle disease/injury, or intestinal ischemia/infarction Hi LDH-1: RBC disease or testicular tumors Hi LDH-4: Pancreatitis

Prothrombin time (PT)	12–15 sec. Full anticoagulant therapy: 1.5–3 × control	**Critical:** > 20 sec.	Hi: Liver disease, hereditary factor deficit, Vitamin K deficiency, bile duct obstruction, Coumadin OD (PT), heparin (PTT), DIC, massive blood transfusion, salicylate intoxication Low: Not significant for PT
Partial thrombo-plastin time (PTT) Activated PTT (aPTT)	60–70 seconds 30–40 seconds Anticoagulant therapy: 1.5–3 × control	**Critical:** PTT > 100 sec., aPTT > 70 sec.	PTT: Early DIC, extensive cancer
Pancreas: Lipase	0–160 U/L (method dependent)		Hi: Pancreatitis, pancreatic cancer or pseudocyst, acute cholecystitis, cholangitis, duct obstruction, renal failure, bowel obstruction/ infarction, salivary gland inflammation/tumor, peptic ulcer disease Low: Not significant

Table 5-13 (continued)

Tests	Normal Range	Critical Values	Comments
Amylase	0–130 U/L; lower for newborns, slightly higher in pregnancy or elders		Hi: Pancreatitis, GI disease (perforation, obstruction), cholecystitis, mumps, ruptured ectopic pregnancy, renal failure, DKA, pulmonary infarction, after endoscopic retrograde pancreatography Low: Hemolytic anemia, chronic blood loss, chronic renal failure
Diabetes mellitus: Blood sugar	70–110 mg/dl; increased for elders	**Critical:** < 40 and > 400 mg/dl	Hi: DM with poor control, all causes of high blood sugar, postsplenectomy, pregnancy Low: Hemolytic anemia, chronic blood loss, chronic renal failure
Glycosylated hemoglobin	4–6% Good diabetic control: 7% Fair diabetic control: 10%		Hi: DM with poor control, all causes of high blood sugar, postsplenectomy, pregnancy Low: Hemolytic anemia, chronic blood loss, chronic renal failure

Poor diabetic control: 13–20%
Affected by long-term variations. Takes 3 weeks after sustained elevation and 4 weeks after low values to change.

Cardiac creatine kinase (CK, CPK) and isoenzymes (CK-MM, CK-MB, CK-BB)

Male: 5–55 U/L
Female: 5–35 U/L
CK-MM: 100%
CK-MB: 0%
CK-BB: 0%
Elevates in 4–8 hours, peaks 12–36 hours, lasts 72 hours. CK-MB 86% specific to MI

Hi: CK-BB: CNS disease, trauma, ECT therapy, adenocarcinoma, pulmonary infarction

Hi: CK-MB: Acute MI, cardiac surgery, defibrillation, myocarditis, ventricular dysrhythmias, cardiac ischemia

Hi: CK-MM: Rhabdomyolysis, muscular dystrophy, myositis, recent surgery or trauma, electromyography, IM injections, delirium tremens, malignant hyperthermia, recent

Table 5-13 (continued)

Tests	Normal Range	Critical Values	Comments
Toxic screens	*Acetaminophen:* Levels increase up to 96 hours. Symptoms of hepatic toxicity: Treat with Mucomyst. Salicylates: 150 mg/kg dose. Rx: Gastric lavage, activated charcoal, alkalization of serum & urine, correct fluid &		seizures, ECT therapy, shock, hypokalemia, hypothyroidism Low: Not significant Nursing history: Time of ingestion, amount, Rx prior to arrival, prior medical history, pregnancy status, current signs and symptoms, risk factors (varies with substance). Treatment: Induced emesis is rarely used and should not be used in many situations. Gastric lavage and activated charcoal: Effective up to 6 hours for selected substances. Cathartics effective for selected substances after 6 hours. Dialysis necessary for some levels of some substances.

electrolyte imbalance, hemodialysis in extremes.

Ibuprofen: > 300 mg/kg dose

Rx: Gastric lavage, activated charcoal

Calcium channel antagonists: Symptoms wax & wane for at least 24 hours.

Rx: lavage, activated charcoal, pacing, calcium, catecholamines

General care: ABCs, VS, safety, education for prevention.

Hi glucose: Isopropyl alcohol, iron

Low glucose: Acetaminophen, methanol, insulin, ETOH

Red urine: Hematuria, myoglobinuria, pyrvinium, Dilantin, phenothiazine, mercury, lead, food pigment in beets and blackberries

Brown/red-brown urine: Porphyria, urobilinogen, nitrofurantoin, furazolidone, metronizole, aloe, seaweed

Orange urine: Refampin, phenazopyridine (Pyridium), sulfasalazine (Azulfidine)

Radiographic meds: Chloral hydrate, heavy metals, iron, phenothiazine, enteric-coated tablets

Table 5-13 (continued)

Tests	Normal Range	Critical Values	Comments
	Cyclic anti-depressants: S&S may peak in under 60 minutes. Serum levels may be false low. Rx: Gastric lavage, activated charcoal, cardiac antidysrhythmics, alkalization of serum, fluid support. *Digoxin:* Peaks 30 min. to 12 hours post ingestion. Rx: Lavage, activated charcoal,		Breath odor: Alcohol: Ethanol, chloral hydrate, phenols Acetone: Acetone, salicylate, isopropyl alcohol Bitter almond: Cyanide Coal gas: Carbon monoxide Garlic: Arsenic, phosphorus. Organophosphate Nonspecific: Consider inhalant abuse Oil of wintergreen: Methyl salicylates

correct electrolyte imbalances, pacing, cardiac antidysrhythmics. Antidote: Digoxin immune Fab (Digibind).

Theophylline: Risk of seizures for serum levels > 20 mg/ml. Rx: Lavage, activated charcoal, hemodialysis.

Iron: > 20 mg/kg toxic dose. 300 mg/kg lethal dose. Persists up to 96 hours. Rx: Emesis, lavage, bowel irrigation,

Table 5-13 (continued)

Tests	Normal Range	Critical Values	Comments
	chelation, gastric surgery to remove bezoar. *Lead:* Usually secondary to pica. Also high lead content in many "street drugs." Rx: Whole bowel irrigation & cathartics, chelation therapy for levels > 45 mcg/dl. *Pesticides:* Rx: Decontamination. Many have antidote of at-		

ropine or prali-
doxime. Protect
care staff.

*Petroleum
distillates:*
Symptoms as in-
halation injury.
Rx: intubation,
ventilation, de-
contamination.

Alcohol (ETOH):
Toxic > 300%.
Ingestion of
1 ml/kg results
in toxicity in 2
hours.
Rx: ABCs

Cocaine: Signifi-
cant cardiac
symptoms in-
cluding acute
MI up 14 days
after ingestion.

Table 5-13 *(continued)*

Tests	Normal Range	Critical Values	Comments
	Rx: Lavage, activated charcoal, MgSO$_4$ for dysrhythmias, benzodiazepines for seizures & agitation. Also give Narcan for commonly associated opiate abuse. *Narcotics/opiates:* Rx: ABCs *Narcan inhalants:* Rx: ABCs, O$_2$, support ventilation *Jimsonweed:* Rx: Gastric lavage,		

activated charcoal, physostigmine in severe anticholinergic toxicity.

CBC:

Red blood cells (RBCs)

Male: 4.5–6 × 10^6/µl

Female: 4.5 × 10^6/µl

Hi: Erythrocytosis, congenital heart disease, COPD, polycythemia vera, severe dehydration, hemoglobinopathies

Low: Anemia, hemoglobinopathies, cirrhosis, hemolytic anemia, hemorrhage, disease, normal pregnancy (dilutional), rheumatoid-vascular-collagen diseases, lymphoma, multiple myeloma, leukemia, Hodgkin's disease

RBC Indices

Mean corpuscular volume (MCV)

82–98 µl

Hi: Pernicious anemia, folic acid deficiency, antimetabolite therapy, alcoholism, chronic liver disease

Low: Iron deficiency, thalassemia, chronic illness

Table 5-13 *(continued)*

Tests	Normal Range	Critical Values	Comments
Mean corpuscular hemoglobin (MCH)	27–33 pg		Hi: Macrocytic anemia Low: Macrocytic anemia, hypochromic anemia
Mean corpuscular hemoglobin concentration (MCHC)	32–36%		Hi: Spherocytosis, intravascular hemolysis, clod agglutinins Low: Iron deficiency anemia, thalassemia
Hemoglobin (HgB)	Male: 13.5–18 g/dl Female: 12–16 g/dl		Low: Anemia, hemoglobinopathy, cirrhosis, hemorrhage, dietary deficiency, bone marrow failure, prosthetic valves, renal disease, normal pregnancy (dilutional), rheumatoid-vascular-collagen diseases, lymphoma, multiple myeloma, leukemia, Hodgkin's disease. Hi: Erythrocytosis, congenital heart disease, severe COPD, polycythemia vera, severe dehydration

Hematocrit (Hct)	Male: 40–54%	Low: (same as hemoglobin)
	Female: 38–47%	Hi: (same as hemoglobin)
Platelets (thrombo-cytes)	150,000–400,000/μl	Low: Hypersplenism, hemorrhage, immune thrombocytopenia, leukemia and other myelofibro-sis disorders, thrombotic thrombo-cytopenia, Grave's disease, inherited disorders, DIC, systemic lupus erythematosus, pernicious anemia, hemolytic anemia, cancer chemotherapy, infection
		Hi: Malignant disorders, poly-cythemia vera, postsplenectomy syndrome, rheumatoid arthritis, iron deficiency anemia, following hemorrhagic anemia, immune re-sponse to heparin (white clot syndrome)

Table 5-13 *(continued)*

Tests	Normal Range	Critical Values	Comments
Leucocytes (WBCs)	4,000–11,000/µl		Low: Drug toxicity, bone marrow failure, overwhelming infections, dietary deficiency, autoimmune disease, hypersplenism Hi: Infection or inflammation, leukemic neoplasias, other malignancy, trauma, stress, hemorrhage, tissue necrosis, dehydration, thyroid storm, steroid use
WBC differential	Neutrophils 50–70%	**Critical:** Absolute neutrophil count (ANC) < 1000/mm^3 ANC = WBC × (neutrophils + bands)/100	Low neutrophils: Neutropenia, aplastic anemia, dietary deficiency, overwhelming sepsis (accompanied at first by increased bands and then by decreased), viral infections, radiation therapy, Addison's disease, drug therapy

Lymphocytes
20–40%

Monocytes
4–8%

Hi neutrophils: Neutrophilia, stress, acute bacterial infection (usually with increased bands), myelocytic leukemia, trauma, Cushing's syndrome, rheumatic fever, thyroiditis, rheumatoid arthritis, ketoacidosis, gout, eclampsia

Low lymphocytes: Leukemia, sepsis, immunodeficiency disease, lupus erythematosus, late stage HIV, drug therapy, radiation therapy, nutrition deficit

Hi lymphocytes: Chronic bacterial infection, viral infection, lymphocytic leukemia, multiple myeloma, mononucleosis, radiation, hepatitis

Low monocytes: Prednisone

Hi monocytes: Chronic inflammatory disorders, viral infections, tuberculosis, chronic ulcerative colitis, parasites (malaria)

Table 5-13 *(continued)*

Tests	Normal Range	Critical Values	Comments
	Eosinophils 2–4%		Low eosinophils: Increased adreno-corticoid production
			Hi eosinophils: Parasitic infections, allergic reactions, eczema, leukemia, autoimmune disease
	Basophils 0–2%		Low basophils: Acute allergy, hyperthyroidism, stress
			Hi basophils: Myeloproliferative disease, leukemia
	Bands (immature neutrophils) 0%		Low bands: Normal; in combination with low neutrophils, exhausted immune system
			Hi bands: Bacterial infection, severe inflammation, stress, trauma, hemorrhage
Culture & Sensitivity	No growth Normal flora		

Cultures for sexually transmitted diseases (STDs)	Preliminary reports: 24 hours
	Bacterial cultures: 48–72 hrs
	Fungus & tuberculosis: 6–8 weeks
	Microscopic examination of vaginal, urethral, anal, or throat cultures
	Organisms:
	  Gonorrhea
	  Chlamydia
	  Herpes
	    genitalis
	  Syphilis
	  Hepatitis virus
	  HIV
	  Trichomonas
	  Scabies
	  Lice
	  Chancroid
		Undiagnosed STDs in pregnancy can cause conjunctivitis, pneumonia, neonatal blindness, neonatal neurologic injury, or death to the infant during birth	Normal is absence of any designated organisms. If organisms are present, treat with sensitivity-specific antibiotics.

Obtaining and Processing Specimens for Culture and Sensitivity

1. Blood: Follow policies and procedures for the facility in which you are practicing. Usual practice is to:
   a. Clean site with iodine solution.
   b. Draw specimens from two sites.
   c. Change needles prior to injecting into culture bottles or vials.
   d. Clean tops of bottles or vials with iodine solution.
   e. Transport to lab within 30 minutes.
2. Wound:
   a. Thoroughly irrigate wound with sterile saline and dry with sterile gauze.
   b. Use sterile cotton swab to depress center of wound tissue until swab is wet; two swabs are preferred.
   c. For large wounds, culture several areas with particular attention focused on areas with increased exudates.
   d. Do *not* sample wound edges.
3. Throat:
   a. Swab posterior pharynx and areas of inflammation, exudate, or ulceration.
   b. Use two sterile swabs if possible.
   c. Send to lab within 30 minutes.
4. Sputum:
   a. Collect first morning specimen.
   b. Have patient rinse mouth with water prior to coughing.
   c. Specimen must be deep lung cough, not saliva.
   d. Send to lab within 30 minutes.
5. Stool:
   a. Can be collected randomly
   b. Only a small amount (no more than an inch) is needed.
   c. There should be *no urine* in the specimen.
   d. Can be collected from the glove used in a rectal exam
   e. Send to lab as soon as collected.

Nursing Priorities

1. Obtain cultures when the results would alter care and treatment
2. If the culture is done on an invasive device such as a central line catheter, a Foley catheter, chest tube, drain, or other device, culture only when there are signs of infection and the results can guide choice and course of antibiotics.
3. When clinical signs of infection exist (e.g., exudates, inflammation, WBC changes, or elevated temperature), place patient on isolation while waiting for C & S results.
4. Use standard precautions in the care of all patients and in obtaining all specimens.

Human Development

The dimensions of growth and development in human beings include cognitive development, personal-social-emotional development, developmental tasks, and physical development (growth charts for birth through young adulthood are found on pages 570–576):

Cognitive: Changes in the intellectual processes of thinking, learning, remembering, judging, problem solving, and communicating. Both heredity and the developmental processes are included.

Personal-social-emotional: The development of attachment, security, trust, affection, and love as well as emotions, feelings, and temperament. It includes such concepts as self, autonomy, stress, acting-out behaviors, the socialization process, moral development, and relationships with family and peers.

Developmental Tasks: A combination of living, growing, and individual needs. This creates a *task* that arises at specific periods and, when successfully achieved, leads to happiness, a sense of accomplishment, and success with later tasks. Likewise, failure in the task leads to individual unhappiness, disapproval by society, and greater difficulty with later tasks.

Physical: Genetic factors, physical growth of all parts/systems of the body, motor development and associated changes, and some related topics such as sexual functioning.

Physical Development

Infancy

See gestational age charts (p. 570).

Development is cephalocaudal (begins with the head and proceeds downward)
See head circumference and growth charts (pp. 571–576)
Physical findings:
- Prone position: pelvis high, knees under the abdomen
- Supine: arms and legs flexed
- Head lags when pulled to a sitting position; fully rounded back

Average weight gain is 3–5 oz weekly until 6 months. There is very rapid growth in this period and for the first year.
Infants communicate by crying.

Early Childhood

The Denver Developmental Screening Tool (DDST) was designed at the University of Colorado Health Science Center and first published in 1967. A standardized test (DDST2), it is administered to well children between birth and 6 years of age using standard test materials consisting of a ball of red wool, a box of raisins, a rattle with a handle, a small bottle, a bell, a tennis ball, and 8 1-inch blocks. Test results fall into four categories: personal-social, fine motor adaptive, language, and gross motor movement. Denver Developmental Materials, Inc. www.denverii.com

Table 5-14 Development During Infancy and Early Childhood

2 months	Lifts head for short periods when prone. Visually follows moving objects
	Smiles and frowns
	Coos
3 months	Turns back to side
	Sits with support
	Can focus on own hands
	Recognizes parent
	Communicates by crying and squealing
4 months	Turns back to prone position
	Lifts head and chest 90° and bears weight on forearms
	When sitting, holds head up
	Reaches for objects, not usually successfully
	Grasps objects with both hands
	Places hands to his or her mouth
	Plays with his or her fingers
	Laughs aloud
	Makes consonant sounds
5 months	Turns from abdomen to back
	Holds object in one hand and reaches for another object with other hand
	Plays with toes
	Puts feet into mouth
6 months	Sits alone; leans forward on both hands
	Reaches for and grasps objects with whole hand
	Extends arms when he or she wishes to be picked up
	Searches for lost objects (briefly)
	First fear of strangers appears
	Brief episodes of peek-a-boo
	Begins to make wordlike sounds
	Birth weight has doubled
	Average weekly gain is 3–5 oz during 6–18 mos.

Table 5-14 (*continued*)

	Begins teething
7 months	Begins to crawl
	Bears weight on feet when placed upright
	Transfers object from one hand to other
8 months	Pulls to standing position
	Sits alone without support
	Releases object intentionally
	Picks objects up with fingers
	More obvious stranger anxiety
	Says *dada* without meaning
9 months	Walks sideways while holding on
	Crawls a lot
	Can bang two blocks together
	Attempts to feed self
	Searches for objects
10 months	May begin to walk
	May begin to climb
	Pulls to standing position
	Makes pincer grasp with hand
	Demonstrates dominance of one hand
	Plays pat-a-cake
	Initiates peek-a-boo game
	May say 1 or 2 words meaningfully
11 months	Cooperates in putting on clothes
	Attempts use of spoon at meals
	Follows simple direction
	Understands the word *no*
	Shakes head *no*
12 months	Walks alone or with a parent holding on hand
	Falls frequently while learning walking
	Drinks from a cup
	Points with one finger
	Can pull off socks

	Birth weight has tripled
	Birth length has increased by 50%
15 months	Walks without assistance
	Pulls or pushes toys
	Throws ball overhanded
	Stacks blocks at least 2 blocks high
	Uses crayons or pencil
18 months	Runs clumsily
	Jumps with both feet
	Stacks blocks 3–4 high
	Motor development of some anal and urinary sphincters
	Says about 10 words
2 years	Runs well
	Climbs stairs with both feet on each step
	Attains consistent bladder and bowel control
	Names some familiar objects words
	Combines 2–3 words into phrases
	Has vocabulary of approximately 300 words
	Weighs about 4 times birth weight
	Weight gain is 4–6 lb/yr
	Has attained about $\frac{1}{2}$ expected adult height
	Picks up object from floor without falling
	Points to objects upon request
	Can turn pages
	Knows own name and sex
	Cuts milk teeth
Early childhood (3 to 5 years)	**Large muscle motor development** **Three years** Jumps 12 in Balances on one foot Hops up to three times Catches ball using body Climbs stairs, alternating feet Rides a tricycle Can push a wagon while using one foot

Table 5-14   (*continued*)

Four years

Broad jumps 15–24 inches

Hops up to six times

Catches a ball

Five years

Broad jumps 28–36 inches

Can skip

Hops on one foot (up to 16 times)

Catches a small ball—hands only

Walks downstairs unaided, using alternating feet

Can walk a balance beam

Small muscle motor development

Three years

Copies a circle

Draws a straight line

Eats with a spoon

Smears paint

Can pour from a pitcher

Four years

Draws shapes and simple stick figures

Draws a person

Dresses self

Makes crude letters

Can build buildings with blocks

Use scissors to cut along a line

Five years

Copies squares

Strings beads

Fastens visible buttons

Fastens zipper

May be able to tie shoelaces

Further Physical Development

Refer to growth charts (pp. 570–576).

In the childhood years, growth is more linear. There are wide individual differences in growth patterns. Superior nutrition and health care promote taller children. This is a socio-cultural phenomenon; for example, middle class children eat better than lower socioeconomic group children. Not all body parts grow at the same rate. Growth proceeds from the head to the toe or downward (cephalocaudal principle).

The following table discusses three of these major areas by age group from birth to death and is divided in the following way:

Infancy (the first 2 years)
Early childhood (3 to 5 years)
Middle childhood (6 to 11 years)
Adolescence (12 to 19 years)
Early adulthood (20 to 29 years)
Middle adulthood (30 to 59 years)
Late adulthood (60 years and over)

Table 5-15   Development Through the Life Span

Infancy to Two Years

Cognitive Development	Personal-Social-Emotional Development	Developmental Tasks
• Through senses and action, begin to develop an understanding of symbols and objects • Cooing and babbling lead to language, one and two words • Learning capacity, recognition, and memory from birth	• Sense of self, self-recognition and gender awareness develop gradually • Temperament becomes basis of personality • Conflict between trust versus mistrust • Social from birth • Attachment to caregiver (7 mos.) then separation and stranger anxiety • Social skills with parents and peers; simple play; focuses on the family	• Learn to take solid foods • Learn to walk • Learn to talk

Early Childhood (2–5 years)

Cognitive Development	Personal-Social-Emotional Development	Developmental Tasks
• Egocentric in thinking, heavily influenced by perception rather than by the logic and reality of the situation • Memory ability increases; strategic and recall still limited • Major advances in understanding symbolic thinking, language, and vocabulary growth	• Ego begins to develop, superego in the later period • Rapid development of gender roles • Beginning internalization of moral standards toward the end of this period, but still fairly egocentric • Family relationships central to child's social life • Increased ability to cooperate with others and to participate in social play • First exposure to school at the end of this period • Conflicts of autonomy versus shame and initiative versus guilt	• Learns to control the elimination of body wastes • Learns sex differences and sexual modesty • Forms concepts about and learns language to describe social and physical reality • Begins to read • Learns to distinguish right from wrong and begins to develop a conscience

Table 5-15 *(continued)*

	Middle and Late Childhood (6–11 years)	
Cognitive Development	**Personal-Social-Emotional Development**	**Developmental Tasks**
• Can apply logic to physical objects but not to abstract ideas	• Libido dormant and child associates with same sex peers	• Learns physical skills necessary for ordinary games
• Increased use of rehearsal as a memory strategy; recall performance improves	• Main conflict of industry vs. inferiority	• Builds wholesome attitudes toward the self as a growing organism
• IQ scores stabilize	• Personality stable	• Learns to get along with peers
• Continued growth of vocabulary; pronunciation improves	• Strong gender role behavior	• Learns appropriate sex-linked social roles
• Reading and writing skills develop	• Internalizing moral standards increases, usually focused on consequences to self	• Develops functional reading, writing, and calculating skills
	• Close same sex friendships forming	• Develops concepts needed in everyday living
	• Play is primarily organized games with rules	• Develops conscience, morality, and values
	• School and television important socializing agents	• Achieves personal independence
		• Develops attitudes toward social groups and institutions

Adolescence (12–19 years)

Cognitive Development	Personal-Social-Emotional Development	Developmental Tasks
• Sophisticated cognitive skills, particularly in areas of expertise • Develops thinking that is relativistic and pragmatic	• Libido emerges; ego functions according to reality principle, balancing the demands of the id and superego • Conflict focuses on identity vs. role confusion • Identity formation, including sexual, political, ethnic, and religious identities, begins in earnest and will continue into early adulthood • Moral reasoning focuses on judgments of others and social standards • Peer involvement and conformity peaks • Increased autonomy from parents	• Achieves new and more mature relationships with peers of both sexes • Achieves a sex-appropriate social role • Learns to accept one's physique and uses the body effectively • Achieves emotional independence from parents and other adults • Prepares for marriage and family life • Prepares for an economic career • Acquires values and an ethical system as a guide to behavior; develops an ideology

Table 5-15 *(continued)*

	• Advanced schooling and careers explored	• Desires and achieves socially responsible behavior
	Early Adulthood (20–30 years)	
Cognitive Development	**Personal-Social-Emotional Development**	**Developmental Tasks**
• Develops sophisticated cognitive skills, especially in areas of expertise • Develops thinking that is relativistic and pragmatic	• Psychosocial conflict focused on intimacy vs. isolation • Work continues on identity achievement • Moral reasoning grounded in social standards and on judgment of others • Personality fairly stable • Divergence of family roles by gender • Careers begun and job changes common • Romantic relations form; marriage and family formation common	• Selects mate • Learns to live with a marriage partner • Starts a family • Rears children • Manages a house • Begins an occupation • Takes on civic responsibility • Finds a congenial social group

- Period of marked change, high risk of divorce and psychological problems

Middle Adulthood (40–64 years)

Cognitive Development	Personal-Social-Emotional Development	Developmental Tasks
• Stable intellectual functioning	• Conflict focused on generativity vs. stagnation	• Helps teenage children become responsible and happy adults
• Peak expertise and creativity	• Continued personality stability	• Achieves adult social and civic responsibility
• Perceptual skills begin to decline	• Midlife transition possible for some, but not for most	• Reaches and maintains satisfactory performance in an occupation or career
• Well-maintained knowledge-based performance	• Gender roles more similar for spouses	• Develops adult leisure activities
• Some increased interference in word recall	• Children have left home, and grandparenting begins	• Relates to spouse as a person
	• High levels of responsibility for younger and older generations	• Accepts and adjusts to physical changes of middle age
	• Career stability and peak productivity	• Adjusts to aging parents

Table 5-15 *(continued)*

	Late Adulthood (65 years and older)	
Cognitive Development	**Personal-Social-Emotional Development**	**Developmental Tasks**
• Declines in cognition common, but not inevitable	• Psychosocial conflict is focused on integrity vs. despair	• Adjusts to decreasing physical strength and health
• Learning slows, use of memory strategies and recall decline	• Maintains core personality traits, self-esteem, and levels of life satisfaction	• Adjusts to retirement and reduced income
• Recognition, memory, and language skills well maintained in normal aging	• Maintains sense of self through selective optimization with compensation	• Adjusts to death of spouse
• Intellectual skills decline if not used and practiced	• Continued close ties to family and friends	• Establishes an explicit affiliation with one's age group
	• Smooth transition to retirement	• Establishes satisfactory living arrangements
	• High marital satisfaction among married couples	
	• Adjusts to death of spouse, especially women	

Sexual Development

Many male babies have erections, often occurring during feeding and sleep, and not necessarily due to penile stimulation. Female infants have sexual responses as evidenced by the presence of vaginal secretions and clitoral erection during the first 24 hours of life. In the first year of life, infants discover their bodies. During this exploration, they randomly touch their genitals and discover that touching is pleasurable.

Preschool children are curious, in general, and explore their bodies. Both boys and girls are fascinated with toilet training and curious about the differences between boys and girls. They peek at one another's bodies. Although this behavior is fairly common and normal, it is a concern when older children are involved with the younger children. Children should be taught to report sexual requests from older children or adults to the parents or responsible adult, particularly when there are requests to take off clothes or to touch genitals.

Children are interested in physical sexual development, human reproduction, and sexual intercourse. The wonder of a child is the ability to ask open and detailed questions about sexuality; and sometimes this makes adults and older children uncomfortable. To teach children about sexuality prior to puberty is a positive and constructive opportunity.

Table 5-16 Sexual Development

Time	Girls	Boys
Onset (as early as 9 years)	Ovarian enlargement begins	Testicular enlargement begins
	Breasts develop to "bud" stage	Seminiferous tubules canalize
	Fine, downy, straight pubic hair appears	Primary spermatocytes appear
		Fine, downy, straight pubic hair appears
A year or more later	Pigmentation of the areolae	Secondary spermatocytes present
	Pubic hair now coarser and curling	Progressive enlargement of penis
		Pubic hair now coarser and curling
A year or more later	Relative increase beginning in pelvis diameter	Enlargement in larynx beginning
	Menarche; first cycles may not produce ova	First ejaculation
A year or more later	Full reproductivity	Mature spermatozoa
	Sweat and sebaceous glands are active	Axillary hair present
		Sweat and sebaceous glands are active

Theories of Development

Freud—Psychosexual Theory of Development

Freud established the relationship between sexuality and personality. He used the term *psychosexual* to describe any sensual pleasure. This particularly applies to childhood when certain areas of the body assume significance as new areas of sensual pleasure.

Oral stage (birth to 1 year): The major source of pleasure for infants is oral, such as sucking, biting, chewing, and vocalizing. Infants may prefer one over the other, and this preference may indicate personality development.

Anal stage (1 to 3 years): As sphincter muscles develop and children are able to control (expel or withhold) fecal matter, pleasure centers develop in the anal region. Approaches taken to toilet training can impact personality development.

Phallic stage (3 to 6 years): During this stage, the genitals, which are increasingly sensitive, capture the interest of the child. Differences in the sexes are recognized and are accompanied with curiosity about the dissimilarities. This is the period identified by Freud as Oedipal and Electra complexes with a focus on penis envy and castration anxiety. These concepts evoke some controversy today.

Latency period (6 to 12 years): During this period, children continue to grow and expand previously learned and acquired skills and traits. Physical and psychic energy are focused on knowledge acquisition and vigorous physical activity or play.

Genital stage (age 13 and over): This remaining state begins with puberty, the production of sexual hormones, and maturation of the reproductive system. Genital organs become the major source of sexual pleasure and tension. The adolescent also focuses on relationship formation and prepares for more permanent relationship, i.e., marriage. Genital sexual pleasure continues throughout adulthood, into advanced years.

PART 5

Table 5-17	Erik Erikson's Psychosocial Theory of Development	
0–1 yrs.	Trust vs. distrust	Learns to trust caregivers for feedings, protection, comfort, and love; and distrust if needs are not met
1–2 yrs.	Autonomy vs. shame & doubt	Gains some physical control over elimination, feeds self, explores world; plays alone vs. developing shame about abilities
3–5 yrs.	Initiative vs. guilt	Motor and intellectual abilities continue to increase, and child assumes more responsibility for initiating and carrying out a plan; if thwarted, child feels guilt for misbehavior
6–11 yrs.	Industry vs. inferiority	Learns to meet the needs of home and school; developing self-worth due to accomplishments and positive interactions vs. feeling inferior due to negative interactions
12–19 yrs.	Identity vs. role confusion	Develops a strong sense of self or becomes confused about roles and identity
20s–30s	Intimacy vs. isolation	Develops close relationships with others or remains isolated from others
40s–50s	Generativity vs. stagnation	Assumes responsibility and adult roles in the family (teaching and nurturing the next generation), in community and work vs. becoming personally impoverished, self-centered & stagnant
60s & over	Integrity vs. despair	Evaluates life and accepts life as opposed to a state of despair regarding an inability to create meaning in one's life

Table 5-18   Piaget's Cognitive Theory of Development

0–2 yrs.	Sensorimotor stage	Learns to coordinate sensory experiences with physical motor actions. Learns how far to reach to get the ball, how to move head to follow a moving object.
2–7 yrs.	Preoperational stage	Acquires language; can manipulate symbols in the environment. Can deal with symbols of the world, but cannot perform reversible mental operations.
7–11 yrs.	Concrete operational stage	Shows capacity for logical reasoning for things actually experienced. Can do mental operations. Can use hierarchical classifications, class inclusion relationships, serialization (grouping objects in order), symmetry, and reciprocity (two brothers are brothers to each other).
11 yrs. & up	Formal operational stage	Begins to think in abstract terms. Uses systematic prepositional logic; solves hypothetical problems and draws conclusions. Uses inductive reasoning and deductive reasoning to construct and test theories. Can use algebraic symbols and metaphoric speech. Can move from what is real to what is possible.

Albert Bandura—Social Learning Theory

Children learn by observing the behavior of others and modeling this behavior, e.g., a child learns to play baseball by watching others and then tries to imitate or model what was seen. Children learn about behavior that is both positively and negatively rewarded by observing. Thus the principles of vicarious reinforcement and punishment emerge.

Abraham Maslow—Hierarchy of Needs Theory, Humanistic Psychology

Human behavior can be explained as motivation to satisfy needs including physiological needs, safety needs, love and belongingness needs, esteem needs, and self-actualization needs (and they are arranged in this order). The survival need of food, water, and protection from harm come first. When these needs are met, we can then direct attention to such things as love, acceptance, and belonging. After these needs are met, we can then address needs such as self-esteem. If we grow up well-fed, safe, loved, and respected, we are more likely to be self-actualized as a person. Maslow believed self-actualization to be the highest need and ultimate accomplishment in life.

Characteristics of self-actualization include:

- Self-acceptance and the acceptance of others just as they are
- Spontaneity
- Problem centered vs. self-centered
- Detachment with a need for privacy
- Autonomous and independent
- Fresh appreciation of people and things
- Profound mystical or spiritual experiences
- Strong sense of social interest in humans
- Strong intimate relationships with a few special and loved people vs. superficial relationships with many
- No confusion between means and ends

- Philosophical rather than hostile sense of humor
- Very creative
- Resistance to cultural conformity

Carl Rogers—Personal Growth Theory

People who are given freedom and emotional support to grow can develop into fully functioning human beings. With an accepting and understanding environment, people will solve their own problems and reach their goals. Each person has two major aspects, one is the way you perceive yourself to be, the other is the ideal self or what you would like to be. We receive parental approval and love when we comply with their specific and rigid conditions. As we fail to live up to the conditions and high standards, we are often criticized, rejected, and punished, and thus may develop low self-esteem, devalue our true selves, and lose ourselves.

To counteract a poor self-image, a person needs unconditional positive regard (or love, approval, companionship, and support of others). A healthy person is one who has achieved congruence between the real self and the ideal self and thus is free from internal conflict and anxiety.

References

Illingworth, R. S. (1994). *Basic developmental screening 0–4 years.* Boston: Blackwell Scientific.

Rice, F. P. (1992). *Human development: A life-space approach.* New York: MacMillan.

Wong, D. L., Hockenberry-Eaton, M., Wilson, D., Winkelstein, M. L., Ahmann, E., & DiVito-Thomas, P. A. (1999). *Waley and Wong's nursing care of infants and children.* St. Louis, MO: Mosby.

Cameron, N. (2002). *Human growth and development.* London: Academic Press.

Sinclair, D. (1989). *Human growth after birth* (5th ed.). Oxford: Oxford Medical.

PART 5

Growth Charts

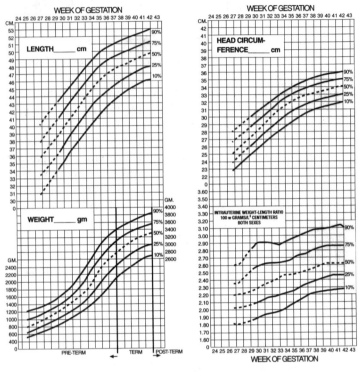

Symbols: X - 1st Exam O - 2nd Exam

Adapted from Lubchenco LO, Hansman C, and Boyd E: *Pediatr.* 1966;37:403; Battaglia FC, and Lubchenco LO: *J Pediatr.* 1967;71:159.

LB146 REV 6/04   ©1988, 1992, 1997, 1999 Mead Johnson & Company, Evansville, Indiana 47721 U.S.A.

Figure 5-19 Classification of newborns based on maturity and intrauterine growth. Courtesy of Mead Johnson Nutritionals.

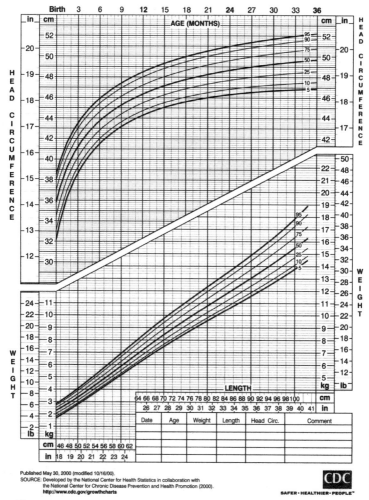

Figure 5-20 Birth to 36 months: Boys head circumference-for-age and weight-for-length percentiles. *Source:* CDC.

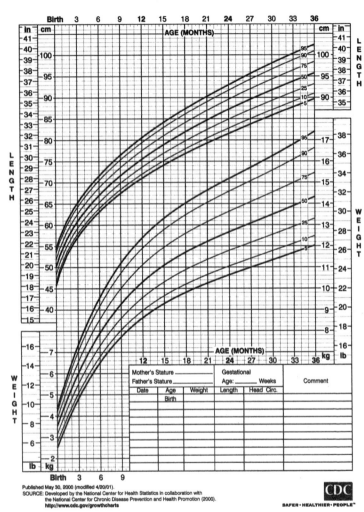

Figure 5-21   Birth to 36 months: Boys length-for-age and weight-for-age percentiles. *Source:* CDC.

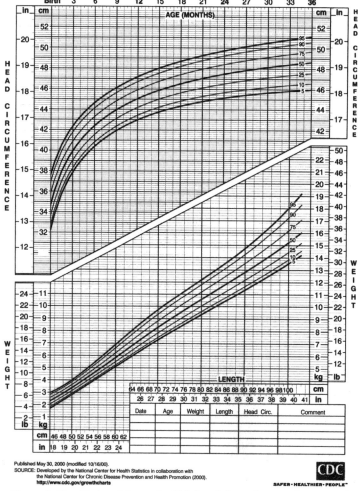

Published May 30, 2000 (modified 10/16/00).
SOURCE: Developed by the National Center for Health Statistics in collaboration with
the National Center for Chronic Disease Prevention and Health Promotion (2000).
http://www.cdc.gov/growthcharts

CDC
SAFER·HEALTHIER·PEOPLE™

Figure 5-22 Birth to 36 months: Girls head circumference-for-age and weight-for-length percentile. *Source:* CDC.

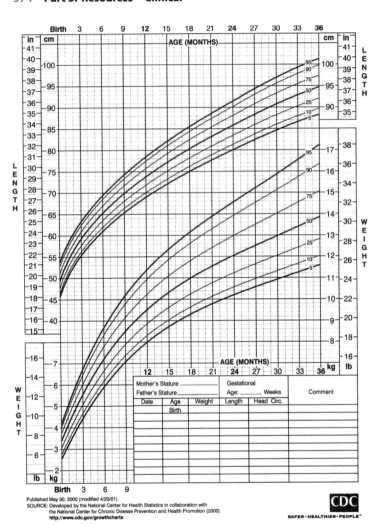

Figure 5-23 Birth to 36 months: Girls length-for-age and weight-for-age percentiles. *Source:* CDC.

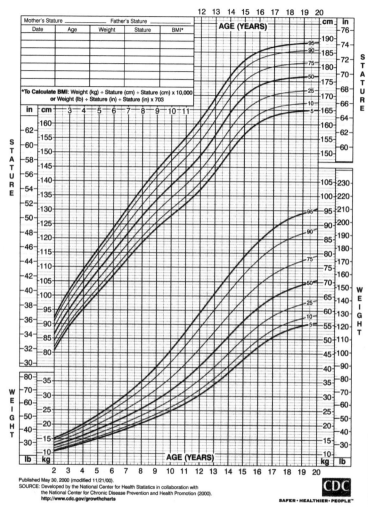

Figure 5-24 2 to 20 years: Boys stature-for-age and weight-for-age percentiles. *Source:* CDC.

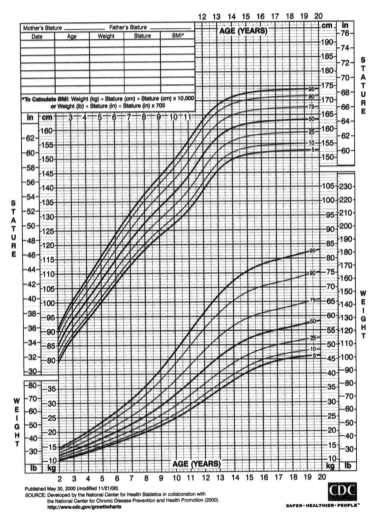

Figure 5-25 2 to 20 years: Girls stature-for-age and weight-for-age percentiles. *Source:* CDC.

NANDA-I Diagnoses Examples

Activity intolerance
Anxiety
Body image, disturbed
Breastfeeding, ineffective
Confusion, acute
Dentition, impaired
Development, risk for delayed
Falls, risk for
Fatigue
Gas exchange, impaired
Grieving, anticipatory
Infection, risk for
Knowledge, deficient (specify)
Nutrition: imbalanced, more than body requirements
Pain, chronic
Parenting, risk for impaired
Post-trauma syndrome
Skin integrity, impaired
Sleep deprivation
Spiritual distress
Urinary elimination, impaired
Violence: other-directed, risk for
Wandering

Source: North American Nursing Diagnosis Association-International (NANDA-I). (2005). *Nursing diagnoses: Definitions and classification 2005–2006.* Philadelphia: Author.

Nutrition

This section is designed to be a quick reference of very commonly prescribed diets and foods eaten throughout the United States. The diets are general descriptions of the most commonly prescribed in health care organizations. Because this is such an evolving field, check with your health care organization's nutrition manual or nutritionist for current practices based on research. If a food is not a fresh food, the label becomes a critical source of information for fats, carbohydrates, proteins, minerals, and vitamins. Because food additives may not be strongly regulated, these should be considered carefully.

Currently, there is considerable controversy surrounding the nature of the balance of types of foods to be ingested (for example, high carbohydrates versus high protein), the influence that knowing calories has to an overall healthy diet, and the use of natural versus supplemental vitamins and minerals. Therefore, you will not see diagrams or charts recommending specific types of foods or reference to selections from certain food groups. A list is included of the recommended levels of primary sources for common vitamins and minerals.

Cultural considerations are important in understanding patients' eating habits and food preferences. For example, caribou is commonly eaten by Native Alaskans; pork is avoided by those of the Jewish faith; and the growing population of people classified as Hispanic derives from no one country of origin so eating habits and food preferences cannot be described consistently for patients with that cultural heritage. Food needs change over the life span. When adolescents are experiencing growth spurts, they may consume calories far exceeding the recommended dietary levels. In the elderly, especially for those who are also sedentary, the calories needed are far less. In either case, appropriate nutrients are needed to maintain wellness.

Each of the food items listed below is described in its pure form, in other words, it is listed in its most natural state without additives such as flavorings, tenderizers, sauces, or toppings. Considerable research has been done in the past several years about nutritional values, quantities, and diets. Nutritional guidelines for normal, healthy diets continue to evolve so no one guideline appears here. Further, to be sure of a given product's ingredients and nutritional value, consult the product information. If patients frequent fast-food restaurants, most now offer brochures of nutritional values to help determine what composes a specific food.

Because obesity is a major health issue in the United States, it is important to compare the actual serving size with the designated quantity here due to the tendency to serve large portions. Although it is important to be concerned with the overabundance of food intake, it is equally important to be concerned with insufficient intake, especially of needed nutrients.

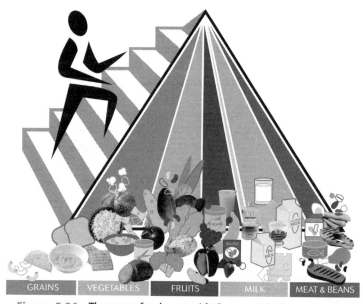

Figure 5-26 The new food pyramid. *Source:* U.S. Department of Agriculture, www.mypyramid.gov.

PART 5

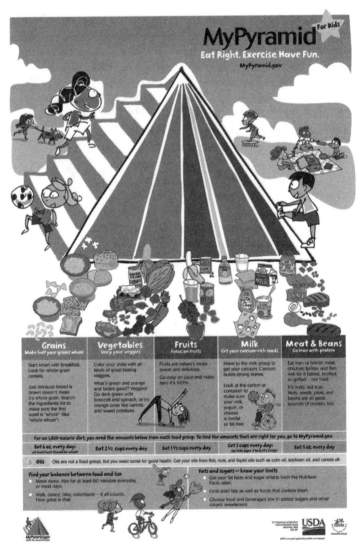

Figure 5-27   Food pyramid guide for young children. *Source:* U.S. Department of Agriculture, www.mypyramid.gov.

Table 5-19   Recommended Daily Allowances for Vitamins and Minerals

Vitamin	Women	Men	Adults
A	700 micrograms	900 micrograms	
D			5 micrograms; 10 for 50–70 years old; 15 for over 70 years old
E			15 milligrams
K	90 micrograms	120 micrograms	
B₁	1.1 milligrams	1.2 milligrams	
B₂	1.1 milligrams	1.3 milligrams	
Niacin	14 milligram NE (niacin equivalent)	16 milligram NE (niacin equivalent)	
Pantothenic acid			5 milligrams
Biotin			30 micrograms
B₆	51 years old + 1.5 milligrams	51 years old + 1.7 milligrams	1.3 milligrams until 51 years old
Folate			400 micrograms DFE (dietary folate equivalent)
B₁₂			2.4 micrograms
C	75 milligrams*	90 milligrams*	*Smokers: add 35 milligrams
Choline	425 milligrams	550 milligrams	
Mineral			
Sodium			2400 milligrams
Potassium			3500 milligrams

Table 5-19   *(continued)*

Vitamin	Women	Men	Adults
Chloride			3400 milligrams
Calcium			1000 milligrams up to 50 years old, 1200 milligrams thereafter
Phosphorus			700 milligrams
Magnesium	310 milligrams until 30 years old; 320 milligrams thereafter	400 milligrams until 30 years old; 420 milligrams thereafter	
Iron	18 milligrams until 50 years old; 8 milligrams thereafter	8 milligrams	
Zinc	8 milligrams	11 milligrams	
Selenium			55 micrograms
Iodine			150 micrograms
Copper			900 micrograms
Manganese	1.8 milligrams	2.3 milligrams	
Fluoride	3 milligrams	4 milligrams	
Chromium	30 micrograms up to 50 years old; 20 micrograms thereafter	35 micrograms up to 50 years old; 25 micrograms thereafter	
Molybdenum			45 micrograms

Source: Insel, P., Turner, R. E., & Ross, D. (2003). *Discovering nutrition.* Sudbury, MA: Jones and Bartlett.

Table 5-20 The Six Classes of Nutrients

Nutrient Class	Major Roles in the Body	Rich Food Sources
Carbohydrates	Energy	Grain products, beans, vegetables, fruits, honey, and candy
Lipids	Triglycerides: energy Cholesterol: certain steroid hormones, bile production, skin maintenance, vitamin D synthesis, and nerve function	Vegetable oils, margarines, fatty meats, cheeses, cream, butter, and fried foods
Proteins	Growth, repair, and maintenance of all cells; production of enzymes, antibodies, and certain hormones	Dried beans, peas, nuts, soy products, meats, shellfish, fish, poultry, eggs, and dairy products (except cream and butter)
Vitamins	Metabolism, reproduction, development, and growth	Widespread in foods: nuts, beans, peas, fruits and vegetables, whole grains, meats
Minerals	Metabolism, development, and growth	Widespread in foods: nuts and whole grains; meats, fish, and poultry; dairy products; fruits and vegetables
Water	Essential for life: many chemical reactions require water; it helps maintain normal body temperature, and dissolves and transports nutrients	Water, nonalcoholic and caffeine-free beverages, fruits, vegetables, and milk (nearly every food contributes water to the diet)

Source: Alters, S., & Schiff, W. (2006). *Essential concepts for healthy living* (4th ed.). Sudbury, MA: Jones and Bartlett.

PART 5

Table 5-21   Common Sources of Nutrients

Fat Soluble Vitamins

A:

Liver	Spinach	Collard greens
Carrots	Watermelon	Tomatoes
Cantaloupe		

D:

| Whole milk | Sardines | Anchovies |

E:

| Wheat germ | Nuts | Whole grains |

K:

| Green tea | Dark green vegetables | Cauliflower |

Water Soluble Vitamins

B_1:

| Wheat germ | Pork | Legumes |

B_2:

| Milk | Eggs | Peanuts |
| Leafy green vegetables | | |

B_3:

| Meats | Legumes | Brewer's yeast |

B_4:

| Liver | Whole grains | Potatoes |

B_{12}:

| Meats | Milk products | Eggs |

Folic Acid:

| Legumes | Dark green vegetables | |

C:

| Citrus fruits | Tomatoes | Strawberries |
| Leafy green vegetables | | Broccoli |

Minerals

Potassium:

| Bananas | Apricots | Citrus fruits |
| Milk | Meats | Legumes |

Table 5-21 (*continued*)

Sodium:		
Table salt		
Calcium:		
Milk Products	Tofu	Salmon
Dark green vegetables		
Fiber:		
Wheat germ	Bran	Oatmeal
Cabbages	Apples	Brown rice
Peas	Citrus fruits	Beans

Table 5-22 Selected Nutrients of Commonly Consumed Foods

Item & Quantity	Calories	Fat (g)	Protein (g)	CHO (g)	Ca (mg)	Iron (mg)	Na (mg)	K (mg)	Vit. A (IU)	Vit. C (IU)
Apple, 1 med	80	tr	tr	22	10	0.2	tr	160	70	8
Apple pie, 1 slice	410	18	3	60	13	1.6	476	126	50	2
Applesauce, 1 c	100	tr	tr	28	7	0.3	5	183	70	3
Apricot, 3 med	51	tr	1	12	15	0.6	1	314	2770	11
Asparagus, 4 spears	25	tr	1	3	14	0.4	2	186	500	16
Avocados, 1 med	324	30	4	12	19	2	21	1097	1060	14
Bacon, 3 slices	110	9	6	tr	2	0.3	303	92	0	6
Bagel, plain, toasted	194	1.1	7.4	38	12.5	2.5	379	72	0	0
Banana, 1	105	1	1	27	7	0.4	1	451	90	10
Beans, pea, 1 c	225	1	15	40	95	5.1	13	790	0	0
Beans, pinto, 1 c	265	1	15	49	86	5.4	3	882	tr	0
Beef patty, lean 6 oz	460	32	42	0	18	3.6	130	512	tr	0
Beef patty, reg 6 oz	490	36	40	0	18	4.2	140	496	tr	0
Beef roast, rel. lean 6 oz	405	24	46	0	10	3.2	100	616	tr	0

Biscuits, (mix) 1	95	3	2	14	58	0.7	262	56	20	tr
Bologna, 2 slices	180	16	7	2	7	0.9	581	103	0	12
Bread, multigrain, 1 slice	65	1	2	12	27	0.8	106	56	tr	tr
Bread, white, 1 slice	65	1	2	12	32	0.7	129	28	tr	tr
Brownie, 1 (1.5" × 1.5")	100	4	1	16	13	0.6	59	50	70	tr
Butter, 1 Tbsp.	100	11	tr	tr	27	0.2	933	29	13,460	0
Carrots, 1	30	tr	1	7	19	0.4	25	233	20,250	7
Chicken, fried, 1/2 breast	365	18	35	13	28	1.8	385	281	90	0
Chicken, baked, 1/2 breast	140	3	27	0	13	0.9	64	220	20	0
Corn on the cob, 1 ear	85	1	3	19	2	0.5	13	192	170	5
Croissant, 1	235	12	5	27	20	2.1	452	68	50	0
Donut, glazed, 1	235	13	4	26	17	1.4	222	64	tr	0
Eggs, whole, 1 raw	80	6	6	1	28	1.0	69	65	260	0

Table 5-22 (continued)

Item & Quantity	Calories	Fat (g)	Protein (g)	CHO (g)	Ca (mg)	Iron (mg)	Na (mg)	K (mg)	Vit. A (IU)	Vit. C (IU)
Grapefruit, ½	40	tr	1	10	14	0.1	tr	167	10	41
Grapes, white seedless, 10	35	tr	tr	9	6	0.1	1	93	40	5
Ham, cooked, 2 slices	105	6	10	2	4	0.6	751	189	0	16
Hot dog, 1	145	13	5	1	5	0.5	504	75	0	12
Lettuce, iceberg 1 wedge	20	tr	1	3	26	0.7	12	213	450	5
Milk, whole, 1 c	150	8	8	11	291	0.1	120	370	310	2
Orange, 1 med	60	tr	1	15	52	0.1	tr	237	270	70
Orange juice, 1 c (from frozen)	110	tr	2	27	22	0.2	2	473	190	97
Peach, 1 med	35	tr	1	10	4	0.1	tr	171	470	6
Peanuts (oil), 1 c	840	71	39	5	24	0.5	122	199	0	0
Peas, frozen, 1 c	125	tr	8	23	38	2.5	139	269	1,070	16
Popcorn, air popped, 1 c	30	tr	1	6	1	0.2	tr	20	10	0

Food										
Pork chop, pan fried, 1	335	27	21	0	4	0.7	64	323	10	tr
Potato, baked, 1 med	220	tr	5	51	20	2.7	16	844	0	26
Potato chips, 10	105	7	1	10	5	0.2	94	260	0	8
Potatoes, French fried, 10	110	4	2	17	5	0.7	16	229	0	5
Potatoes, mashed with butter and milk, 1 c	225	9	4	32	103	0.5	697	489	380	20
Rice, white, 1 c	225	tr	4	50	21	1.8	0	57	0	0
Salmon, canned, 3 oz	120	5	17	34	167	0.7	443	307	60	0
Strawberries, fresh, 1 c	45	1	1	10	21	0.6	1	247	40	84
Steak, sirloin, 6 oz	480	30	46	0	18	5.2	106	612	tr	0
Tomato, 1 med	25	tr	1	5	9	0.6	10	255	1,390	22
Trout, broiled, 3 oz	175	9	21	tr	26	1.0	122	297	230	1
Tuna, canned (water), 3 oz	135	1	30	0	17	0.6	468	255	110	0

Table 5-23 Commonly Prescribed or Used Diets

Type	Restrictions	Patient Problem/Condition	Example of Restriction
Regular	No restrictions	State of wellness	None
Clear liquid	Nontransparent/translucent liquids	Initial recovery from severe nausea and vomiting; recovery from surgery	Milk, cream soups
Full liquid	No soft or solids; may include eggs	Transition from clear liquid	Mashed potatoes, soups with meat and pasta additions
Soft	No solids; typically mild in seasonings	Difficulty swallowing and chewing	Meats that are not pureed, crunchy vegetables
Mechanical soft/edentulous	Nothing that hasn't been ground or pureed unless it is soft or liquid	Difficulty chewing, including lack of teeth/dentures	Steak, chicken, crusty bread

Bland	No spicy foods	GI irritation	Pepper, jalapeños,
Low calorie	Fats and foods high in fats	Overweight	Butter, eggs, cheese, cream
High calorie	Any low-calorie food	Underweight	Diet drinks, skim milk
High fiber	Fats and processed foods	GI disease	Baked desserts, highly processed foods
Diabetic	Few restrictions; focus is on balance of food groups	Diabetes	Sugar-intense foods, sole food category
High protein	Carbohydrates	Overweight, healing process, underweight	Breads, desserts, sugar-intense foods
Low fat	Dairy products unless with reduced fat	Diseases associated with heart, liver, and gallbladder	Cheese, whole milk, ice cream (unless reduced fat)
Low cholesterol	Meat and cheese	Hypercholesteremia	Beef, pork, cheese
Low sodium	No salt, even during cooking	Renal and heart disease	No salt present

Table 5-23 *(continued)*

Type	Restrictions	Patient Problem/Condition	Example of Restriction
Kosher	No non-Kosher meat; no milk at same meal as meat	Religious	Organ meat, shellfish
Lacto-ovo vegetarian	No meat or meat products or fish	Religious or food preference	Beef, pork, chicken, fish
Lacto-vegetarian	No meat or meat products or fish or eggs	Religious or food preference	Beef, pork, chicken, fish, eggs
Vegan	No meat or meat products or fish, no eggs, and no dairy products	Religious or food preference	Beef, pork, chicken, fish, eggs, milk, cottage cheese
DASH (dietary approaches to stop hypertension)	Sodium-, fat- and cholesterol-rich foods	Stage I hypertension	Most snack products (high in sodium), highly processed foods
Renal	Low protein (in symptomatic patients)	Protein sources must be high biologic value	Meat, fish, poultry, dairy products

Nutritional Support

Nutritional support should be provided in the most appropriate manner possible. This means that if the GI tract is functioning, oral supplements would be best. If oral is not appropriate for some reason, then tube feedings are the next best choice. If the GI tract is not functioning, some form of parenteral supplement is appropriate (for example, PPN or TPN). If the tract is not functional for a longer period of time, a directly implanted tube such as a gastrostomy or jejunostomy tube is appropriate.

The amount of supplement is determined based on the individual's needs. A specific nutritional consultation is appropriate, especially for longer-term use.

To determine the desired rate of flow for an established tube feeding, divide the total number of calories to be delivered in a designated time period by the designated time period (for example, 1000 cal (at 1 cal/cc) in 12 hours is approximately 83 cc per hour).

The General Rules of Tube Support

Irrespective of the kind of tube used, the following list of precautions should be used. Note: Many institutions require visualization of placement after initial insertion and require detailed measures to determine ongoing tube placement.

- Use small bore feeding tubes for patient comfort.
- Use sanitary techniques.
- Check the tube upon insertion and before feedings or medication administration to be sure of patency and position.
- Tape nasogastric tubes to avoid irritation to the nares.
- Keep the head of the bed elevated 30° to 45° during and after a feeding to prevent any aspiration (not necessary with jejunostomy).
- Use room temperature fluids.

- Irrigate the feeding tube frequently with clear water if no automatic water flush is available by enteral pump. (200 cc for nasogastric and 100 cc for a G tube is considered safe.) Should be ordered by physician, nurse practitioner, or physician's assistant.
- Irrigate the tube with clear water before and after administering anything (formula or medications) and after aspirating gastric contents.
- Use slow rates to administer feedings, especially at first.
- Maintain accurate fluid records.
- Monitor fluid and electrolyte data.

Determining BMI (Body Mass Index)

Body mass index (BMI) has become the standard for checking for underweight and overweight conditions. Because the number one health concern in the country is obesity, nurses need to be able to calculate BMIs. Please visit 🖰 www.cdc.gov/nccdphp/dnpa/bmi/calc-bmi.htm for an online calculator.

The following information is derived from government Web sites to provide the most official data about BMI.

BMI for Adults
The BMI Formula

If you are unable to use the BMI calculator, or if you are interested in how BMI is calculated, here are the mathematical formulas. You can calculate BMI using English measure (feet, inches, and pounds), or metric (meters, centimeters, and kilograms).

English Formula   Body mass index can be calculated using pounds and inches with this equation:

$$\text{BMI} = \left(\frac{\text{Weight in pounds}}{(\text{Height in inches}) \times (\text{Height in inches})} \right) \times 703$$

For example, a person who weighs 220 pounds and is 6 feet 3 inches tall has a BMI of 27.5.

$$\frac{220 \text{ lbs.}}{(75 \text{ inches}) \times (75 \text{ inches})}) \times 703 = 27.5$$

Metric Formula   Body mass index can also be calculated using kilograms and meters (or centimeters):

$$\text{BMI} = \frac{\text{Weight in kilograms}}{(\text{Height in meters}) \times (\text{Height in meters})}$$

or

$$\text{BMI} = \left(\frac{\text{Weight in kilograms}}{(\text{Height in centimeters}) \times (\text{Height in centimeters})} \right)$$
$$\times 10,000$$

For example, a person who weighs 99.79 kilograms and is 1.905 meters (190.50 centimeters) tall has a BMI of 27.5.

$$\frac{99.79 \text{ kg}}{(1.905 \text{ m}) \times (1.905 \text{ m})} = 27.5$$

BMI and Disease Risk for Adults

Body mass index, or BMI, is the measurement of choice for many physicians and researchers studying obesity. BMI uses a mathematical formula that takes into account both a person's height and weight. BMI equals a person's weight in kilograms divided by height in meters squared ($\text{BMI} = \text{kg/m}^2$).

Table 5-24   Risk of Associated Disease According to BMI and Waist Size

BMI		Waist less than or equal to 40 in. (men) or 35 in. (women)	Waist greater than 40 in. (men) or 35 in. (women)
18.5 or less	Underweight	—	N/A
18.5–24.9	Normal	—	N/A
25.0–29.9	Overweight	Increased	High
30.0–34.9	Obese	High	Very high
35.0–39.9	Obese	Very high	Very high
40 or greater	Extremely obese	Extremely high	Extremely high

BMI for Children and Teens

BMI is used differently with children than it is with children and teens, body mass index is used to assess underweight, overweight, and risk for overweight. Children's body fatness changes over the years as they grow. Also, girls and boys differ in their body fatness as they mature. This is why BMI for children, also referred to as BMI-for-age, is gender and age specific. BMI-for-age is plotted on gender specific growth charts. These charts are used for children and teens 2–20 years of age. For the 2000 CDC growth charts and additional information, visit the CDC's National Center for Health Statistics Web site at ⌐ www.cdc.gov/nchs.

Each of the CDC BMI-for-age gender specific charts contains a series of curved lines indicating specific percentiles. Healthcare professionals use the following established percentile cutoff points to identify underweight and overweight children.

Underweight   BMI-for-age < 5th percentile
At risk of overweight   BMI-for-age ranges from 85th percentile to < 95th percentile
Overweight   BMI-for-age ≥ 95th percentile

BMI decreases during the preschool years, then increases into adulthood. The percentile curves show this pattern of growth.

Looking at the BMI for a boy as he grows, even though his BMI changes, he remains at the 95th percentile BMI-for-age.

Table 5-25   Example BMI of Growing Boy

Age	BMI	Percentile
2 years	19.3	95th
4 years	17.8	95th
9 years	21.0	95th
13 years	25.1	95th

PART 5

Notice how the boy's BMI declines during his preschool years and increases as he gets older.

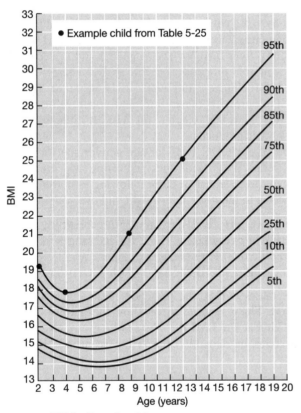

Figure 5-28   BMI for Boys: 2 to 20 years.

Why Is BMI-for-Age a Useful Tool?

BMI-for-age is used for children and teens because of their rate of growth and development. It is a useful tool because:

- BMI-for-age provides a reference for adolescents that can be used beyond puberty.
- BMI-for-age in children and adolescents compares well to laboratory measures of body fat.
- BMI-for-age can be used to track body size throughout life.

References

Centers for Disease Control and Prevention [CDC]. (2006). BMI—body mass index: About BMI for adults. Retrieved March 6, 2006, from http://www.cdc.gov/nccdphp/dnpa/bmi/adult_BMI/about_adult_BMI.htm

CDC. (2006). BMI—body mass index: About BMI for children and teens. Retrieved March 6, 2006, from http://www.cdc.gov/nccdphp/dnpa/bmi/childrens_BMI/about_childrens_BMI.htm

Hammer, L. D., Kraemer, H. C., Wilson, D. M., Ritter, P. L., & Dornbusch, S. M. (1991). Standardized percentile curves of body-mass index for children and adolescents. *American Journal of Disease of Child, 145,* 259–263.

Pietrobelli, A., Faith, M. S., Allison, D. B., Gallagher, D., Chiumello, G., & Heymsfield, S. B. (1998). Body mass index as a measure of adiposity among children and adolescents: A validation study. *Journal of Pediatrics, 132,* 204–210.

PART 6

Resources—Professional

Code of Ethics for Nurses

1. The nurse, in all professional relationships, practices with compassion and respect for the inherent dignity, worth, and uniqueness of every individual, unrestricted by considerations of social or economic status, personal attributes, or the nature of health problems.
2. The nurse's primary commitment is to the patient, whether an individual, family, group, or community.
3. The nurse promotes, advocates for, and strives to protect the health, safety, and rights of the patient.

4. The nurse is responsible and accountable for individual nursing practice and determines the appropriate delegation of tasks consistent with the nurse's obligation to provide optimum patient care.

5. The nurse owes the same duties to self as to others, including the responsibility to preserve integrity and safety, to maintain competence, and to continue personal and professional growth.

6. The nurse participates in establishing, maintaining, and improving health care environments and conditions of employment conducive to the provision of quality health care and consistent with the values of the profession through individual and collective action.

7. The nurse participates in the advancement of the profession through contributions to practice, education, administration, and knowledge development.

8. The nurse collaborates with other health professionals and the public in promoting community, national, and international efforts to meet health needs.

9. The profession of nursing, as represented by associations and their members, is responsible for articulating nursing values, for maintaining the integrity of the profession and its practice, and for shaping social policy.

Source: Reprinted with permission from American Nurses Association, *Code of Ethics for Nurses with Interpretive Statements,* © 2001 Nursesbooks.org, American Nurses Association, Washington, DC.

Standards of Nursing Practice

Standards of Practice

Standard 1: Assessment
The nurse collects patient health data pertinent to the patient's health or the situation.

Standard 2: Diagnosis
The registered nurse analyzes the assessment data to determine the diagnoses or issues.

Standard 3: Outcomes Identification

The registered nurse identifies expected outcomes for a plan individualized to the patient or the situation.

Standard 4: Planning

The registered nurse develops a plan that prescribes strategies and alternatives to attain expected outcomes.

Standard 5: Implementation

The registered nurse implements the identified plan.

Standard 5A: Coordination of Care

The registered nurse coordinates care delivery.

Standard 5B: Health Teaching and Health Promotion

The registered nurse employs strategies to promote health and a safe environment.

Standard 5C: Consultation

The advanced practice registered nurse and the nursing role specialist provide consultation to influence the identified plan, enhance the abilities of others, and effect change.

Standard 5D: Prescriptive Authority and Treatment

The advanced practice registered nurse uses prescriptive authority, procedures, referrals, treatments, and therapies in accordance with state and federal laws and regulations.

Standard 6: Evaluation

The registered nurse evaluates progress toward attainment of outcomes.

Standards of Professional Performance

Standard 7: Quality of Practice

The registered nurse systematically enhances the quality and effectiveness of nursing practice.

Standard 8: Education

The registered nurse attains knowledge and competency that reflects current nursing practice.

Standard 9: Professional Practice Evaluation

The registered nurse evaluates one's own nursing practice in relation to professional practice standards and guidelines, relevant statutes, and rules and regulations.

Standard 10: Collegiality

The registered nurse interacts with and contributes to the professional development of peers and colleagues.

Standard 11: Collaboration

The registered nurse collaborates with patients, families, and others in the conduct of nursing practice.

Standard 12: Ethics

The registered nurse integrates ethical provisions in all areas of practice.

Standard 13: Research

The registered nurse integrates research findings into practice.

Standard 14: Resource Utilization

The registered nurse considers factors related to safety, effectiveness, cost, and impact on practice in the planning and delivery of nursing services.

Standard 15: Leadership

The registered nurse provides leadership in the professional practice setting and the profession.

Source: Reprinted with permission from American Nurses Association, *Nursing: Scope and Standards of Practice,* © 2003 Nursesbooks.org., American Nurses Association, Washington, DC.

Principles for Nurse Staffing

Introduction

Adequate nurse staffing is critical to delivery of quality patient care. Identifying and maintaining the appropriate number and mix of nursing staff is a problem experienced by nurses at every level in all settings. Regardless of organizational mission, tempering the realities of cost containment and cyclical nursing shortages with the priority of safe, quality care has been difficult, in part, because of the paucity of empirical data to guide decision making. Since 1994, the recognition of this critical need for such empirical data has driven many American Nurses Association (ANA) activities, including identification of nursing-sensitive indicators, establishment of data collection projects using these indicators within the State Nurses Associations (SNAs), and the provision of ongoing lobbying at federal and state levels for inclusion of these data elements within state and national data collection activities. In 1996, the Institute of Medicine produced its report *The Adequacy of Nurse Staffing in Hospitals and Nursing Homes* (Wunderlich et al., 1996) in which it too recognized the need for such data. Despite these efforts, heightened and more immediate attention to issues related to the adequacy of nurse staffing is needed to assure the provision of safe, quality nursing care.

Policy Statements

- Nurse staffing patterns and the level of care provided should not depend on the type of payer.
- Evaluation of any staffing system should include quality-of-work life outcomes as well as patient outcomes.
- Staffing should be based on achieving quality of patient care indices, meeting organizational outcomes, and ensuring that the quality of the nurse's work life is appropriate.

Principles

The nine principles identified by the expert panel for nurse staffing and adopted by the ANA Board of Directors on November 24, 1998, are listed below.

1. Patient care unit related
   a. Appropriate staffing levels for a patient care unit reflect analysis of individual and aggregate patient needs.

   b. There is a critical need to either retire or seriously
      question the usefulness of the concept of nursing hours
      per patient day (HPPD).
   c. Unit functions necessary to support delivery of quality
      patient care must also be considered in determining
      staffing levels.
2. Staff related
   a. The specific needs of various patient populations should
      determine the appropriate clinical competencies re-
      quired of the nurse practicing in that area.
   b. Registered nurses must have nursing management sup-
      port and representation at both the operational level
      and the executive level.
   c. Clinical support from experienced RNs should be read-
      ily available to those RNs with less proficiency.
3. Institution/organization related
   a. Organizational policy should reflect an organizational
      climate that values registered nurses and other employ-
      ees as strategic assets and exhibit a true commitment to
      filling budgeted positions in a timely manner.
   b. All institutions should have documented competencies
      for nursing staff, including agency or supplemental and
      traveling RNs, for those activities that they have been
      authorized to perform.
   c. Organizational policies should recognize the myriad
      needs of both patients and nursing staff.

Source: Reprinted with permission from American Nurses Association, *Principles for Nurse Staffing,* © 1999, Nursesbooks.org, American Nurses Association, Washington, DC.

Bill of Rights for Registered Nurses

Registered nurses promote and restore health, prevent illness, and protect the people entrusted to their care. They work to alleviate the suffering experienced by individuals, families, groups, and communities. In so doing, nurses provide services that maintain respect for human dignity and embrace the uniqueness of each patient and the nature of his or her health problems, without restriction in regard to social or economic status. To maximize the contributions nurses make to society, it is necessary to protect the dignity and autonomy of nurses in the workplace. To that end, the American Nurses Association has established that the following rights must be afforded:

1. Nurses have the right to practice in a manner that fulfills their obligations to society and to those who receive nursing care.
2. Nurses have the right to practice in environments that allow them to act in accordance with professional standards and legally authorized scopes of practice.
3. Nurses have the right to a work environment that supports and facilitates ethical practice, in accordance with the Code of Ethics for Nurses and its interpretive statements.
4. Nurses have the right to freely and openly advocate for themselves and their patients, without fear of retribution.
5. Nurses have the right to fair compensation for their work, consistent with their knowledge, experience, and professional responsibilities.
6. Nurses have the right to a work environment that is safe for themselves and their patients.
7. Nurses have the right to negotiate the conditions of their employment, either as individuals or collectively, in all practice settings.

Source: Reprinted with permission from American Nurses Association, *American Nurses Association's Bill of Rights for Registered Nurses*, © 2001 Nursesbooks.org., American Nurses Association, Washington, DC.

Professional Organizations

Organizations and Their Web Sites

Academy of Medical-Surgical Nurses
    http://www.medsurgnurse.org
Air and Surface Transport Nurses Association
    http://www.astna.org
American Academy of Ambulatory Care Nursing
    http://www.aaacn.org
American Academy of Nurse Practitioners
    http://www.aanp.org
American Academy of Nursing
    http://www.aannet.org
American Assisted Living Nurses Association
    http://www.alnursing.org
American Association for the History of Nursing
    http://www.aahn.org
American Association of Colleges of Nursing
    http://www.aacn.nche.edu
American Association of Continuity in Care
    http://www.continuityofcare.com
American Association of Critical Care Nurses
    http://www.aacn.org
American Association of Diabetes Educators
    http://www.aadenet.org
American Association of Legal Nurse Consultants
    http://www.aalnc.org
American Association of Neuroscience Nurses
    http://www.aann.org
American Association of Nurse Anesthetists
    http://www.aana.com
American Association of Occupational Health Nurses
    http://www.aaohn.org
American Association of Office Nurses
    http://www.aaon.org

American Association of Spinal Cord Nurses
http://www.aascin.org
American College of Cardiovascular Nursing
http://www.accn.net
American College of Nurse Midwives
http://www.acnm.org
American College of Nurse Practitioners
http://www.nurse.org/acnp
American Holistic Nurses Association
http://www.ahna.org
American Nephrology Nurses Association
http://anna.inurse.com
American Nurses Association
http://www.nursingworld.org
American Nurses Credentialing Center
http://www.nursecredentialing.org
American Nursing Informatics Association
http://www.ania.org
American Organization of Nurse Executives
http://www.aone.org
American Psychiatric Nurses Association
http://www.apna.org
American Public Health Association
http://www.apha.org
American Society of Ophthalmic Registered Nurses
http://webeye.ophth.uiowa.edu/asorn
American Society of Pain Management Nurses
http://www.aspmn.org
American Society of Perianesthesia Nurses
http://www.aspan.org
American Society of Plastic Surgical Nurses
http://www.aspsn.org
Association of Child Neurology Nurses
http://www.acnn.org

Association of Nurses in AIDS Care
   http://www.anacnet.org
Association of Pediatric Oncology
   http://www.apon.org
Association of Perioperative Registered Nurses
   http://www.aorn.org
Association of Rehabilitation Nurses
   http://www.rehabnurse.org
Association of Women's Health, Obstetric, and Neonatal Nurses
   http://www.awhonn.org
Case Management Society of America
   http://www.cmsa.org
Dermatology Nurses Association
   http://www.dnanurse.org
Development Disabilities Nurses Association
   http://www.ddna.org
Emergency Nurses Association
   http://www.ena.org
Endocrine Nurses Society
   http://www.endo-nurses.org
Home Healthcare Nurses Association
   http://www.hhna.org
Hospice and Palliative Nurses Association
   http://www.hpna.org
Infusion Nurses Society
   http://www.ins1.org
International Council of Nurses
   http://www.icn.ch
National Association of Clinical Nurse Specialists
   http://www.nacns.org
National Association of Hispanic Nurses
   http://www.thehispanicnurses.org
National Association of Neonatal Nurses
   http://www.nann.org

National Association of Nurse Massage Therapists
http://www.nanmt.org
National Association of Orthopedic Nurses
http://www.orthonurse.org
National Association of Pediatric Nurse Practitioners
http://www.napnap.org
National Association of School Nurses
http://www.nasn.org
National Black Nurses Association
http://www.nbna.org
National Association of Neonatal Nurses
http://www.nann.org
National Association of School Nurses
http://www.nasn.org
National Council of State Boards of Nursing
http://www.ncsbn.org
National Gerontological Nursing Association
http://www.ngna.org
National League for Nursing
http://www.nln.org
National Nursing Staff Development Organization
http://www.nnsdo.org
National Organization for Associate Degree Nursing
http://www.noadn.org
National Organization of Nurse Practitioner Faculties
http://www.nonpf.com
National Student Nurses Association
http://www.nsna.org
Oncology Nursing Society
http://www.ons.org
Sigma Theta Tau, International
http://www.nursingsociety.org
Society of Gastroenterology Nurses and Associates
http://www.sgna.org

Society of Pediatric Nurses
http://www.pedsnurses.org
Society of Urologic Nurses and Associates
http://suna.inurse.com
Society for Vascular Nursing
http://www.svnnet.org
The American Association of Nurse Attorneys
http://www.taana.org
Transcultural Nursing Society
http://www.tcns.org
Wound, Ostomy and Continence Nurses Society
http://www.wocn.org

Organizational and Professional Acronyms and Credentials

AA: Alcoholics Anonymous
AAA: Area Agencies on Aging
AAACE: American Association of Adult and Continuing
   Education
AAAS: American Association for the Advancement of Science
AACHP: American Association for Comprehensive Health
   Planning
AACN: American Association of Colleges of Nursing
AACN: American Association of Critical-Care Nurses
AAFP: American Academy of Family Practitioners
AAHPERD: American Alliance for Health, Physical Education,
   Recreation, and Dance
AAMC: American Association of Medical Colleges
AAMR: American Association on Mental Retardation
AAN: American Academy of Nursing
AANA: American Association of Nurse Anesthetists
AAP: American Academy of Pediatrics
AAPC: American Association of Pastoral Counselors
AAPD: American Academy of Pediatric Dentists
AAPH: American Association of Partial Hospitalization

AARP: American Association for Retired Persons
AART: American Association for Respiratory Therapy
AART: Association for the Advancement of Rehabilitation Technology
AAS: Associate of applied science
ABPTS: American Board of Physical Therapy Specialists
ACA: American Counseling Association
ACALD: Association for Children and Adults with Learning Disabilities
ACCD: American Coalition of Citizens with Disabilities
ACCH: Association for the Care of Children's Health
ACCME: Accreditation Council for Continuing Medical Education
ACCP: American College of Chest Physicians
ACDD: Accreditation Council on Services for People with Developmental Disabilities
ACF: Administration for Children and Families
ACHCA: American College of Health Care Administrators
ACIP: Advisory Committee on Immunization Practices
ACNP: Acute care nurse practitioner
ACOG: American College of Obstetricians and Gynecologists
ACOTE: Accreditation Council for Occupational Therapy Education
ACPE: Accreditation Commission for Pharmaceutical Education
ACRE: American Council on Rural Education
ACRM: American Congress of Rehabilitation Medicine
ACRN: AIDS certified registered nurse
ACS: American Cancer Society
ACSM: American College of Sports Medicine
ACTG: AIDS clinical trial group
ACYF: Administration on Children, Youth, and Families
ADA: American Dietetic Association
ADD: Administration on Developmental Disabilities
ADHA: American Dental Hygienists Association

ADN: Associate degree of nursing; also associate director of nursing

ADRDA: Alzheimer's Disease and Related Disorders Association

AERA: American Educational Research Association

AF: Arthritis Foundation

AFH: American Federation of Hospitals

AFL-CIO: American Federation of Labor and Congress of Industrial Organizations

AFT: American Federation of Teachers

AGA: American Geriatric Association

AGHE: Association for Gerontology in Higher Education

AGS: American Geriatrics Society

AHA: American Hospital Association

AHCA: American Health Care Association

AHNA: American Holistic Nurses Association

AHPA: Arthritis Health Professional Association; or American Herbal Products Association

AHRQ: Agency for Healthcare Research and Quality, DHHS

AICPA: American Institute of Certified Public Accountants

AICR: American Institute for Cancer Research

AIHA: American International Health Alliance

AJN: *American Journal of Nursing*

AMA: American Medical Association

AMDA: American Medical Directors Association

AMEND: Aiding Mothers Experiencing Neonatal Death

AMH: Accreditation Manual for Hospitals (JCAHO)

ANA: American Nurses Association

ANCC: American Nurses Credentialing Center

ANDMCN: American Nursing Division of Maternal Child Nursing

ANF: American Nurses Foundation

ANM: Assistant nurse manager

ANP: American Nurses Publishing

ANP: Adult nurse practitioner

ANSI: American National Standards Institute

AOA: Administration on Aging, DHHS
AOA: American Optometric Association
AOA: American Osteopathic Association
AOCN: Advanced oncology certified nurse
AONE: American Organization of Nurse Executives (affiliated
  with the AHA)
AOPA: American Orthotic and Prosthetic Association
AORN: Association of Perioperative Registered Nurses
APN: Advanced practice nurse (e.g., nurse practitioner, nurse–
  midwife, nurse anesthetist, clinical nurse specialist)
APON: Association of Pediatric Oncology Nurses
APNP: Advanced practice nurse prescriber
APRN: Advanced practice registered nurse
APS: Adult Protective Services
AOTA: American Occupational Therapy Association
APA: American Psychiatric Association
APA: American Psychological Association
APHA: American Public Health Association
APTA: American Physical Therapy Association
ARC: Association for Retarded Citizens
ARCA: American Rehabilitation Counseling Association
ARF: Association of Rehabilitation Facilities
ARNP: Advanced registered nurse practitioner
ASA: American Society on Aging
ASAE: American Society of Association Executives
ASAHP: American Society of Allied Health Professions
ASHA: American Speech-Language-Hearing Association
ASHT: American Society of Hand Therapists
ASI: Assessment Systems, Inc.
ASN: Associate in science of nursing
ASPA: Association of Specialized and Professional AC Creditors
ASPN: Associated Science of Practical Nursing
ASTM: American Society for Testing and Materials
AT: Art therapist
ATLS: Advanced trauma life support

AWHONN: Association of Women's Health, Obstetric, and
   Neonatal Nurses

BAA: Bachelor of applied arts in nursing
BC: Board certified (at ANCC, this implies a bachelor of science
   or higher degree)
BC/BS: Blue Cross/Blue Shield Association
BCPE: Board for Certification in Professional Ergonomics
BHP: Bureau of Health Professions (DHHS)
BLS: Bureau of Labor Statistics (DOL)
BOC: Board of Commissioners (JCAHO)
BSN: Bachelor of science in nursing

C: Certified, frequently refers to a generalist level and to a nurse
   without a bachelor's degree
CAAHEP: Commission on Accreditation of Allied Health
   Education Programs
CAHEA: Committee on Allied Health Education and
   Accreditation (AMA)
CAN: Center for American Nurses
CAPA: Certified ambulatory perianesthesia nurse
CAPTE: Commission on Accreditation in Physical Therapy
   Education
CARF: Commission on Accreditation of Rehabilitation Facilities
CARN: Certified addictions registered nurse
CARN-AP: Certified addictions registered nurse, advanced
   practice
CBO: Congressional Budget Office
CBE: Certified breastfeeding educator
CCB: Child Care Bureau
CCD: Consortium for Citizens with Disabilities
CCCN: Certified continence care nurse
CCES: Council of Childbirth Education Specialists
CCHP: Certified correctional health professional
CCM: Certified case manager

CCNS: Certified clinical nurse specialist
CCRN: Certified critical care registered nurse
CCR&R: Child Care Resource and Referral Agency
CCS: Certified coding specialist
CCS: Crippled Children Services
CCTC: Certified clinical transplant coordinator
CCY: Coalition for Children and Youth
CDAC: Certified drug and alcohol counselor
CDC: Centers for Disease Control and Prevention
CDDN: Certified developmental disabilities nurse
CDE: Certified diabetes educator
CDMS: Certified disability management specialist
CDONA/LTC: Certified director of nursing administration in
    long-term care
CEC: Council for Exceptional Children
CEN: Certified emergency nurse
CENA: Certified enterostomal therapy nurse
CFNP: Certified family nurse practitioner
CFRN: Certified flight registered nurse
CGA: Certified gastroenterology associate
CGN: Certified gastroenterology nurse
CGRN: Certified gastroenterology registered nurse
CHES: Certified health education specialist
CHF: Coalition for Health Funding
CHHA/CHS: Council of Home Health Agencies and
    Community Health Services (NLN)
CHN: Community health nurse
CHPN: Certified hospice and palliative nurse
CHRN: Certified hyperbaric registered nurse
CHT: Certified hemodialysis technician
CHTRN: Certified hyperbaric technological registered nurse
CIC: Certified in infection control
CIMS: Coalition for Improved Maternity Services
CIS: Communities in Schools
CLEAR: Clearinghouse on Licensure, Enforcement, and
    Regulation

CLNC: Certified legal nurse consultant

CM: Certified midwife (lay)

CMA: Constituent member association (of ANA)

CMT: Certified medical transcriptionist

CMCN: Certified managed care nurse

CMDSC: Certified medical doctors coordinator

CME: Council on Medical Education (AMA)

CMS: Centers for Medicare and Medicaid Services, DHHS (formerly Health Care Financing Administration)

CNA: Certified nursing administrator; also certified nurse's aide

CNA: Canadian Nurses Association

CNAA: Certified nurse administrator, advanced (master's degree)

CNA-A: Certified nursing assistant, advanced

CNLCP: Certified nurse life care planner

CNE: Chief nurse executive; also certified nurse educator

CNM: Certified nurse midwife

CNN: Certified nephrology nurse; or certified neonatal nurse

CNNP: Certified neonatal nurse practitioner

CNO: Chief nursing officer

CNOR: Certified nurse, operating room

CNPE: Congress on Nursing Practice and Economics (ANA)

CNRN: Certified neuroscience registered nurse

CNS: Certified nurse specialist (master's-prepared)

CNSD: Certified nutrition support dietician

CNSN: Certified nutrition support nurse

COA: Certified ophthalmic assistant

COC: Commission on Certification (ANCC)

COCN: Certified ostomy care nurse

COHN: Certified occupational health nurse

COHN/CM: Certified occupational health nurse/case manager

COHN-S: Certified occupational health nurse, specialist

COHN-S/CM: Certified occupational health nurse, specialist case manager

COM: Commission on Magnet Recognition Program (ANCC)

COMT: Certified ophthalmic medical technologist
CON: College of Nursing
COPA: Council on Postsecondary Accreditation
CORE: Commission on Rehabilitation Education
COT: Certified ophthalmic technician
COTA: Certified ophthalmic technician assistant
CPAN: Certified post-anesthesia nurse
CPDN: Certified peritoneal dialysis nurse
CPFT: Certified pulmonary function technician
CPHQ: Certified professional in health care quality
CPN: Certified pediatric nurse
CPNA: Certified pediatric nurse associate
CPNL: Certified practical nurse, long-term care
CPNP: Certified pediatric nurse practitioner
CPON: Certified pediatric oncology nurse
CPS: Child Protective Services; or Canadian Paediatric Society
CPSC: Consumer Product Safety Commission
CPSN: Certified plastic surgical nurse
CPTC: Certified procurement transplant coordinator
CRA: Certified retinal angiographer
CRN: Certified rehabilitation nurse; also certified radiology
    nurse
CRNA: Certified registered nurse anesthetist
CRNFA: Certified registered nurse, first assistant
CRNI: Certified registered nurse, intervenous
CRNL: Certified registered nurse, long-term care
CRNO: Certified registered nurse in ophthalmology
CRNP: Certified registered nurse practitioner
CRRN: Certified rehabilitation registered nurse
CRRN-A: Certified rehabilitation registered nurse, advanced
CRTT: Certified respiratory therapy technician
C-SPI: Certified specialist in poison information
CS: Certified specialist; or clinical specialist
CSA: Certified surgical assistant
CSG: Council of State Governments

CSN: Children's Safety Network
CSN: Certified school nurse
CSS: Children's Specialty Services
CTN: Certified transcultural nurse
CUA: Certified urologic associate
CUCNS: Certified urologic clinical nurse specialist
CUNP: Certified urologic nurse practitioner
CUPA: Certified urologic physician assistant
CURN: Certified urologic registered nurse
CVN: Certified vascular nurse
CWCN: Certified wound care nurse
CWLA: Child Welfare League of America
CWPA: Commission on Workplace Advocacy

DAHEA: Division of Allied Health Education and Accreditation
   (AMA)
DAHP: Division of Associated Health Professions (DHHS)
DEA: Drug Enforcement Agency
DHHS: Department of Health and Human Services
DNC: Dermatology nurse, certified
DO: Doctor of osteopathy
DOE: Department of Education
DOL: Department of Labor
DNHW: Department of National Health and Welfare (Canada)
DSHEA: Dietary Supplement Health and Education Act
DSMOs: Data Standards Maintenance Organizations
DTR: Dietetic technician, registered

ECELS: Early Childhood Education Linkage System
ECI: Early childhood intervention
EdD: Doctorate of education
EDP: Emergency department physician
EFA: Epilepsy Foundation of America
EFNEP: Expanded Food and Nutrition Education Program
EHA: Education of Handicapped Act

EHAB: Ethics and Human Rights Advisory Board
EMFP: Ethnic Minority Fellowship Program
EMT-1: Emergency medical technician, basic; also abbreviated
EMT-B
EMT-P: Emergency medical technician, paramedic

FAAN: Fellow, the American Academy of Nursing
FAH: Federation of American Hospitals
FAHD: Forum on Allied Health Data
FAO: United Nations Food and Agriculture Organization
FDA: Food and Drug Administration (DHHS)
FEC: Federal Election Commission
FEHBP: Federal Employees Health and Benefits Program
FEMA: Federal Emergency Management Agency
FM: Financial Management Department
FTC: Federal Trade Commission
FNC: Family nurse clinician
FNP: Family nurse practitioner
FPNP: Family planning nurse practitioner
FUSA: Families United for Senior Action

GAO: Government Accounting Office
GMENAC: Graduate Medical Education National Advisory
Committee
GN: Graduate nurse (nursing school graduate; has yet to pass li-
censing exam)
GNP: Gerontological nurse practitioner
GPN: General pediatric nurse
GSA: Gerontological Society of America
GU: Generations United

HCPAC: Health Care Professionals Advisory Committee (AMA)
HCPDG: Health Care Professionals Discussion Group
HFMA: Healthcare Financial Management Association
HHA: Home health aide

HHS: U.S. Department of Health and Human Services
HIAA: Health Insurance Association of America
HMHB: Healthy Mothers, Healthy Babies Coalition
HMO: Health maintenance organization
HNC: Holistic nurse, certified
HOME: Home Observation for Measurement of the
    Environment
HPNEC: Health Professions and Nursing Education Coalition
HRA: Health Resources Administration (DHHS)
HRSA: Health Resources and Services Administration
    (DHHS)
HSF: Health Services Foundation
HSQB: Health Standards and Quality Bureau (HCFA)
HTL: Healing Touch International

IBFAN: International Baby Food Action Network
ICEA: International Childbirth Education Association
ICI: ANCC Institute for Credentialing Innovation
ICN: Infection control nurse
ICN: International Council of Nurses
ICP: Infection control practitioner
IDEA: Individuals with Disabilities Education Act
IHS: Indian Health Service
ILCA: International Lactation Consultants Association
IOM: Institute of Medicine
IRB: Institutional Review Board (for research proposals)
IRS: Internal Revenue Service
IRSG: Insurance Rehabilitation Study Group
ISO: International Standards Organization
ISONG: International Society of Nurses in Genetics
ISQua: The International Society for Quality in Health Care,
    Inc.

JCAHO: Joint Commission on Accreditation of Healthcare
    Organizations

JOGNN: *Journal of Obstetric, Gynecologic and Neonatal Nursing*

LCCE: Lamaze certified childbirth educator
LDA: Learning Disabilities Association
LLI: LaLeche League International
LNC: Legal nurse consultant
LNCC: Legal nurse consultant, certified
LOINC: Logical Observation Identifier Names and Codes
LPC: Licensed professional counselor
LPN: Licensed practical nurse
LPT: Licensed psychiatric technician
LRCT: Licensed respiratory care technician
LRCP: Licensed respiratory care practitioner
LVN: Licensed vocational nurse (equivalent to LPN)

MCH: Maternal and Child Health (DHHS)
MCHB: Maternal and Child Health Bureau (DHHS)
MDAA: Muscular Dystrophy Association of America
MICN: Mobile intensive care nurse
MN: Master's in nursing
MPH: Master's in public health
MPI: Meeting Planners International
MRC: Medical Research Council
MSN: Master's in science of nursing

NA: Nurse aide (without certification)
NACCRRA: National Association of Child Care Resource and
    Referral Agencies
NADT: National Association for Drama Therapy
NAEYC: National Association for Education of Young Children
NAF: Nursing's Agenda for the Future
NAHB/NRC: National Association of Home Builders/National
    Research Center
NAHC: National Association for Home Care
NAHHA: National Association of Home Health Agencies

NAIP: National Association of Inpatient Physicians

NAMI: National Alliance for the Mentally Ill

NAMME: National Association of Medical Minority Educators

NAMT: National Association for Music Therapy

NANDA-I: North American Nursing Diagnosis Association International

NANN: National Association of Neonatal Nurses

NAPHS: National Association of Psychiatric Health Systems

NAPNAP: National Association of Pediatric Nurse Associates and Practitioners

NAPSO: National Alliance of Pupil Service Organizations

NARA: National Association of Rehabilitation Agencies

NARC: National Association for Retarded Citizens

NARF: National Association of Rehabilitation Facilities

NAS: National Academies of Science

NASA: National Aeronautics and Space Agency

NASDSE: National Association of State Directors of Special Education

NASL: National Association for Long-Term Care

NASMHPR: National Association of State Mental Health Program Directors

NASN: National Association of School Nurses

NASUA: National Association of State Units on Aging

NASW: National Association of Social Workers

NCAHE: National Commission on Allied Health Education

NCBFE: National Center for a Barrier-Free Environment

NCC: Nationally certified counselor

NCCAM: National Center for Complementary and Alternative Medicine

NCCNHR: National Citizens Coalition for Nursing Home Reform

NCD: National Council on Disability

NCDB: National Center for Drugs and Biologics

NCDC: National Center for Disease Control

NCDPEH: National Coalition for Disease Prevention and
Environmental Health
NCEA: National Center for Elder Abuse
NCEMCH: National Center for Education in Maternal and
Child Health
NCES: National Center for Education Statistics (DHHS)
NCHC: National Council on Health Care Technologists
NCHCA: National Commission for Health Certifying Agencies
NCHHA: National Council of Homemakers and Home Health
Aides
NCHP: National Council for Health Planning
NCHPEG: National Coalition for Health Professional
Education in Genetics
NCHS: National Center for Health Statistics (DHHS)
NCIL: National Council on Independent Living
NCMRR: National Center for Medical Rehabilitation Research
NCNQ: National Center for Nursing Quality
NCOA: National Council on Aging
NCPCA: National Committee to Prevent Child Abuse
NCPIE: National Council of Patient Information and
Education
NCSBN: National Council of State Boards of Nursing
NCSL: National Conference of State Legislatives
NCSN: National certified school nurse
NCVHS: National Committee on Vital and Health Statistics
NDTA: Neurodevelopmental Treatment Association
NGNA: National Gerontological Nursing Association
NHANES: National Health and Nutrition Examination Society
NHC: National Health Council
NHLA: National Health Lawyers Association
NHO: National Hospice Organization
NHTSA: National Highway Traffic Safety Administration
NIA: National Institute on Aging
NIAAA: National Institutes on Alcohol Abuse and Alcoholism
(Public Health Service)

NIC: Nursing Intervention Classification

NICCYD: National Information Center for Children and Youth with Disabilities

NICN: Neonatal intensive care nurse

NIDA: National Institute of Drug Abuse

NIDRR: National Institute on Disability and Rehabilitation Research

NIDSEC: Nursing Information Data Set Evaluation Center

NIH: National Institutes of Health

NIHR: National Institute of Handicapped Research

NIMH: National Institute of Mental Health

NINR: National Institute for Nursing Research

NLN: National League for Nursing

NLRB: National Labor Relations Board

NMHA: National Mental Health Association

NMSS: National Multiple Sclerosis Society

NNP: Neonatal nurse practitioner

NP: Nurse practitioner

NP-C: Nurse practitioner, certified

NPP: Psychiatric nurse practitioner

NPSRC: National Professional Standards Review Council

NQF: National Quality Forum

NRA: National Rehabilitation Association

NRA: Nurse Reinvestment Act

NRC: National Research Council

NRCA: National Rehabilitation Counseling Association

NRTI: National Rehabilitation Training Institutes

NUCEA: National University Continuing Education Association

NVOILA: National Voluntary Organizations for Independent Living for the Aging

OAA: Older Americans Act

OAM: Office of Alternative Medicine

OB/GYN: Obstetrics and gynecology

OBRA: Omnibus Budget Reconciliation Act
OCN: Oncology certified nurse
OCR: Office of Civil Rights
OE: Office of Education
OGNP: OB/GYN nurse practitioner
OH: Office of the Handicapped
OIG: Office of the Inspector General
OMAR: Office of Medical Applications and Research
OMB: Office of Management and Budget (Executive Office of the President)
OMH: Office of Minority Health
ONC: Orthopedic nurse, certified
OPM: Office of Personnel Management
OPRR: Office for Protection from Research Risks (DHHS)
ORHP: Office of Rural Health Policy
ORWH: Office of Research on Women's Health
OSEP: Office of Special Education Programs
OSERS: Office of Special Education and Rehabilitation Services (DOE)
OSG: Office of the Surgeon General
OSHA: Occupational Safety and Health Administration
OTA: Office of Technology Assessment
OTR: Occupational therapist, registered
OVR: Office of Vocational Rehabilitation
OWH: Office of Women's Health (DHHS)

PA: Physician assistant (nonphysician primary care providers)
PA-C: Physician assistant, certified
PAHO: Pan American Health Organization
PATH: Partners for Appropriate Technology for the Handicapped
PCPD: President's Committee on People with Disabilities
PhMRA: Pharmaceutical Manufacturers and Research Association
PHN: Public health nurse
PHS: Public Health Service

PMHNP: Psychiatric-mental health nurse practitioner (ANCC)
PNP: Pediatric nurse practitioner
PPO: Preferred provider organization
PPS: Prospective payment system
PROPAC: Prospective Payment Assessment Commission
PRRB: Provider Reimbursement Review Board
PRSA: Public Relations Society of America
PSRO: Professional Standards Review Organization
PTAC: Professional and Technical Advisory Committee
    (JCAHO)
PVA: Paralyzed Veterans of America

RCN: Royal College of Nurses (UK)
RCNA: Royal College of Nurses, Australia
RN: Registered nurse
RNA: Registered nurse's assistant
RNAC: Registered nurse assessment coordinator
RN,BC: Registered nurse, board certified (ANCC credential for
    BSN prepared certificants)
RN,C: Registered nurse, certified (ANCC credential for
    ADN/diploma prepared certificants)
RN,CS: Registered nurse, certified specialist (credential for cer-
    tified NP/CNS; ANCC is now using APRN,BC)
RNFA: Registered nurse, first assistant
RNR: Registered nurse recruiter
RPFT: Registered pulmonary function technician
RSA: Rehabilitation Services Administration (DOE)
RSVP: Retired Senior Volunteer Program
RT: Respiratory technician

SAM: Society for Adolescent Medicine
SAMHSA: Substance Abuse and Mental Health Service
    Administration (DHHS)
SBON: State board of nursing (regulates nursing practice)
SISSC: Special Interest Section Steering Committee

SN: Student nurse
SNAP: Society of National Association Publications
SON: School of Nursing
SSA: Social Security Administration (DHHS)

TASH: The Association for Persons with Severe Handicaps
TNCC: Trauma nurse core curriculum
TNS: Trauma nurse specialist
TRB: Transportation Research Board

UAN: United American Nurses (ANA's collective bargaining
    unit)
UAP: Unlicensed assistive personnel
UCPA: United Cerebral Palsy Association
UNAIDS: Joint United Nations Programme on HIV/AIDS
UNICEF: United Nation's Children's Fund
UNO: United Network for Organ Sharing
USDA: United States Department of Agriculture
USDA/FCS: United States Department of Agriculture, Food,
    and Consumer Service
USDHHS: United States Department of Health and Human
    Services
USFDA: United States Food and Drug Administration
USP: United States Pharmacopeia
USPHS: United States Public Health Service
USPSTF: United States Preventive Services Task Force

VA: Department of Veterans Affairs
VA DM&S: Veterans Administration Department of Medicine
    and Surgery
VDRL: Venereal Disease Research Laboratory
VEWAA: Vocational Evaluation and Work Adjustment
    Association (NRA)
VNA: Visiting Nurse Association
VNS: Visiting Nurse Service

WABA: World Alliance for Breastfeeding Action
WCPT: World Confederation of Physical Therapists
WFOT: World Federation of Occupational Therapists
WHCOA: White House Conference on Aging
WHIF: Washington Health Issues Forum
WHNP: Women's health care nurse practitioner
WHO: World Health Organization
WIC: Women in Communication; or Women, Infants, & Children (food program)
WMA: World Medical Association
WMD: Weapons of mass destruction
WOCN: Wound, ostomy, and continence nurse
WPA: Workplace advocacy
WPSIS: Work Programs Special Interest Section (AOTA)

Symbols Common to Health Care

Symbols, like abbreviations, can easily be misread and misinterpreted. Their use is discouraged, and many healthcare organizations are prohibiting or limiting their use. However, it is still possible to find these symbols in use in some practice sites. *Use caution* in interpreting them for purposes other than general comprehension of a situation.

↑	Increase
↓	Decrease
→	Leading to, causes
°	Degree
1°	Degree, primary; first degree
2°	Degree, secondary; second degree
3°	Degree, tertiary; third degree
@	At
α	Alpha
β	Beta
Δ	Delta, change, or heat
n	Sample size
N	Population size
π	Pi, 3.1416, ratio of circumference of a circle to diameter of circle
+	Plus, excess, positive
−	Minus, deficiency, negative
±	Plus or minus, nondefined exactness
≈	About, approximate, approximately equal

=	Equals, equal to
≠	Not equal to
>	Greater than
≥	Greater than or equal to
≯	Not greater than
<	Less than
≤	Less than or equal to
≮	Not less than
∨	Systolic blood pressure
∧	Diastolic blood pressure
∞	Infinity
Σ	Sum
%	Percent
:	Ratio, is to (equation)
∴	Therefore
c̄	With
s̄	Without
ō	None, no
#	Number, pound
/; ÷	Per, divided by
×	Times, multiplied by
′	Minutes
″	Seconds
♂, □	Male
♀, ○	Female
♏	Minim
ʒ	Dram
℥	Ounce
℞	Prescription
η, μ	Millimicron, nanometer
μg	Microgram
ā	Before
p̄	After
s̈s	One half

C°   Centigrade, Celsius
F°   Fahrenheit
Q   Sitting
φ   Standing
○—   Lying

A P P E N D I X B

Acidosis/Alkalosis

Table B-1 Metabolic Acidosis and Alkalosis

	Acidosis	**Alkalosis**
Signs and symptoms	Conscious Lethargy Kussmaul's respirations Fruity breath Decreased muscle tone Decreased deep tendon reflexes	Irritable Confused Decreased respiratory rate and depth Possible hyperactive reflexes Possible arrhythmias
Lab	ABG: • pH below 7.35 • Urine pH below 6 • Bicarb below 24 mEq/L • Partial pressure CO_2 decreased	ABG: • pH above 7.45 • Urine pH above 7 • Bicarb above 29 mEq/L
Treatment	IV NA bicarb For diabetic acidosis: insulin and fluids	KCL and NS

Table B-2   Respiratory Acidosis and Alkalosis

	Acidosis	**Alkalosis**
Signs and symptoms	Headache Dyspnea Diaphoresis Nausea and vomiting Bounding pulse Rapid, shallow respirations Restlessness and confusion Asterixis and decreased reflexes	Light headedness Parasthesia Anxiety Rapid breathing Possible tetany
Lab	ABG: • PCO_2 increased above 45 mmHg • pH below normal • HCO_3 normal (acute); elevated (chronic)	ABG: • PCO_2 decreased below 35 mmHg • pH increasing (acute); normal (chronic)
Treatment	Bronchodilators Oxygen Remedy the underlying cause	Rebreathing Sedatives Remedy the underlying cause

Table B-3 Changes in Acid–Base and Common Compensation

Type of Acid–Base Disorder	H+	pH	HCO$_3$	PCO$_2$	Common Compensation
Normal	37–43	7.35–7.45	22–26	35–45	
Acidosis: Metabolic	Elevated	Lowered	Lowered	Lowered	PCO$_2$ decreased 11 to 13 mmHg for every 10 mmol increase in HCO$_3$
Acidosis: Respiratory	Elevated	Lowered	Elevated	Elevated	Acute: HCO$_3$ increased 1 mmol for every 10 mmHg elevation in PCO$_2$ Chronic: HCO$_3$ increased 3.5 mmol for every 10 mmHg elevation in PCO$_2$

Alkalosis: Metabolic	Lowered	Elevated	Elevated	Elevated	PCO_2 increased 6 to 7 mmHg for every 10 mmol increase in HCO_3
Alkalosis: Respiratory	Lowered	Elevated	Lowered	Lowered	Acute: HCO_3 decreased 2.5 mmol for every 10 mmHg decrease in PCO_2 Chronic: HCO_3 decreased 5 mmol for every 10 mmHg decrease in PCO_2

Sources: The Merck Manual, 18th edition, Holloway's Nurse's Fast Facts, and Peterson's Just the Facts.

Index

INDEX